# Making Data Talk

# Making Data Talk

## Communicating Public Health Data to the Public, Policy Makers, and the Press

David E. Nelson
Bradford W. Hesse
Robert T. Croyle

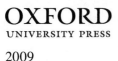

## OXFORD
UNIVERSITY PRESS

2009

# OXFORD

UNIVERSITY PRESS

Oxford University Press, Inc., publishes works that further
Oxford University's objective of excellence
in research, scholarship, and education.

Oxford  New York
Auckland  Cape Town  Dar es Salaam  Hong Kong  Karachi
Kuala Lumpur  Madrid  Melbourne  Mexico City  Nairobi
New Delhi  Shanghai  Taipei  Toronto

With offices in
Argentina  Austria  Brazil  Chile  Czech Republic  France  Greece
Guatemala  Hungary  Italy  Japan  Poland  Portugal  Singapore
South Korea  Switzerland  Thailand  Turkey  Ukraine  Vietnam

Copyright © 2009 by Oxford University Press, Inc.

Published by Oxford University Press, Inc.
198 Madison Avenue, New York, New York 10016
www.oup.com

Library of Congress Cataloging-in-Publication Data

Nelson, David E., M.D.
Making data talk: communicating public health data to the public, policy makers, and the press/
David E. Nelson, Bradford W. Hesse, Robert T. Croyle.
p. ; cm.
Includes bibliographical references.
ISBN 978-0-19-538153-5
1. Communication in public health. 2. Health education.   I. Hesse, Bradford W. II. Croyle, Robert T.
III. Title.
[DNLM: 1. Health Education—methods. 2. Public Health. 3. Information Dissemination—methods.
WA 590 N425m 2009]
RA423.2.N45 2009
613—dc22                                                                        2008033685

9 8 7 6 5 4 3 2 1
Printed in the United States of America
on acid-free paper

**Disclaimer**

The findings and conclusions in this book are those of the authors and do not necessarily represent the views of the Centers for Disease Control and Prevention or the National Institutes of Health.

*This book is dedicated to the loving memory
of Claire Emily Nelson (1989–2005). To paraphrase
Benjamin Franklin's epitaph for his son, she was the
delight of all who knew her.*[1]

[1] Isaacson W. *Benjamin Franklin: An American Life*. New York, N.Y.: Simon & Schuster; 2003.

# Foreword

Without question, communicating scientific information, and in particular, scientific data, to lay audiences is difficult. I routinely observe the struggles faced by scientists, public health practitioners, clinicians, and many others who attempt to convey "the numbers" to persons from all walks of life. Indeed, there is a growing need to make key public health data available, but they must be selected and presented in a manner that is to be understandable, have meaning, and help people answer the critical question "so what?"

Other authors have attempted to provide recommendations about one aspect of data communication, such as visual data presentation, but they have not taken into account the totality of communication processes in public health and the many factors that influence it. This book appropriately emphasizes the importance of data selection, recognizes that presentation extends beyond visual modalities, and points out the need for careful integration of words, symbols, and numbers. I was particularly pleased that the Drs Nelson, Hesse, and Croyle highlight the often hidden roles that communicators' values, ethics, and assumptions play in data selection and presentation, the reality that presenting more data is rarely better, and sometimes the "best" data to present are no data at all.

Although substantial advances have occurred as the result of specialization within scientific fields, a major drawback of specialization is the distance it creates within and across disciplines, which can prevent cross-fertilization of research ideas and methodologies. An additional challenge is that, unfortunately, researchers and practitioners in public health and related fields often live in parallel universes and do not regularly communicate with each other. As demonstrated by many initiatives sponsored by governmental and non-governmental organizations, there is a great interest and recognized value for transdisciplinary work to establish networks across fields. In the field of health communication, transdisciplinary efforts are needed not only across traditional scientific disciplines, but also from practitioners and experts trained in related fields, such as the graphic arts and rhetoric.

I believe this book reflects a careful synthesis of research from many disciplines, resulting in knowledge advancement, yet with practical implications and advice for data communicators working in the trenches.

Furthermore, this volume represents a concrete example of the tremendous value that a transdisciplinary effort can have in increasing knowledge about communication for public health practice. You will find the content scientifically sound, easy to read, and practical. It is a significant achievement and a contribution to literature and regularly and consistently following its principles will help you improve your communication skills.

Jay M. Bernhardt, PhD, MPH
Director, National Center for Health Marketing
Centers for Disease Control and Prevention (CDC)
Atlanta, GA

# Preface

We wrote this book with two main purposes in mind: (a) to summarize and synthesize research on the selection and presentation of data pertinent to public health, and (b) to provide practical suggestions, based on this research summary and synthesis, on how scientists and other public health practitioners can better communicate data to the public, policy makers, and the press in typical real-world situations. Because communication is complex and no one approach works for all audiences, we emphasize how to communicate data "better" (and in some instances, contrast this with how to communicate data "worse"), rather than attempting a cookbook approach. We include many case studies and other examples to illustrate major points and actual situations whenever possible. We summarize key principles and recommendations at the end of each chapter.

Although this book discusses many general characteristics and specific recommendations about communicating data, it is based on five overarching themes that can help public health scientists and practitioners make better choices. The first theme is to raise awareness of the many factors and complexities that need to be considered, and the possible choices to be made, when selecting and presenting data. It will become painfully obvious that it is not as easy as simply "showing audiences data, and hoping that the numbers will speak for themselves."

The second theme is that there is a close and inseparable relationship between data selection and presentation with the purpose for communication, intended audience(s), and the context in which communication occurs. As discussed in Chapter 2, the four purposes for communicating public health information with lay audiences are to increase knowledge (educate with no intent to influence), instruct, facilitate informed decision making, and persuade. These purposes involve critical value and ethical decisions. Given that data selection and presentation are closely tied to purpose, audience(s), and context, selection of data is inevitable: decisions must be made to present certain data and to use certain presentation formats at the exclusion of other data or formats.

The third theme is that data should be used to support a science-based storyline. Storyline, as defined in this book, refers to the conclusion, based upon the current state of scientific knowledge drawn about a specific aspect of a public health topic, that scientists or public health practitioners want lay audiences to understand. Storylines can vary widely, depending on the amount of research and level of consensus among scientists. Storylines may lead to communication messages designed for lay audiences with a straightforward persuasive purpose (e.g., these data show why it is important to engage in regular hand washing to prevent infectious disease transmission), to increase knowledge with no intent to persuade (e.g., these data illustrate a scientific finding or trend that is important knowledge about public health), or for an informed decision-making purpose (e.g., these data demonstrate why it is important to you to consider this information and these sources prior to making a personal health decision).

The fourth theme is that data need to be used ethically and in such a manner as to maximize their impact and effectiveness to increase audience understanding. This means selecting and presenting data that are most likely to resonate with intended audiences for the desired communication purpose and storyline. Our explicit assumption is that readers of this book are "honest brokers" who would like to communicate public health data and other information to lay audiences in an ethical manner, not simply "cherry picking" data from research studies or surveillance systems that most easily demonstrate the key point(s) they wish to convey.

Finally, the fifth theme is that selecting and presenting data to lay audiences needs to avoid unintended consequences. Presenting inappropriate or poorly selected data may result in lay audiences failing to attend to messages (e.g., not recognizing important points or being distracted), becoming overly fearful, "underconcerned" about public health problems, or in some other way misunderstanding the key storyline. This theme emphasizes the important role that formative and other types of evaluation research play in public health communication, broadly, and in data communication, specifically.

We did not attempt to conduct an in-depth review of all the research that bears on data communication, as doing so would require a multivolume set of books. Much research has been done, and many books written, for example, about risk communication in public health and about decision making in clinical settings. In contrast, there is a paucity of research for some topics, such as communicating data to policy makers. For areas such as these, we had to rely on information based on the experiences of practitioners ("expert opinion") and research on related topics. Thus, we believe this book may best be considered a metareview of research-based recommendations from seminal books, reviews, and research articles, supplemented by the practice-based recommendations of experts.

Now for caveats and disclaimers. One of our biggest challenges was the large number of fields in which relevant research has been conducted. They included anthropology, business, communication, computer science, economics, education, epidemiology, genetic counseling, health education/ health promotion, informatics, journalism, law, mathematics, medicine, nursing, political science, psychology, sociology, and the visual arts. If nothing else, our review of these literatures confirmed what many others before us have learned: (a) many, many factors influence whether a communication effort or activity is successful with a given audience, and (b) communication is as much an art as a science. It was a humbling experience!

We do not consider ourselves expert in all these areas. Our background and experience are primarily in the fields of communication, epidemiology, medicine, public health, and social psychology. For subject areas that we knew less well, we solicited recommendations about key research from experts in these areas. We realize that it is likely that we failed to cite some classic studies or explore avenues of research that would have provided additional insights. We apologize in advance for any omissions.

The book chapters can be broadly divided into four areas. Chapter 1 provides an introduction and background information about the challenges involved in communicating quantitative public health data. Chapters 2–4 provide an overview of communication, how people process and understand data, and the palette of options for data presentation, drawing heavily from the fields of psychology and communication. Readers most interested in practical application may be tempted to skip these chapters, but we encourage all to read these chapters, as they provide the rationale for better communication practices and include many practical examples.

Chapters 5–7 are the third part of the book. They integrate material from previous chapters and contain recommendations and extensive examples about communicating data to lay audiences in more common public health situations (Chapter 5), as well as in more specialized circumstances (e.g., outbreaks or crises [Chapter 6] or advocacy [Chapter 7]). The final chapter (Chapter 8) contains suggestions for future directions in data communication.

We hope this book will stimulate interest among public health practitioners, scholars, and students to more seriously consider ways they can understand and improve communication about data and other types of scientific information with the public, policy makers, and the press. We are confident that improved communication about data to lay audiences will increase the chance that evidence-based scientific findings play a greater role in improving the public's health.

David E. Nelson
Bradford W. Hesse
Robert T. Croyle

# Acknowledgments

We wish to thank the many people who helped make this book a reality. Claudia Parvanta provided the genesis of the idea of the book. Jeffrey House and Carrie Pedersen, formerly of Oxford University Press, believed in our book concept and gave us critical support along the way.

Many others helped in the development of this book by reviewing earlier drafts or contributing in some other way. They include June Bancroft, Jay Bernhardt, Bob Brewer, Ross Brownson, Linda Cameron, Janet Croft, Donna Garland, Bridget Grant, Kurt Greenlund, Beth Haslett, Rick Hull, Lloyd Johnston, Mary Grace Kovar, Gary Kreps, Lore Lee, Stephen Marcus, Grant Martin, Robert Nicholson, Charles Pavitt, Elizabeth Perse, Geraldine Perry, Sam Posner, Pat Remington, Barbara Reynolds, Jeff Sacks, Wendy Samter, Mary Schwarz, Nancy Signorielli, Jessica Spraggins, Anne Turner, Marsha Vanderford, and K. (Vish) Viswanath.

We give special thanks to Christine Theisen of Matthews Media, who provided invaluable editing services and ideas along the way and who helped in so many ways to improve the final product.

Finally, we acknowledge the invaluable support of our families and friends. Anne Turner, Shay and Peter Fontana, Grant Nelson, Hayley Nelson, and Dale Nelson provided much moral support, understanding, and patience. Nicola and Brent Hesse, James and Jyl Alexander, and a host of important others showed a remarkable degree of support to a process that invariably intruded into vacations and family time.

# Contents

# Making Data Talk

# 1

# Introduction

Why does it matter how health and science issues are reported?...
It matters because misleading information is potentially dangerous:
It can even cost lives.

The Royal Institution of Great Britain. *Guidelines on
Science and Health Communication*[1]

## Background

Regardless of the issue, the ultimate goal of public health is to apply the "art
and science of preventing disease, prolonging life, and promoting health"
to the focused goal of saving and improving lives.[2] To achieve this goal,
public health practitioners, health care professionals, research scientists, and
even organizational administrators often find themselves in the position of
having to communicate data to lay audiences. In fact, whether the purpose
of messages is to increase knowledge, instruct, facilitate informed decision
making or persuade, effective communication is probably *the* major public
health intervention; this has been described as the act of "treating people
with information."[3]

Communicating health and scientific information, whether it occurs in
one-on-one counseling situations or as part of state or national campaigns,
is especially difficult with any lay audience not well versed in science or
mathematics, be they individuals within the general public, policy makers,
or members of the media. Nevertheless, because communication serves to
help translate scientific findings into public health practice, we argue that
there is a strong and ethical obligation for scientists, health care providers,

advocates, organizations, and others in public health to ensure that results are communicated in ways that are more likely to have beneficial effects.

This is not to say that scientists must always take primary responsibility for communicating directly to public audiences, as government and non-government institutions can serve important roles in communicating with lay audiences, as of course, do health care providers.[4-7] Skilled science and health writers from the journalistic community endorse the same values for contributing to the public welfare as do many scientists.[8]

Problems occur, however, when the scientific community opts out of its communication role with lay audiences. This can lead to the public "marketplace" of ideas being influenced by individual biases and by market and other societal forces,[9-11] as well as the glut of information on health topics now available to information-seeking lay audiences on the Internet and via other sources and the difficulties they can face sifting through it.[12] For example, research has generally shown an inverse relationship between the number of newspaper stories published on specific health topics and the importance of these topics as public health concerns: more coverage is given to rare or anomalous events (e.g., alleged adverse effects of vaccines or natural disasters) than to findings with greater relevance to a larger number of people from a population perspective (e.g., preventing heart disease).[13-15]

The focus of this book is on selecting and communicating quantitative data, that is, numbers from scientific research, public health surveillance, and other sources in ways lay audiences can understand. Unfortunately, examples of poor communication of data abound—on Web sites, in written materials (e.g., reports, brochures), during oral presentations, and during media interviews, leaving many people awash in a morass of confusing "data smog."[16]

Box 1.1 is an example of what happens when scientific data concerning potential dioxin exposure were poorly communicated to lay audiences. By comparison, the clear presentation of state trends in obesity using maps (Box 1.2 and Figure 1.1) demonstrates the positive role that effectively communicating data to both lay and scientific audiences can play in raising awareness about this problem.

Situations in public health and clinical health care environments commonly arise where it is necessary to communicate scientific data to lay audiences.[17-25] Breast and prostate cancer screening recommendations,[26-29] the folic acid fortification of bread policy to reduce the risk of neural tube birth defects (Box 1.3),[30] vaccine safety (Box 1.4),[31-34] genetic testing,[35, 36] infectious disease outbreaks,[37, 38] occupational or environmental exposures,[39-42] and individual-level medical care decision making about treatment options for coronary heart disease[43-45] are just a few of many examples.

Understanding quantitative information is difficult for most people and communicating complex information is a challenge.[46] Few public health

**Box 1.1** Trying to explain research on dioxin

Dioxin is the general term used to describe a class of chemicals, the most potent being 2,3,7,8-tetrachlorodibenzo-*p*-dioxin. Dioxin is a chemical contaminant that occurs as a result of manufacturing insecticides, disinfectants, and herbicides, the most well known being Agent Orange, which was used during the Vietnam War. Scientific consensus about the level of health risks, such as cancer or birth defects, associated with dioxin has been elusive, but in the late 1970s and early 1980s there was widespread concern about its toxicity and extensive media coverage about these issues.

In 1984, dioxin was found in a Pennsylvania campsite that had been used by thousands of Boy Scouts 3 years earlier at their National Jamboree. The Dow Chemical Company has for decades been a major manufacturer of chemical products (including the herbicide Agent Orange) that result in the creation of dioxin. Although Dow had nothing to do with the contamination found at the Boy Scout campsite, because of the company's extensive experience with the chemical, leaders at the company were contacted for some explanation about dioxin and health risks.

At public hearings, Dow scientists and other representatives attempted to educate the public about dioxin by describing, in detail, several technical aspects of dioxins (e.g., chemical structures and varieties), emphasizing that toxicity varies depending on which specific chemical individuals are exposed. At one point, chemists at Dow attempted to reduce public concerns by pointing out that dioxin could be found in the exhaust pipes of cars and cigarette smoke.

Based on their research, Dow scientists became convinced that low-level dioxin exposure was not a health hazard to humans. Dow's corporate executive officer attempted to communicate these findings broadly to the public through the news media. During a morning television show appearance, he stated the company scientists' conclusions about the safety of dioxin but failed to provide any data or other supportive evidence for his conclusions.

The news media and public perceived that Dow, out of self-interest, was defending dioxin, and that the company failed to appreciate the anger and fear stemming from the seriousness of the health concerns, the uncertainty, and the involuntary nature of the public's exposure. Concerns about the health effects of dioxin exposure, especially among Vietnam veterans, continued for many years. This and many other examples of communication in acute situations (Chapter 6) demonstrate the many factors and aspects involved in communication that transcend simply "showing and explaining the data."

Source: Bond GG. Dioxin: A case study. *Am J Ind Med.* 1993;23(1): 177–182. Friedman SM, Dunwoody S, Rogers CL, eds. *Communicating Uncertainty: Media Coverage of New and Controversial Science.* Mahwah, N.J.: Lawrence Erlbaum; 1999.

---

**Box 1.2** Mapping the obesity epidemic

CDC scientists have collected state-specific data on the prevalence of adult obesity through the Behavioral Risk Factor Surveillance System (BRFSS) since the 1980s. Typically, data from surveillance systems such as the BRFSS are presented in table format, include specific multiple data points or, less frequently, utilize visual modalities such as line graphs or bar charts.

In a 1999 article published in *JAMA*, Mokdad and colleagues used a different approach to help audiences easily grasp the rapid increase, and extent, of obesity in the United States without relying on data-rich but cognitively challenging tables. They used a series of color-coded maps for the years 1991, 1993, 1995, and 1998 to demonstrate, at a glance, the increase in adult obesity prevalence by state.

These, and subsequent state obesity maps (Figure 1.1), have had a broad appeal for both scientific and lay audiences alike. They have been presented not only at many scientific conferences, but also to local, state, and federal policy-maker audiences and to the press, and have no doubt helped to raise awareness of the obesity problem in the United States and elsewhere. CDC's obesity maps have been widely adopted by others and republished on several organizational and other types of Web sites.

Source: Centers for Disease Control and Prevention. *U.S. Obesity Trends, 1985–2006: Centers for Disease Control and Prevention*; 2007. Mokdad AH, Serdula MK, Dietz WH, Bowman BA, Marks JS, Koplan JP. The spread of the obesity epidemic in the United States, 1991–1998. *JAMA.* 1999;282(16):1519–1522. Harvard School of Public Health. *Nutrition Source: Healthy Weight*; 2006. Tooele County (Utah) Health Department. *Obesity Epidemic*; 2006.

---

practitioners have a good understanding of how lay audiences consider public health issues or the health-related decision-making processes that they use,[47, 48] and rarely do they receive education or training about how to communicate scientific findings to lay audiences.[49–54]

Scientists who conduct research on communicating quantitative findings to lay audiences are scattered across disciplines, so research that shows how best to communicate quantitative data is rarely synthesized, nor does it reach those who could best utilize it. Kahneman and Tversky's groundbreaking research on judgment and decision making under uncertainty was originally published in the 1970s and early 1980s.[55, 56] To take one specific research finding, Tversky and Kahneman found that the way data are framed, that is, whether the same data are presented in terms of losses or gains (e.g., probability of mortality versus the probability of survival), has a strong influence on decision making among scientific and lay audiences.[56, 57] Their research,

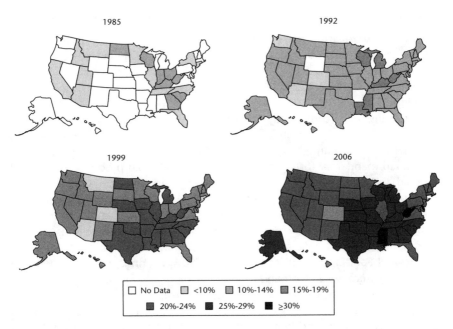

**Figure 1.1** U.S. state trends in obesity prevalence, 1985–2006. (Source: Centers for Disease Control and Prevention. *U.S. Obesity Trends, 1985–2006: Centers for Disease Control and Prevention*; 2007.)

along with that of many others, has important implications for communicating data and other forms of scientific information to lay audiences, but is not widely known by public health scientists and professionals beyond those explicitly trained in the behavioral sciences. As a result, the same communication mistakes are often unnecessarily repeated.

This is not to suggest, however, that this or any other book provides a sure formula for selecting or presenting scientific findings to the public, policy makers, or the press. Nothing can replace the importance of a careful analysis of intended audiences, contexts, and other factors that can influence the communication process (Chapters 2 and 3). There is, however, sufficient research to guide public health practitioners on how to better select and ethically present quantitative data to different lay audiences, as well as recommendations on what to avoid. Studying this book can lead to substantial improvement in learning and performing these important, yet often neglected, skills.

## Definitions

Terms and categories such as audiences; communication; data, public health, and science have different meanings for different people. Below are the definitions for terms used throughout this book.

**Box 1.3** Advocating for a national policy to increase folic acid consumption to reduce neural tube birth defects

The case of folic acid fortification provides an example of communicating public health data primarily toward policy makers. Research over many years consistently demonstrated that the risk of neural tube defects, such as spina bifida, was substantially lower among pregnant women who consumed higher levels of folic acid. Many scientists recommended mandatory fortification of certain cereal grain products, such as bread and flour, with folic acid on a national basis as the best approach for preventing neural tube defects, that is, a policy intervention. These efforts eventually resulted in an extensive debate in the scientific community about the pros and cons of fortification because some persons who consume too much folic acid will develop pernicious anemia.

Several Food and Drug Administration (FDA) hearings were held, with scientists from several organizations, including the Centers for Disease Control and Prevention and other federal health agencies, presenting evidence that higher levels of folate helped prevent neural tube defects, as well as the risks and benefits of a fortification policy. These included recommendations, based on scientific research, about the level of folic acid fortification that would maximize the protective effects for reducing the risk of neural tube defects and minimize the increase in pernicious anemia.

The arguments in favor of fortification were successful, as in March 1996 the FDA issued regulations requiring that manufacturers of certain enriched cereal-grain products fortify them with 140 µg of folic acid per 100 g of product by January 1998. Subsequent research has estimated the benefits of this folic acid fortification policy to be a reduction in the rate of neural tube birth defects of 20–30% after the policy was implemented.

Source: Lumley J, Watson L, Watson M, Bower C. Periconceptional supplementation with folate and/or multivitamins for preventing neural tube defects. *Cochrane Database Syst Rev.* 2001;CD001056. Centers for Disease Control and Prevention. Spina bifida and anencephaly before and after folic acid mandate: United States, 1995–1996 and 1999–2000. *MMWR.* 2004;53:362–365. Grosse SD, Waitzman NJ, Romano PS, Mulinare J. Reevaluating the benefits of folic acid fortification in the United States: Economic analysis, regulation, and public health. *Am J Public Health.* 2005;95(11):1917–1922. Mills JL, Signore C. Neural tube defect rates before and after food fortification with folic acid. *Birth Defects Res Part A Clin Mol Teratol.* 2004;70(11):844–845. U.S. Food and Drug Administration. Food standards: Amendments of standards of identity for enriched grain products to require addition of folic acid. *Fed Reg.* 1996;8781–8797.

**Box 1.4** Challenging vaccine safety

Advances in vaccine development have led to dramatic declines in morbidity and mortality from diphtheria, tetanus, and many other infectious diseases. What used to be widespread support among lay audiences for new vaccines has not been nearly as universal in recent years, however. For example, an increased risk of intussusception (the slide of one part of the intestine into another part) among infants receiving rotavirus immunizations in 1999 led to a multistate investigation and eventual discontinuation of the use of this vaccine.

Controversy also developed in the late 1990s concerning the presence of mercury-containing preservative (thimerosal) in childhood vaccines, with some people attributing autism to vaccines despite scientific evidence to the contrary.

There are organizations and individuals that routinely challenge public health scientists about vaccine-related issues. Scientists and public health practitioners face questions about vaccines in a manner similar to those involved with certain occupational, environmental health, and cancer screening and treatment controversies. This requires better understanding of audiences to more effectively communicate with lay audiences. Public health practitioners can assume that their research findings on immunizations will continue to be challenged by some lay audience members.

Source: Centers for Disease Control and Prevention. Achievements in public health, 1900–1999: Impact of vaccines universally recommended for children—United States, 1900–1998. *MMWR*. 1999;48:243–248. Danovaro-Holliday MC, Wood AL, LeBaron CW. Rotavirus and the news media, 1987–2001. *JAMA*. 2002;287(11):1455–1462. Halsey NA. Limiting infant exposure to thimerosal in vaccines and other sources of mercury. *JAMA*. 1999;282(18):1763–1766. Allen A. *Vaccine: The Controversial Story of Medicine's Greatest Lifesaver*. New York, N.Y.: Norton; 2007.

## Audiences

The three lay audiences emphasized throughout this book are the general public, policy makers, and the press. More specifics about lay audiences are included in Chapter 2. Classifying lay audiences in this manner is useful for practical purposes,[58, 59] especially given that they have different roles and none of the three are very familiar with, nor do they have a good understanding of, science or mathematics.[60, 61]

The *general public*, sometimes referred to in the plural as "publics,"[6] are individuals within the population at large. "General public" is really a misnomer, as there are many different publics because of the heterogeneity inherent across groups or populations of people, for example, by age, past experience, culture, or level of involvement.

*Policy makers* consist of administrators and elected officials with the authority to make decisions about laws, regulations, policies, programs, or resources that affect the health of populations.[62, 63] They not only include publicly elected officials and high level administrators within the executive branch of federal, state, and local governments, but also private policy makers, such as high level officials within private corporations, institutions (e.g., foundations), and insurance companies, who make public health-related decisions. Some policy makers may be public health practitioners or scientists themselves, but the vast majority will have backgrounds in other fields and may have responsibilities in areas outside the public health arena.

The *press*, which will be used interchangeably with the words *news media*, *journalist*, and *reporter*, comprises persons who obtain or report news for magazines, newspapers, television, radio, news wire services (e.g., the Associated Press), or Internet news sites. Journalists are typically either general reporters, who cover many topic areas, or specialized reporters, who limit their scope of work to one or a few areas.[50, 54] Journalists are an important audience, as they function as intermediaries in communicating public health information to the public and policy makers and play a key role in defining which issues or topics are more important (Agenda setting) and how they are presented (Framing).[64, 65]

## Communication

Communication is difficult to define. It depends on three aspects: intentionality, verbal or nonverbal messages, and whether messages intended for audiences are received.[66] In this book, communication is considered to be the process by which verbal or visual messages are intentionally transmitted by sources (senders) through channels, and that are received by intended audiences. *Information* consists of the messages transmitted or made available to lay audiences.

Although this book emphasizes communicating quantitative data, there is some overlap with general recommendations about communicating information, and this body of work will be cited as needed. A good understanding of the information environment, audiences, communication purpose, and context of specific situations is essential and are expanded upon further in the next few chapters. Readers desiring a broader overview of communicating health information, including planning, message development, and evaluation are referred to several references listed at the end of this chapter.[67–74]

Data, Public Health, and Science

The terms *data*, *numbers*, and *findings* will be used interchangeably in this book. They refer to numbers, mathematical operations, or statistical or scientific calculations or mathematical terms commonly used in public health research or surveillance (quantitative data). These types of data can generally be placed into one of five broad classifications: simple numbers and basic mathematical calculations, intermediate mathematical operations, complex mathematical operations, statistical uncertainty and significance testing, and specialized concepts or calculated values (Table 1.1).

Simple numbers and basic mathematical operations are taught in elementary school.[75–77] Intermediate mathematical operations are typically taught in middle or high school mathematics courses.[75] Complex mathematical operations are much more advanced and are likely to be familiar only to those with coursework or training in more advanced mathematical or scientific undergraduate or graduate courses (e.g., statistics, chemistry, or epidemiology).

Statistical uncertainty and statistical testing are also unlikely to be familiar to most lay audiences. Several specialized concepts or calculated values used in public health, that is, attributable risk, cost-effective measures (to name but a few of many) are likely to be familiar only to persons trained within specific public health or other fields, such as economics.

*Public health* refers to major topic areas and disciplines that are most commonly under the purview of persons employed in government agencies, nongovernmental organizations, or research institutions concerned with population-based health. Broad topic areas typically cover certain types of

**Table 1.1 Classification of quantitative data with examples from statistics and epidemiology**

| Classification | Examples |
|---|---|
| Simple numbers and basic mathematical calculations | Integers, decimals, fractions; addition, subtraction, multiplication, division, rounding |
| Intermediate mathematical operations | Percentage, ratio (e.g., odd ratios or relative risk), rate, average, probability |
| Complex mathematical operations | Regression analysis, correlation analysis, specificity, sensitivity, false positive, power calculations, number needed to treat |
| Statistical uncertainty and significance testing | Variance, confidence intervals, $p$ values |
| Specialized concepts or calculated values | Attributable risk/attributable fraction, age or other type of adjusted value, life expectancy, years of potential life lost (YPLL), quality-adjusted life years (QALY), risk assessment, risk benefit, economic discount rate, cost effectiveness |

infectious diseases (including vaccine-preventable diseases), chronic diseases, substance abuse, health care services, environmental and occupational health, natural disasters, genetics, injury, reproductive health, maternal and child health, mental health, and oral health.[19]

*Public health practitioner* refers to individuals who conduct the daily work of public health on the front lines of local, state, and federal health departments,[78] as well as persons who function in similar or related roles in private or nonprofit organizations or institutions (e.g., hospital infection control employees). This book stresses communication in public health rather than in clinical settings such as health or medical clinics. However, some of the relevant research comes from clinical studies[79, 80] and many public health practitioners provide clinical services. The principles and recommendations about data communication covered in this book are applicable in the clinical environment; indeed, such settings have the added benefit of allowing practitioners the opportunity for direct two-way communication. For readers specifically interested in broader aspects of communication, decision making, and decision aids in health care environments, recommended references are included at the ends of chapters.

*Science* refers to knowledge, especially of facts, principles, or theories, gained through systematic study, using methodologies generally agreed upon by others within their respective fields,[81] that is, a body of knowledge and generalized truths surrounding phenomena based primarily on hypotheses and deductions.[58, 59] Science is heavily based on the mathematical principles and analyses of quantitative and qualitative data. A wide variety of scientific and related disciplines contribute to public health, from areas such as epidemiology, the social sciences (e.g., psychology, communication, anthropology), laboratory sciences (e.g., microbiology, toxicology), the "hard" sciences (e.g., physics, chemistry), mathematics, and direct health care–related areas such as medicine, dentistry, and nursing. Scientists function as both knowledge producers and knowledge validators.[58, 59] In this book, *scientists* are individuals whose primary job consists of conducting research or public health surveillance, or synthesizing research or surveillance findings.

## Why Communicating Scientific Findings to Lay Audiences Is Often Necessary

More details are provided about the fundamentals of communication in Chapter 2, but it is first necessary to ask the question "Why should public health scientists and practitioners present the details of scientific findings to lay audiences?" In reality, there are times, such as in emergency or natural disaster situations, when it is not necessary to communicate data, especially initially. Lay audiences, for example, will usually have high levels of trust for governmental messages concerning protective actions to take in the event of natural disasters (e.g., tornadoes or blizzards) and are not likely to care about research data demonstrating the effectiveness of such recommendations. In these instances, communicating the gist of a protective message in a clear and precise way is exactly what the public needs.

The main reason to communicate data is because audiences want to know the reasons why individuals or policy makers should believe or do what scientists recommend; surveillance or research data can provide that justification. Scientific findings in public health that are communicated to lay audiences usually have an applied or practical application, and if not directly persuasive, attempt to influence people's thinking.

For many major public health issues, particularly those that are well established and nonacute in nature, lay audiences have preexisting beliefs, attitudes, values, or behaviors; they are also influenced by structural or external factors that, directly or indirectly, have some bearing on their decisions to accept the information that scientists provide to them or recommendations scientists make (Chapters 2 and 3).[47] Lay audiences may not be convinced to change their thinking based solely on the expertise or authority of public health scientists or practitioners without being provided a rationale for how scientists reached their conclusions. Data, then, can provide the evidence to justify conclusions or recommendations of scientists.[82–84]

Because of the ongoing expansion of the scientific knowledge base resulting from research, new prevention and treatment options will be developed that require decision making by the public and policy makers. For example, the completion of the human genome project[85] will undoubtedly result in the development of new genetic screening tests.[86–88] These will provide communication challenges for both public heath scientists and practitioners to explain testing to lay audiences.

The sheer amount of health information readily available through the Internet, television, and print media is of highly variable quality. There are tens of thousands of health-related Web sites,[89] and public health topics are commonly covered by multiple information sources (see Chapter 2). Careful and effective explanation of scientific findings can potentially help to counter sources that are less trustworthy.

In many situations, regardless of the level of scientific evidence, the credibility of scientists or their organizations, and the strength of communication efforts, scientific findings may play a minor or even no role in influencing lay audiences, particularly in advocacy situations (Chapter 7). Realistically, scientific findings are just one of many factors considered by lay audiences. Good or "better" communication is not a panacea, nor a solution to every challenge in public health (or other areas of life, for that matter). For many public health issues, people (including scientists) have strongly held attitudes or beliefs and will dismiss messages that challenge or run counter to them (worldviews; see Chapter 2).[90] Such attitudes or beliefs can have a strong, yet often hidden, influence on the effectiveness of communication efforts that involve data selection and presentation to lay audiences.

This is not to suggest, however, that scientific data have no role in influencing lay audiences.[84] Failure to communicate relevant scientific findings or to communicate these findings at all to such audiences, especially findings with strong scientific consensus, poorly, prevents scientific evidence from having any opportunity to play a role in improving the public's health.

## Scientists, Scientific Culture, and Implications for Communicating with Lay Audiences

Kuhn[81] recognized that scientists share a common culture. The scientific disciplines typically use their own distinctive terminology, with terms such as "surveillance," "risk," and "cohort" having specific meanings for scientists that differ from those of lay audiences. To better understand some of the reasons why scientists have difficulty translating their findings to lay audiences, it is useful to review scientific culture, ways of thinking, how scientists explain findings to each other, and also to contrast these with lay audiences not trained in the sciences (Table 1.2).

There are several "givens" in scientific culture that influence scientists' ways of thinking and communicating. As part of scientific training and immersion in their fields, scientists adopt certain common viewpoints and approaches.[81, 91] There is strong agreement among scientists as to what constitutes better or worse examples of data sources, study designs, statistical tests, and generalizability of findings that provide "sufficient scientific evidence" for an assertion or recommendation.[92–94] These rules and ways of conducting science are

**Table 1.2 Contrasts between scientists and lay audiences**

|  | Scientists | Lay audiences |
|---|---|---|
| Sources and definition of acceptable evidence | Narrow | Broad |
| Belief in rational decision making | Strong | Variable |
| Acceptance of uncertainty | High | Low |
| Level of interest in scientific topic | High | Medium to low[a] |
| Quantitative and science literacy | High | Low |
| Ability and interest in reviewing extensive amounts of data | High |  |

*Note*: [a]Except for audience members with high levels of involvement for a specific issue.

generally so well accepted that most scientists are oblivious to the fact that they belong to a distinct culture with such rules,[81] failing to recognize that others may think differently about what constitutes evidence, let alone sufficient evidence, for influencing beliefs, attitudes, values, or behaviors.

## Rational Decision Making

Most scientists are strong believers in the "rational decision-making" model.[58, 59, 95, 96] This model assumes that people make decisions based on careful weighing of information from sources they deem as credible (i.e., scientists). Scientists share this belief in rational decision making with persons in other fields, such as economists and computer scientists.[97] Other types of information from "less credible" sources are criticized or discounted by scientists if they do not conform to the rules agreed upon within the science culture.[98]

The rational decision-making model is not commonly used by most lay audience members for health or other topics.[95, 96] People use many heuristics (shortcuts), often relying on faulty reasoning and intuition when making decisions, rather than carefully weighing evidence.[55, 90] Scientists' belief in rational decision making may lead them to mistakenly believe that simply providing more data or citing more scientifically credible studies will be more persuasive when communicating information to lay audiences. The public may not have much interest in the foundations of those arguments, though, and will listen instead to what the gist of the message may mean for them.

## An Acceptance of Uncertainty

Scientists generally acknowledge that science does not definitively prove that something is "true"; instead, theories or explanations that cannot be falsified, based on previous work and scientific consensus, are considered to be tentatively "correct."[98] There is always some level of uncertainty in science, not only concerning theories or hypotheses, but also about quantitative data, as demonstrated by the inclusion of confidence intervals and concerns about validity and representativeness of study populations.

New findings add to the knowledge base for a subject area and are considered within the context of previous work. Scientific theories, understanding, and explanations change as new knowledge is gained—previously accepted explanations, including those extensively disseminated to lay audiences and accepted for years, can be discarded or replaced because of new scientific discoveries or explanations.[81] Perhaps the classic public health example is "miasma theory," which was developed in the nineteenth century. This theory suggested that poor environments, such as foul-smelling odors, caused illness and disease. This theory was discarded and generally replaced by the microbiological "theory" after the discovery of the *Tubercle bacillus* and other microorganisms.[99] A more recent example was the discovery that peptic ulcers are caused by *Helicobacter pylori*, a bacterium, rather than emotional stress, as was thought for many years.[100]

## Intrinsic Interest in the Subject Matter

Scientists are specialists in their fields, regardless of whether they focus exclusively on one disease (or behavior or mechanism) or more broadly focus on a topic within their field, such as an infectious disease. This specialization can lead scientists to be especially enthusiastic about their subject area(s) of interest and fail to recognize that others may be much less interested (or uninterested) because of their lack of involvement with the subject.[101]

For the majority of people in the United States, health issues are of moderate-to-low interest.[6] In reality, unless audiences are involved with a particular health topic in some way,[101] efforts are needed to gain their attention (Chapters 2–5). This can be difficult, as people use mental "filters" to screen information to avoid attending to messages of little interest to them.[46, 102, 103] A further challenge is that people in the United States and other industrialized countries live in an information-rich environment, surrounded by mass media and commercial messages, and thus are exposed to literally hundreds of messages each day competing for their attention.[104]

## Sharing Information with Lay Audiences

Within the scientific community, transparency in information sharing is considered of strong value.[105] However, when asked to translate their findings to a lay audience, many scientists assume that communication should be one-way, that is, they provide their expertise to "less knowledgeable" persons[49, 106–108] who are expected to act in accordance with what scientists recommend (Chapter 2). Although this is true in some instances in public health (especially when new diseases or conditions are discovered), a one-way view of communication can lead scientists to have unrealistic expectations about how much power they have to persuade others. With the widespread availability of information to lay audiences through the Internet, and the increased use of a shared or informed decision-making model by lay audiences and health experts,[109, 110] scientists who adhere to the one-way communication model and who attempt to communicate scientific findings to lay audiences (especially to policy makers or journalists) can become disillusioned if they believe that their "scientific evidence," or the contextual limitations or caveats they provide are discounted or disregarded altogether.[26, 111]

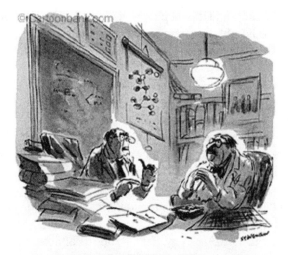

"One thing I'll say for us, Meyer—we
never stooped to popularizing science."

**Figure 1.2** Source: Cartoonbank.

In fact, one of the unanticipated consequences of the information age is that it has opened up an entirely new level of discourse between scientists and the public. In previous decades, scientists were cautioned away from communicating too much with the public as "popularizing" their research might prove damaging to their career (Figure 1.2). With the arrival of the Internet, individual citizens have been encouraged by public policy to take full advantage of the research and knowledge accumulated through scientific endeavors.[112] Professional organizations, such as the American Medical Association, have recognized the influx of lay traffic to their Web sites and have responded by posting information that is easily consumable by lay audiences. Interest in eHealth[113] and eGovernment[114, 115] has prompted discussions of how to put scientifically based evidence directly into the hands of consumers. Newspapers such as *USA Today*® have won awards for making statistical charts and graphs easy to read by the general public. Scientists are now being told that communicating with the public is part of their job description and that defending the relevance of scientific work belongs in the general public dialogue.[17]

## Statistical Thinking

Because of their training and experience, scientists are highly literate in science and mathematics and can easily talk in ways that others may not understand—"technical jargon." They may believe that lay audiences are literate in the science and mathematics used in public health research or surveillance, although this is often not the case.[61] Even simple concepts such as percentage can be misunderstood by many lay audiences,[116] let alone probabilistic reasoning or theory development.[117] As a result, scientists and public health practitioners often fail to provide basic background information that can help audiences understand data.

For example, scientific findings in health may not provide "yes or no" (definitive) answers because there is often a continuum along which health risks or benefits may be lesser or greater. This is especially evident in environmental or occupational health, such as when policy recommendations or regulatory standards are being set regarding what constitutes a "safe" or acceptable level for exposure to compounds such as radon or sulfur dioxide, but also occurs for other issues, such as defining recommendations about nutrition or physical activity.[118, 119] Public health practitioners in other areas also struggle with continuous versus dichotomous measures and what recommendations should be made concerning "safe" or "recommended" levels. There remains uncertainty within the scientific community about the level and type of treatment for elevated blood cholesterol,[120] cut-points for laboratory screening of low incident neonatal conditions,[121] and acceptable blood lead levels.[122]

Lay audiences commonly look to experts to provide clear recommendations based on the scientists' expertise.[90] Scientists may not provide definitive explanations or recommendations because of uncertainty, which may exist because of lack of research or absence of consensus among experts, the probabilistic nature of level of individual risk (e.g., estimating that 3 in 1,000 people taking a certain medication will develop a serious side effect but being unable to ascertain which individuals are at highest risk), or when previously well-accepted recommendations change. This inability of scientists to provide definitive answers can cause confusion, anxiety, fear, and anger in lay audiences, and can reduce their trust in scientists and their institutions or organizations.[42, 55, 123] This lack of definitiveness may be especially vexing for policy makers who look to scientists or other experts for answers to complex situations to help guide their decision making.[90]

## Rules of Evidence

What counts as evidence, or "how we know what we know," is referred to as epistemology, and differs between scientists,[58, 98] health care practitioners,[124] and lay audiences. Scientifically trustworthy sources for health information, such as the Centers for Disease Control and Prevention (CDC), the National Institutes of Health (NIH), or scientists employed by major research institutions,[125] are viewed as providing one type of evidence. These scientific sources are likely to be accorded expert status, especially by some policy makers and some journalists. It is not surprising, then, that religiosity and a personal belief in God is higher among lay audiences than among scientists,[126] as most faith-based traditions rely on a completely different approach to what counts as "acceptable evidence" for knowledge and beliefs, typically relying on authority to dictate what is "true" or "not true."[98] These basic epistemological differences help to explain many of the conflicts between science and religion.

Lay audiences, however, rely on many other sources for health information besides scientists and health professionals (Chapters 2 and 7).[39, 58, 127] Personal experience, emotions, interpersonal sources of information such as friends and family, community opinion leaders, economic interests (especially for policy makers), social and cultural realities ("common sense"), television news stories, and fictional accounts (e.g., movies), can also have important influences and constitute acceptable forms of "evidence" for many people.[39, 58, 127]

## Structures for Dialog

When it comes to communicating formally with others in their fields about scientific research, scientists typically use a highly structured approach to creating scientific journal articles, written reports, and presentations for professional conferences that is well understood by other scientists.[128] Depending on the type of study or presentation, a relevant theory or scientific model may be described. In journal articles, work on similar or related topics is reviewed and summarized (Introduction). Definitions, methodology, data sources/data collection, and statistical methods are described (Methods). Findings are described, often in some detail in text, tables, or figures (Results), and statistical uncertainty and statistical testing results are typically included. Finally, the contribution of the research to the scientific literature, comparisons with other research, explanations, study limitations or caveats, and in some instances, implications or recommendations are provided (Discussion).

Given their use and preference for more and new information, and their belief in the value of careful weighing of evidence from multiple perspectives, it is not surprising that scientists may believe that there cannot be too many "data points" on a particular topic. More data are better because they can be used to further demonstrate results and provide a stronger basis for drawing conclusions and making recommendations.

Unfortunately, the "more is better" approach tends to be counterproductive when communicating scientific findings to lay audiences. Not only does this approach assume that audiences are mathematically and scientifically literate, but it also ignores the problem of the limited capacity of most people to process and understand much information, especially complex information, at one time (cognitive overload; Chapter 3). Lay audiences typically want experts to quickly reach the bottom line with their conclusions and recommendations.[129]

## Values and Ethics

It may seem comforting to think that scientists are completely objective when it comes to their understanding, decisions, and actions involving public health issues. However, although scientific methods provide an invaluable framework for description and exploration, scientists are not value free.[58, 59, 81, 130] Indeed, there is ample evidence that most scientists, and the research they conduct, are consonant with broader values and goals within their own societies.[58, 59] Scientists have the same selective exposure and confirmation bias tendencies as everyone else (Chapter 2), preferring to associate with people and be exposed to information that confirms their existing beliefs.

Values and ethics are integral, although often hidden, aspects of scientific decision making.[59, 84, 130–132] These include decisions about (a) whether a health condition or problem exists, (b) definitions that classify individuals or populations as having or not having a health condition or being at high or low risk, (c) funding of research or public health surveillance, (d) data analysis, (e) data interpretation, (f) selecting or omitting findings in reports or other materials (e.g., bias among scientific journal editors against publishing negative research findings[133, 134]), and (g) data presentation.

Much communication in public health involves at least some element of persuasion.[135, 136] This means that should data be selected and presented to lay audiences, they may be chosen (or omitted) or presented in such a way as to maximize, minimize, or ignore certain themes—or attempt to lead audiences to draw certain conclusions.[84, 131, 137, 138] This tendency to strategically "use" data is obvious in advertising and politics,[139–142] but even well-intentioned scientists, practitioners, and others in public health and other fields are not immune.[19, 131, 137, 141, 143]

This does not mean that all scientific data are relative and malleable to suit the purposes of communicators. It does mean that it is important for public health scientists and practitioners to recognize the underlying values behind their messages and communication activities with lay audiences.[132, 142] The selection and presentation of information can have a strong influence on

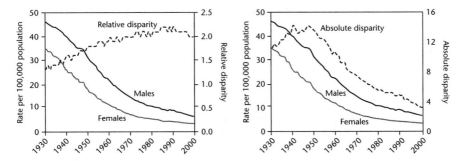

**Figure 1.3** Absolute and relative gender disparities in stomach cancer mortality, United States, 1930–2000. (Source: Harper S, Lynch J. Methods for measuring cancer disparities: Using data relevant to health people 2010 cancer-related objectives. *NCI Cancer Surveillance Monograph Series No. 6.* Bethesda, MD; National Cancer Institute: 2005. NIH Pub. No. 05-5777.)

audiences and their interpretation.[142, 144] Figure 1.3 illustrates the radically different conclusions about gender disparities in trends for stomach cancer[145] that audiences are likely to reach based on whether relative or absolute rate differences are presented. Persons who want to stress that gender disparities have increased over time would be more inclined to use the figure showing relative disparity trends, whereas those who want to emphasize declines in gender disparities would be more inclined to use the absolute disparity trend figure.

Furthermore, because most lay audiences will assume that scientists are experts about public health issues and are trustworthy (expert heuristic; Chapter 3), scientists and others communicating scientific information to lay audiences have an important ethical responsibility. They need to carefully assess whether they are, intentionally or unintentionally, misleading or manipulating audiences through their selection and presentation of data or other types of scientific information.[59, 130–132, 143]

## Conclusion

Communicating scientific findings, including data, to lay audiences is an important, underappreciated, and difficult role for many involved in public health. Effective communication about data can help to improve the health of the public; conversely, not communicating such information accurately, ethically, and effectively can have serious consequences.

Fortunately, there is a substantial amount of research and experience about how to better communicate quantitative findings. Throughout the remainder of this book, we describe the rationale and approaches that can substantially improve the ability of public health scientists and practitioners, along with those primarily involved in direct health care, to better communicate data to lay audiences.

---

**The bottom line**

Communicating quantitative data to lay audiences is possible

The major reason for communicating quantitative data to lay audiences is to provide evidence for the conclusions and recommendations of scientists

Scientists exist in their own culture that strongly believes in rational decision making and may mistakenly assume that lay audiences think the way they do about numbers

The three lay audiences described in this book—the general public, policy makers, and the press—can have different expectations of, and needs for, data in different situations

Understanding the characteristics of the lay audience to which you want to communicate data will give you clues as to the most effective approaches to use

---

## Further Reading

### Public Health Communication Planning

CDC. *CDCynergy, Basic Edition 3.0.* Atlanta, Ga.: Centers for Disease Control and Prevention; 2004.

National Cancer Institute. *Making Health Communication Programs Work.* Washington, D.C.: US Department of Health and Human Services, National Institutes of Health, National Cancer Institute; 2002. NIH Pub. No. 02–5145.

Schiavo R. *Health Communication: From Theory to Practice.* San Francisco, Calif.: Jossey-Bass; 2007.

Witte K, Meyer G, Martell D. *Effective Health Risk Messages: A Step-by-Step Guide.* Thousand Oaks, Calif.: Sage; 2001.

### Ethics and Values

Bayer R, Gostin LO, Jennings B, Steinbock B. eds. *Public Health Ethics: Theory, Policy, and Practice.* New York, N.Y.: Oxford; 2007.

Guttman N. *Public Health Communication Interventions: Values and Ethical Dilemmas.* Thousand Oaks, Calif.: Sage; 2000.

Perloff RM. *The Dynamics of Persuasion: Communication and Attitudes in the 21st Century,* 2nd ed. Mahwah, N.J.: Erlbaum; 2003.

Stone D. *Policy Paradox: The Art of Political Decision Making.* New York, N.Y.: Norton; 2002.

## Scientists and Scientific Culture

Garvin T. Analytical paradigms: The epistemological differences between scientists, policy makers, and the public. *Risk Anal.* 2001;21:443–455.

Gregory J, Miller S. *Science in Public: Communication, Culture, and Credibility.* New York, N.Y.: Plenum Trade; 1998.

Kuhn TS. *The Structure of Scientific Revolutions.* 3rd ed. Chicago, Ill.: University of Chicago Press; 1996.

Pavitt C. *The Philosophy of Science and Communication Theory.* Hauppauge, N.Y.: Nova Science; 2001.

## References

1. The Royal Institution of Great Britain. *Guidelines on Science and Health Communication.* London, England: The Royal Institution of Great Britain; November 2001.
2. Winslow CEA. *The Untilled Fields of Public Health.* [New York]: Health service, New York County chapter, the American Red Cross; 1920.
3. Rothman AJ, Kiviniemi MT. Treating people with information: An analysis and review of approaches to communicating health risk information. *J Natl Cancer Inst Monogr.* 1999;25:44–51.
4. Griffiths F, Convery B. Women's use of hormone replacement therapy for relief of menopausal symptoms, for prevention of osteoporosis, and after hysterectomy. *Br J Gen Pract.* 1995;45(396):355–358.
5. Hesse BW, Nelson DE, Kreps GL, et al. Trust and sources of health information: The impact of the Internet and its implications for health care providers: Findings from the first Health Information National Trends Survey. *Arch Intern Med.* 2005;165(22):2618–2624.
6. Miller JD, Kimmel LG. *Biomedical Communications: Purposes, Methods, and Strategies.* San Diego, Calif.: Academic Press; 2001.
7. Homan JM, McGowan JJ. The Medical Library Association: Promoting new roles for health information professionals. *J Med Libr Assoc.* 2002;90(1):80–85.
8. Viswanath K, Blake K, Meissner H, Hesse BW, Croyle RT. Occupational practices and the making of health news: A national survey of US Health and Medical Science journalists. *Journal of Health Communication.* In press.
9. Davis JJ, Cross E, Crowley J. Pharmaceutical websites and the communication of risk information. *J Health Commun.* 2007;12(1):29–39.
10. Nisbett RE, Borgida E, Crandall R, Reed H. Popular induction: Information is not necessarily informative. In: Carroll JS, Payne JW, eds. *Cognition and Social Behavior.* Vol. 2. Hillsdale, N.J.: Lawrence Erlbaum; 1976:227–236.
11. Nisbet MC, Mooney C. Framing science. *Science.* 2007;316(5821):56.
12. Hoffman J. Awash in information, patients face a lonely, uncertain road. *The New York Times.* August 14, 2005, pp. A1, A18, A19.
13. Frost K, Frank E, Maibach E. Relative risk in the news media: A quantification of misrepresentation. *Am J Public Health.* 1997;87(5):842–845.
14. King's Fund. *Health in the News: Risk, Reporting, and Media Influence.* London, England: King's Fund; 2003.

15. Woloshin S, Schwartz LM. What's the rush? The dissemination and adoption of preliminary research results. *J Natl Cancer Inst.* 2006;98(6):372–373.

16. Shenk D. *Data Smog: Surviving the Information Glut.* New York, N.Y.: Bantam; 1997.

17. Gregory J, Miller S. *Science in Public: Communication, Culture, and Credibility.* New York: Plenum Trade; 1998.

18. Mazur D. *The New Medical Conversation: Media, Patients, Doctors, and the Ethics of Scientific Communication.* Oxford, UK: Rowman & Littlefield; 2003.

19. Nelson DE, Brownson RC, Remington PL, Parvanta C, eds. *Communicating Public Health Information Effectively: A Guide for Practitioners.* Washington, D.C.: American Public Health Association; 2002.

20. Roter D, Hall J. *Doctors Talking with Patients/Patients Talking with Doctors: Improving Health Communication in Medical Visits.* 2nd ed. Westport, Conn.: Praeger; 2006.

21. Rains SA. Perceptions of traditional information sources and use of the World Wide Web to seek health information: Findings from the Health Information National Trends Survey. *J Health Commun.* 2007;12:667–680.

22. Ratzan SC. More evidence of communication for patients—time for action. *J Health Commun.* 2007;12:605–606.

23. Stone JH. Communication between physicians and patients in the era of E-medicine. *N Engl J Med.* 2007;356(24):2451–2454.

24. Hesse BW, Shneiderman B. eHealth research from the user's perspective. *Am J Prev Med.* May 2007;32(5 Suppl):S97–103.

25. LaVenture M. Using the power of googling and health informatics to improve public health practice. *Am J Prev Med.* 2007;33(1):75–76.

26. Fletcher SW. Whither scientific deliberation in health policy recommendations? *Alice in wonderland* in breast cancer screening. *N Engl J Med.* 1997;336(16):1180–1183.

27. National Institutes of Health. *Breast Cancer Screening for Women Ages 40–49.* Bethesda, Md.: National Institutes of Health; 1997.

28. Olesen O, Gotzsche PC. Cochrane review on screening for breast cancer with mammography. *Lancet.* 2001;358:1340–1342.

29. Harris R, Lohr, KN. Screening for prostate cancer: An update of the evidence for the U.S. Preventive Services Task Force. *Ann Intern Med.* 2002;137(11):917–929.

30. Feinleib M, Beresford SAA, Bowman BA, et al. Folate fortification for the prevention of birth defects: Case study. *Am J Epidemiol.* 2001;154(12 Suppl):S60–S69.

31. Colgrave J. *State of Immunity: The Politics of Vaccination in Twentieth-Century America.* Berkeley, Calif.: University of California Press; 2007.

32. Offit PA. Thimerosal and vaccines—a cautionary tale. *N Engl J Med.* 2007;357(13):1278–1279.

33. Thompson WW, Price C, Goodson B, et al. Early thimerosal exposure and neuropsychological outcomes at 7 to 10 years. *N Engl J Med.* 2007;357(13):1281–1292.

34. Baker JP. Mercury, vaccines, and autism: One controversy, three histories. *Am J Public Health.* 2008;98(2):244–253.

35. Julian-Reynier C, Welkenhuysen M, Hagoel L, Decruyenaere M, Hopwood P. Risk communication strategies: State of the art and effectiveness in the context of cancer genetic services. *Eur J Hum Genet.* 2003;11(10):725–736.

36. Koenig BA, Silverberg HL. Understanding probabilistic risk in predisposition genetic testing for Alzheimer disease. *Genet Test.* 1999;3(1):55–63.

37. Gregg MB, ed. *Field Epidemiology.* 3rd ed. New York, N.Y.: Oxford University Press; 2008.

38. Fearn-Banks K. *Crisis Communications: A Casebook Approach.* Mahwah, N.J.: Lawrence Erlbaum; 2002.

39. Johnson JD. *Cancer-Related Information Seeking.* Cresskill, N.J.: Hampton Press; 1997.

40. Sandman PM. *Responding to Community Outrage: Strategies for Effective Risk Communication.* Fairfax, Va.: American Industrial Hygiene Association; 1993.

41. Sandman PM. Crisis communication best practices: Some quibbles and additions. *J Appl Commun Res.* 2006;34:257–262.

42. Bennett P, Calman K, ed. *Risk Communication and Public Health.* New York, N.Y.: Oxford University Press; 1999.

43. Fagerlin A, Wang C, Ubel PA. Reducing the influence of anecdotal reasoning on people's health care decisions: Is a picture worth a thousand statistics? *Med Decis Making.* 2005;25(4):398–405.

44. Ali MJ, Davidoff R. Surgical, medical, and percutaneous therapies for patients with multivessel coronary artery disease. *Curr Cardiol Rep.* 2006;8(4):247–254.

45. Hannan EL, Wu C, Walford G, et al. Drug-eluting stents vs. coronary-artery bypass grafting in multivessel coronary disease. *N Engl J Med.* 2008;358(4):331–341.

46. Albers MJ. *Communication of Complex Information: User Goals and Information Needs for Dynamic Web Information.* Mahwah, N.J.: Lawrence Erlbaum; 2004.

47. Rowan KE. When simple language fails: Presenting difficult science to the public. *J Tech Writ Commun.* 1991;21:369–382.

48. Meyer D, Leventhal H, Guttmann M. Common-sense models of illness: The example of hypertension. In: Salovey P, Rothman AJ, ed. *Social Psychology of Health.* New York, N.Y.: Psychology Press; 2003:9–20.

49. Turney J. Public understanding of science. *Lancet.* 1996;347(9008):1087–1090.

50. Friedman SM, Dunwoody S, Rogers CL, ed. *Scientists and Journalists: Reporting Science as News.* New York, N.Y.: Free Press; 1986.

51. Gastel B. *Presenting Science to the Public.* Philadelphia, Pa.: ISI Press; 1983.

52. Gastel B. *Health Writer's Handbook.* Ames, Iowa: Iowa State University Press; 1998.

53. National Research Council. *Improving Risk Communication.* Washington, D.C.: National Academy Press; 1989.

54. Nelkin D. *Selling Science: How the Press Covers Science and Technology.* New York, N.Y.: W. H. Freeman; 1995.

55. Kahneman D, Slovic P, Tversky A, ed. *Judgment under Uncertainty: Heuristics and Biases.* Cambridge, UK: Cambridge University Press; 1982.

56. Tversky A, Kahneman D. The framing of decisions and the psychology of choice. *Science.* 1981;211:453–458.

57. Plous S. *The Psychology of Judgment and Decision-Making.* New York, N.Y.: McGraw-Hill; 1993.

58. Garvin T. Analytical paradigms: The epistemological distances between scientists, policy makers, and the public. *Risk Anal.* 2001;21(3):443–455.

59. Steinbock B, ed. *The Oxford Handbook of Bioethics.* New York, N.Y.: Oxford University Press; 2007.

60. Cohn V, Cope L. *News and Numbers: A Guide to Reporting Statistical Claims and Controversies in Health and Other Fields.* 2nd ed. Ames, Iowa: University of Iowa; 2001.

61. Weigold ME. Communicating science: A review of the literature. *Science Communication.* 2001;23:164–193.

62. Brownson RC, Malone BR. Communicating public health information to policy makers. In: Nelson DE, Brownson RC, Remington PL, Parvanta C, eds.

*Communicating Public Health Information Effectively: A Guide for Practitioners.* Washington, D.C.: American Public Health Association; 2002:97–114.

63. Remington PL, Ahrens D. Communicating public health information to private and voluntary health organizations. In: Nelson DE, Brownson RC, Remington PL, Parvanta C, eds. *Communicating Public Health Information Effectively: A Guide for Practitioners.* Washington, D.C.: American Public Health Association; 2002:115–126.

64. Dearing JW, Rogers EM. *Agenda-Setting.* Thousand Oaks, Calif.: Sage; 1996.

65. Reese SD, Gandy OH, Grant AE, eds. *Framing Public Life: Perspectives on Our Understanding of the Social World.* Mahwah, N.J.: Lawrence Erlbaum; 2001.

66. Littlejohn SW, Foss KA *Theories of Human Communication.* 9th ed. Belmont, Calif.: Wadsworth; 2007.

67. Centers for Disease Control and Prevention. *CDCynergy,* Basic edition 3.0. In: Centers for Disease Control and Prevention, ed. Atlanta, Ga; 2004.

68. Maibach E, Parrott RL, ed. *Designing Health Messages: Approaches from Communication Theory and Public Health Practice.* Thousand Oaks, Calif.: Sage; 1995.

69. National Cancer Institute. *Making Health Communication Programs Work.* Washington, D.C.: US Department of Health and Human Services, National Institutes of Health, National Cancer Institute; 2002. NIH Pub. No. 02–5145.

70. Rice RE, Atkin CK ed. *Public Communication Campaigns.* 3rd ed. Thousand Oaks, Calif.: Sage; 2001.

71. Schiavo R. *Health Communication: From Theory to Practice.* San Francisco, Calif.: Jossey-Bass; 2007.

72. Thomas RK. *Health Communication.* New York, N.Y.: Springer; 2006.

73. Thompson TL. *Handbook of Health Communication.* Mahwah, N.J.: Lawrence Erlbaum Associates; 2003.

74. Witte K, Meyer G, Martell D. *Effective Health Risk Messages: A Step-by-Step Guide.* Thousand Oaks, Calif.: Sage; 2001.

75. Institute of Education Sciences. *National Assessment of Adult Literacy.* Washington, D.C.: U.S. Department of Education; 2007.

76. Loveless T. Trends in math: The importance of basic skills. *Brookings Review.* 2003;21(4):40–43.

77. National Mathematics Advisory Panel. *Foundations for Success: The Final Report of the National Mathematics Advisory Panel.* Washington, D.C.: U.S. Department of Education; 2008.

78. Stover GN, Bassett MT. Practice is the purpose of public health. *Am J Public Health.* 2003;93(11):1799–1801.

79. Edwards A, Elwyn G. Understanding risk and lessons for clinical risk communication about treatment preferences. *Qual Health Care.* 2001;10(Suppl 1):i9–i13.

80. Edwards A, Elwyn G, Mulley A. Explaining risks: Turning numerical data into meaningful pictures. *BMJ.* 2002;324(7341):827–830.

81. Kuhn TS. *The Structure of Scientific Revolutions.* 3rd ed. Chicago, Ill.: University of Chicago Press; 1996.

82. Corbett E, Connors R. *Classic Rhetoric for the Modern Student.* 4th ed. New York, N.Y.: Oxford University Press; 1999.

83. Parrott R, Silk K, Dorgan K, Condit C, Harris T. Risk communication and judgments of statistical evidentiary appeals. When a picture is not worth a thousand words. *Hum Commun Res.* 2005;32:423–452.

84. Stone DA. *Policy Paradox: The Art of Political Decision Making.* Rev. ed. New York, N.Y.: Norton; 2002.

85. Guttmacher AE, Collins FS. Welcome to the genomic era. *N Engl J Med.* 2003;349(10):996–998.

86. Croyle R, Lerman C. Psychological impact of genetic testing. In: Croyle R, ed. *Psychosocial Effects of Screening for Disease Prevention and Detection.* New York, N.Y.: Oxford University Press; 1995:11–38.

87. Burke W, Psaty BM. Personalized medicine in the era of genomics. *JAMA.* 2007;298(14):1682–1684.

88. Feero WG, Guttmacher AE, Collins FS. The genome gets personal—almost. *JAMA.* 2008;299(11):1351–1352.

89. U.S. Department of Health and Human Services. *Report on Objective 11–4: Estimating the Proportion of Health-Related Websites Disclosing Information that Can Be Used to Assess Their Quality.* Washington, D.C.: U.S. Department of Health and Human Services; 2007.

90. Slovic P, ed. *The Perception of Risk.* Sterling, Va.: Earthscan; 2000.

91. Fox RC. Cultural competence and the culture of medicine. *N Engl J Med.* 2005;353(13):1316–1319.

92. Brownson RC, Baker EA, Leet TL, Gillespie KN. *Evidence-Based Public Health.* New York, N.Y.: Oxford University Press; 2003.

93. Campbell DT, Stanley JC. *Experimental and Quasi-Experimental Designs.* Boston, Mass.: Houghton Mifflin; 1963.

94. Hill AB. The environment and disease: Association or causation. *Proc Res Soc Med.* 1965;58:295–300.

95. Nelkin D. Communicating technological risk: The social construction of risk perception. *Annu Rev Public Health.* 1989;10:95–113.

96. Redelmeier DA, Rozin P, Kahneman D. Understanding patients' decisions: Cognitive and emotional perspectives. *J Am Med Assoc.* 1993;270(1):72–76.

97. Fischhoff B, Bostrom A, Quadrel MJ. Risk perception and communication. *Annu Rev Public Health.* 1993;14:183–203.

98. Pavitt C. *The Philosophy of Science and Communication Theory.* Hauppauge, N.Y.: Nova Science; 2001.

99. Susser M, Susser E. Choosing a future for epidemiology: I. Eras and paradigms. *Am J Public Health.* 1996;86(5):668–673.

100. Moss SF, Sood S. Helicobacter pylori. *Curr Opin Infect Dis.* 2003;16(5):445–451.

101. Petty RE, Cacioppo JT. *Communication and Persuasion: Central and Peripheral Routes to Attitude Change.* New York, N.Y.: Springer-Verlag; 1986.

102. Hastie R, Dawes RM. *Rational Choice in an Uncertain World: The Psychology of Judgment and Decision Making.* Thousand Oaks, Calif.: Sage; 2001.

103. Berry D. *Risk, Communication, and Health Psychology.* Berkshire, UK: Open University Press; 2004.

104. McQuail D. *McQuail's Mass Communication Theory.* 5th ed. London, UK: Sage; 2005.

105. True J. *Finding Out: Conducting and Evaluating Social Research.* 2nd ed. Belmont, Calif.: Wadsworth; 1989.

106. Lum M, Parvanta C, Maibach E, Arkin E, Nelson DE. General public: Communicating to inform. In: Nelson DE, Brownson RC, Remington PL, Parvanta C, eds. *Communicating Public Health Information Effectively: A Guide for Practitioners.* Washington, D.C.: American Public Health Association; 2002:47–57.

107. Wright N, Nerlich B. Use of the deficit model in a shared culture of argumentation: The case of foot and mouth science. *Public Understand Sci.* 2006;15:331–342.

108. Young N, Matthews R. Experts' understanding of the public: Knowledge control in a risk controversy. *Public Understand Sci.* 2007;165:123–144.

109. Briss P, Rimer B, Reilley B, et al. Promoting informed decisions about cancer screening in communities and healthcare systems. *Am J Prev Med.* 2004;26(1):67–80.

110. McNutt RA. Shared medical decision making: Problems, process, progress. *JAMA.* 2004;292(20):2516–2518.

111. Lewenstein BV, Jasanoff S, Markle X. Science and the media. *Handbook of Science and Technology Studies.* London, UK: Sage; 1995:343–361.

112. Hesse BW, Grantham CE. The emergence of electronically distributed work communities: Implications for research on telework. *Electron Net Res Appl Policy.* 1991;1(1):4–17.

113. Atienza AA, Hesse BW, Baker TB, et al. Critical issues in eHealth research. *Am J Prev Med.* 2007;32(5 Suppl):S71-S74.

114. Quantin C, Allaert FA, Fassa M, Riandey B, Avillach P, Cohen O. How to manage secure direct access of European patients to their computerized medical record and personal medical record. *Stud Health Technol Inform.* 2007;127:246–255.

115. Marchionini G, Levin M. Digital Government Information Services: The Bureau of Labor Statistics case. *Interactions.* 2003;4:18–27.

116. Yamagishi K. When a 12.86% mortality is more dangerous than 24.14%: Implications for risk communications. *Appl Cognit Psychol.* 1997;11:495–506.

117. Woloshin S, Schwartz LM, Moncur M, Gabriel S, Tosteson AN. Assessing values for health: Numeracy matters. *Med Decis Making.* 2001;21(5):382–390.

118. Bull FC, Bellew B, Schoppe S, Bauman AE. Developments in national physical activity policy: An international review and recommendations towards better practice. *J Sci Sports Med.* 2004;7(Suppl 1):93–107.

119. O'Dell B. *Handbook of Nutritionally Essential Minerals.* Boca Raton, Fla.: CRC Press; 1999.

120. Frethem A, Williams JW Jr, Oxman AD, Herrin J. The relation between methods and recommendations in clinical practice guidelines for hypertension and hyperlipidemia. *J Fam Pract.* 2002;51(11):963–968.

121. Holtzman NA. Expanding newborn screening: How good is the evidence? *JAMA.* 2003;290(19):2606–2608.

122. Bellinger DC. Lead. *Pediatrics.* 2004;113(4):1016–1022.

123. O'Keefe DJ. *Persuasion: Theory and Research.* Thousand Oaks, Calif.: Sage; 2002.

124. Groopman JE. *How Doctors Think.* Boston, Mass.: Houghton Mifflin; 2007.

125. Payne JG. Oral presentations. In: Nelson DE, Brownson RC, Remington PL, Parvanta C, eds. *Communicating Public Health Information Effectively: A Guide for Practitioners.* Washington, D.C.: American Public Health Association; 2002:141–154.

126. Larson E, Witham L. Leading scientists still reject god. *Nature.* 1998;394:313.

127. Brashers DE, Goldsmith DJ, Hsieh E. Information seeking and avoiding in health contexts. *Hum Commun Res.* 2002;28:258–271.

128. Valiela I. *Doing Science: Design, Analysis, and Communication of Scientific Research.* New York, N.Y.: Oxford; 2000.

129. Hibbard JH, Peters E. Supporting informed consumer health care decisions: Data presentation approaches that facilitate the use of information in choice. *Annu Rev Public Health.* 2003;24:413–433.

130. Coughlin SS, Beauchamp TL. *Ethics and Epidemiology.* New York, N.Y.: Oxford University Press; 1996.

131. Bayer R, Beauchamp DE. *Public Health Ethics: Theory, Policy, and Practice.* Oxford; New York, N.Y.: Oxford University Press; 2007.

132. Guttman N. *Public Health Communication Interventions: Values and Ethical Dilemmas.* Thousand Oaks, Calif.: Sage; 2000.

133. Felson DT, Glantz L. A surplus of positive trials: Weighing biases and reconsidering equipoise. *Arthritis Res Ther.* 2004;6(3):117–119.

134. Kennedy D. The old file-drawer problem. *Science.* 2004;305(5683):451.

135. Witte K. The manipulative nature of health communication research: Ethical issues and guidelines. *Am Behav Sci.* 1994;38(2):285–293.

136. Perloff RM. *The Dynamics of Persuasion: Communication and Attitudes in the 21st Century.* 2nd ed. Mahwah, N.J.: Lawrence Erlbaum; 2003.

137. Adelman C. The propaganda of numbers. *Chronicle of Higher Education.* October 13, 2006:B6–B9.

138. Thornton H. Patients' understanding of risk: Enabling understanding must not lead to manipulation. *BMJ.* 2003;327(7417):693–694.

139. Donahue JM, Cevasco M, Rosenthal MB. A decade of direct-to-consumer advertising of prescription drugs. *NEJM.* 2007;357:673–681.

140. Huff D. *How to Lie with Statistics* (paperback reissue). New York: Norton; 1993.

141. Monmonier MS. *How to Lie with Maps.* 2nd ed. Chicago: University of Chicago Press; 1996.

142. Pratkanis AR, Aronson E. *Age of Propaganda: The Everyday Use and Abuse of Persuasion.* Rev. ed. New York, N.Y.: W.H. Freeman; 2001.

143. Tufte ER. *The Visual Display of Quantitative Information.* 2nd ed. Cheshire, Conn.: Graphics Press; 2001.

144. Rothman AJ, Kiviniemi MT. Treating people with information: An analysis and review of approaches to communicating health risk information. *J Natl Cancer Inst Monogr.* 1999(25):44–51.

145. Harper S, Lynch J. *Methods for Measuring Cancer Disparities: Using Data Relevant to Healthy People 2010 Cancer-Related Objectives.* Bethesda, Md.: National Cancer Institute; 2005. NIH Pub. No. 05–5777.

# 2

## Communication Fundamentals

> Meaning arises only when listeners, readers, or viewers actively
> make sense of what they hear, read, or see. Meaning is not transmit-
> ted by experts so much as it is constructed by audiences.
>
> Lum et al. "General public: Communicating to inform,"
> Communicating Public Health Information Effectively:
> A Guide for Practitioners[1]

### Introduction

Presenting scientific data to audiences is but one aspect of the broader topic
of communication. Before discussing approaches to communicating data to
lay audiences, it is essential to understand the fundamentals of communication. In this chapter, we review these fundamentals and discuss the many
factors that influence communication. We also review the research on the
rationale and value of communicating data to lay audiences.

### Overview of the Basic Communication Model

In the basic model of communication, a source (or sender) uses a channel(s) to send
messages to an audience (receiver) or audiences[2, 3] (Figure 2.1). Sources are the
individuals or organizations that supply messages,[4] and they generally select the
channel(s) through which they attempt to reach audiences with those messages.[4]
Communication channels are often categorized as being interpersonal or mediated; mediated channels can reach larger numbers of people and are further
classified as mass media (e.g., television or radio) or small media (e.g., brochures, posters). Because there is overlap between the terms sources and channels in the communication literature,[4] they are considered together here.

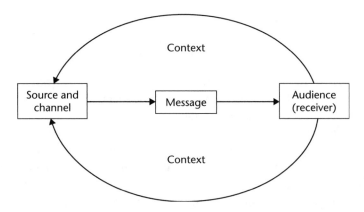

**Figure 2.1** Basic communication model.

Messages are the words, symbols, or pictures used by sources to transmit information.[4] This book primarily concerns approaches to communicating messages that contain quantitative data. An audience can be an individual, group of individuals, or as large as millions of people on an international scale. Note that the curved lines with arrows directly connecting audiences to sources and channels in Figure 2.1 show that audiences are active participants in the entire communication process, capable of seeking information themselves.

Three additional components are important considerations in the basic communication model: purpose, strategy, and context.[3] Purpose is the "why" of communication, that is, what senders intend to accomplish by making messages available to audiences.[5, 6] Strategy refers to an active or passive approach used by senders to gain the attention and interest of audiences about messages.[4, 7] Context consists of individual and environmental factors that may influence audience members' receipt or interpretation of messages (Figure 2.1).

This basic communication model is highly simplistic and may inappropriately imply communication is a one-way process in which experts transmit packets of information to a passive or uninformed audience.[3] Extensive research has shown that people have preexisting ideas about many health topics; they are exposed to, or obtain health information, on their own—they are not simply information recipients but they develop their own understanding and interpretation.[4, 8] Communicating public health information is a two-way process in which senders listen to, and work carefully with, intended audiences to better understand them and obtain their input, with senders making adjustments as necessary.[1]

## Sources and Channels

### Background

Interpersonal sources consist of family members, friends, neighbors, work colleagues, acquaintances in religious, civic, or social organizations, and personal health care providers.[7] Interpersonal communication channels typically involve face-to-face or small group in-person meetings, telephone conversations, oral presentations, correspondence, or email. Mediated sources are more impersonal and involve the use of a communication channel(s) that can reach a larger audience consisting of individuals not usually known to the persons or organizations creating messages. With the exception of tailored communication,[9–11] mediated communication is less personalized and may involve little (if any) two-way communication.[3] The Internet does not easily fit into a category, as it has characteristics of both interpersonal and mediated communication channels.

Although classifying channels of communication is useful for descriptive and planning purposes, they tend to be interrelated. There is much interaction between peoples' interpersonal and mediated sources for health and other types of information[12]; for example, health information received from mass media channels often becomes part of interpersonal communications[4, 13–15] (Box 2.1), which is sometimes referred to as the two-step flow of information.[16]

---

**Box 2.1** Beware the flesh-eating bananas!  An Internet hoax

The development and expansion of the Internet has greatly expanded the size of audiences and the speed by which communication messages flow. Although this expansion of communication has been beneficial in many ways, it has also allowed erroneous health information, which would otherwise have had little credence and be known only to a small number of people, to spread rapidly from interpersonal channels to sometimes a worldwide audience.

One example of this has been false rumors about necrotizing fasciitis. This serious health condition results from bacteria entering the body through a small cut or scratch; as bacteria reproduce, they produce toxins that break down body tissues, which often have to be removed by amputation of affected body areas. Nicknamed by media representatives as "flesh-eating disease," individuals with the condition received extensive, and often tabloid-like, coverage through certain news media venues in the late 1990s.

In 1999, a nonexistent research organization sent emails to some individuals, warning them that persons who ate bananas imported from Costa

*(continued)*

---

Rica could be infected with "flesh-eating disease." There is no association between bananas and necrotizing fasciitis, but the email spread quickly from the originator of the hoax to thousands of individuals in several countries. Believing that the danger was real, the message about Costa Rican bananas was widely forwarded to other email addresses by individuals wanting to warn their friends and loved ones of the alleged danger.

This Internet email hoax spread so rapidly that in January 2000, the Centers for Disease Control and Prevention (CDC) released a statement to try to reassure the public. The statement emphasized that (a) the usual route of transmission for the bacteria is person to person, (b) sometimes causative bacteria can be transmitted through foods but that this was extremely unlikely for necrotizing fasciitis, and (c) the CDC and Food and Drug Administration (FDA) agreed that the bacteria cannot survive long on the surface of a banana.

Flesh-eating banana emails continued to circulate, however, but with variations on the message. Instead of listing the source as a fake research group, email messages purported to be from, or endorsed by, CDC and other reputable federal agencies were circulated. A more recent form of the hoax warned South Africans of the "danger" of eating Costa Rican flesh-eating bananas. Interpersonal communication channels, enhanced and amplified by the Internet and its email capabilities, have kept the urban legend of flesh-eating bananas alive for many years.

Source: Centers for Disease Control and Prevention. *False Internet Report about Bananas*; 2000. Emery D. *The Great Internet Banana Scare of 2000*. About.com; 2000.

Rapid technologic advances have provided myriad ways for people to communicate with each other or seek information.[17–19] There is now widespread use of Web portals, personal digital assistants (PDAs), cellular telephones, digital photography, mapping software, video and audio computerization (e.g., downloading of music or movie clips), electronic games, and virtual computer technology throughout much of the world, which has made unprecedented amounts of information available to the public. From the perspective of communicating data, these advances can provide new and different ways for audiences to visualize and process information (see Chapter 4), potentially changing how people think about health and other issues.[20]

## Availability, Preference, and Credibility

The availability, preference, and credibility of sources are key, interrelated aspects of communication. Source availability, preference, and credibility are often underappreciated by public health practitioners and scientists, and failure to consider all three can lead to ineffective communication regardless of the quality of the message or its presentation.

*Availability* refers to audiences' access to information sources and channels and can be highly variable depending on audience characteristics, such as education or income, and structural factors, such as health insurance status. For example, radio and television are almost universally available in the United States and much of the world,[21, 22] but the availability of Internet services, although increasing, is not as universal.[23, 24] Of special note is that people with lower levels of education, in general, have substantially reduced access to, and thus use, fewer sources of information than do more highly educated persons.[4]

*Preference* refers to where and how audiences like to obtain information, and is related to availability. Preferences vary widely among populations and individuals with differences especially great by education level and age[4, 7, 18, 25, 26] (Box 2.2). Persons with lower levels of education, for example, are more likely to rely on interpersonal sources and television for health information.[4, 25] The widespread diffusion of Internet access has transformed where many people

---

**Box 2.2 Preferences and trust of health sources: The generation gap**

People receive health information from a multiplicity of sources, but most have clear preferences as to what information sources they like to use and trust. Not surprisingly, physicians and other health care providers are widely considered trusted sources of health information. The rise of the Internet with its large number of Web sites, and the extent of information available, however, has changed how people obtain health information. Nevertheless, one clear demographic difference in preferred health information sources is age.

Adults less than 65 years of age, and especially younger adults with higher levels of education, are much more likely to seek and trust health information obtained from the Internet. When they do seek medical care, they prefer a shared decision-making approach, working with their providers to discuss potential courses of action. Increasingly, health care providers report having patients arrive for appointments with pages of Internet printouts and lists of specific questions.

In marked contrast, older adults are more inclined to seek, and have great trust in, information from their health care providers. This probably results, to a large extent, from the long history of paternalism that characterized many physician–patient relationships: the doctor acted

*(continued)*

independently by gathering information, weighing choices, making treatment decisions, and telling patients what to do. Additionally, many older adults have lower levels of education, are not as computer-proficient, and rarely access the Internet.

Source: Arora NK, McHorney CA. Patient preferences for medical decision making: Who really wants to participate? *Med Care*. 2000;38(3):335–341. Hesse BW, Nelson DE, Kreps GL, et al. Trust and sources of health information: The impact of the Internet and its implications for health care providers: Findings from the first Health Information National Trends Survey. *Arch Intern Med*. 2005;165(22):2618–2624. Murray E, Lo B, Pollack L, et al. The impact of health information on the Internet on the physician–patient relationship: Patient perceptions. *Arch Intern Med*. 2003;163(14):1727–1734.

obtain health information.[27–29] Internet use is highest among populations who are younger, highly educated, or who have higher incomes, although differences between demographic groups have narrowed in recent years.[27, 29, 30] However, some older adults strongly prefer to rely on their health care providers for health information and never use Web sites. In reality, most people typically use multiple sources for health information, especially when seeking information that is salient to their immediate needs or concerns.[4, 30]

Preferences for different media have changed over the years. Increasingly, newspaper readers are adults aged 40 years or older with high levels of education.[22] Magazines, radio, and television audiences are highly segmented, with specific publications, genres, and programs produced to appeal to individuals with narrow ranges of interests or tastes.[18, 22, 24, 28, 31, 32]

*Credibility* concerns the believability of sources and is based on two major dimensions: perceived trustworthiness and expertise (Box 2.3).[33–36] A common mental heuristic (shortcut) that people use to determine the believability of a message is their judgment about the credibility of message sources.[33, 34]

The good news for public health practitioners is that educational and occupational credentials, such as advanced academic or professional degrees or having certain job titles (within their area of expertise), increase the credibility of sources among lay audiences.[34, 36] For example, most mainstream health professionals, especially physicians, are perceived as highly credible sources of health information.[37] Research has also shown that the credibility of sources is enhanced when they use credible and relevant citations to support their statements or claims (e.g., in oral presentations or written materials).[34]

Similarly, representatives from many government health agencies, such as the Centers for Disease Control and Prevention (CDC), the National Institutes of Health (NIH), state health departments, and many academic institutions[4, 25] are normally considered to be highly credible, as are persons from well-known

---

**Box 2.3** Using numbers to enhance source credibility

Presenting findings using numbers can have a powerful and persuasive effect on audiences. Early studies in persuasion and communication confirmed the observation that presenting information with a scientific veneer—that is, through numbers and statistics—could enhance an audience's perceptions of credibility for a communicator and the communicator's message.

With an enhanced perception of credibility, an audience is more likely to trust communicators' messages. Subsequent research done in the context of jury deliberations confirmed those early observations. When an attorney or witness brought data-based evidence to bear on the premises of an argument, the argument would be perceived as being more credible and the communicator would be perceived as being more trustworthy than when the premises were presented alone.

Source: Hovland CI, Janis IL, Kelley HH. *Communication and Persuasion: Psychological Studies of Opinion Change.* Westport, Conn.: Greenwood; 1982. Reynolds RA, Reynolds JL. Evidence. In: Dillard JP, Pfau M, eds. *The Persuasion Handbook: Developments in Theory and Practice.* Thousand Oaks, Calif.: Sage; 2002:427–444.

---

voluntary or other health organizations (e.g., the American Cancer Society, March of Dimes).[38, 39] In contrast, representatives from organizations with perceived conflicts of interest or self-serving interests, such as the tobacco industry, are not considered to be credible sources of health information.[34]

But health professionals and organizations are not the only credible sources for health information among lay audiences, as certain interpersonal, Internet, and mass media sources may also be highly trusted.[25] For some people, selected family members, neighbors, worksite colleagues, or community organization leaders may be viewed as highly credible health information sources. There is growing research suggesting that ".gov" Web sites are generally perceived as more credible than ".com" sites[39]; nevertheless, lay users of science, health, and other types of Web sites assess source credibility using many dimensions (e.g., accessibility of the site, ease of navigation) besides organizational reputation or the scientific credentials of cited individuals.[39–42]

## Messages

Much of the theoretical and applied communication literature, including this book, concerns messages, especially message content and presentation, and to a lesser extent, exposure and attention of audiences to messages. Health-related messages are built upon the foundation of science-based storylines.

## Storyline

A storyline, as used throughout this book, refers to the major conclusion(s) based on the review and synthesis of the science that communicators would like audiences to understand, that is, the science-based "bottom line." It represents the current status of scientific knowledge for either a general or a specific aspect of a health topic that scientists or public health practitioners want lay audiences to know. (This definition differs from the more general usage, where storyline usually refers to the plot in a book, dramatic presentation, or movie.)

Science-based storylines vary widely, depending on the type of research and level of consensus among scientists. The strongest types of storylines are based on comprehensive reviews of the scientific evidence, such as those conducted by the Task Force on Community Preventive Services,[43] the U.S. Preventive Services Task Force Guide to Clinical Preventive Services,[44] the Cochrane Collaboration,[45] or some other type of scientifically defensible review process. The easiest storylines are based on "settled science," that is, when there is a clear scientific consensus based on many studies over time, such as the importance of screening for hypertension or immunization against many vaccine-preventable diseases. Such storylines provide a clear rationale for scientists and public health practitioners to communicate messages to lay audiences for the purpose of persuasion or instruction (see discussion on purpose later in this chapter).

But other science-based storylines are not so clear-cut. A review of the science may indicate that there is little or no scientific knowledge at all (e.g., about the potential health effects associated with many environmental chemical exposures), that there are several appropriate "ways" or "options" to address an issue (e.g., coronary artery disease treatment), or that no scientific consensus exists (e.g., screening for prostate cancer). The purposes for communicating messages to lay audiences, in these instances, will be to increase knowledge (with no intent to persuade), or for informed decision making. The key point to remember is that messages about public health topics, first and foremost, must be based on scientific knowledge and understanding.

## Content and Presentation

Much of the practice (and research) in communication concerns message content and presentation to audiences to achieve what communicators hope will be the desired effects.[27, 46, 47] A few of many examples include topics such as the use of different types of appeals for persuasion,[47] visual presentation approaches,[48] and optimal Web site design.[49] Content refers to determining what messages to develop and use, and varies depending on the purpose, audience, and context for communication. Presentation refers to such activities as channel selection (e.g., visual, audio, or written) and the organization and layout of messages. For example, there is an extensive research literature on message argument strength and believability, message appeal (e.g., emotional versus rational), and message tone in the persuasion, debate, and marketing literatures,[27, 34, 46, 47, 50–52] as well as other fields such as health promotion and health education.[53–56] The major emphasis of this book is the selection of content and the presentation of messages containing quantitative data.

## Exposure and Attention

Whatever the purpose for communication, it is necessary that intended audiences be exposed to messages.[5] Although ensuring audiences are adequately exposed to messages seems obvious, it is easy to forget once work begins on content and presentation. Research on health campaigns, for example, has consistently shown that many fail because only a small percentage of intended audience members were exposed to messages.[57] Inadequate message exposure occurs in many other situations, as audiences may not read targeted emails or newspaper articles, or Web sites may be designed in such a way that audiences fail to locate key messages.

Exposure does not guarantee that audiences will attend to messages. Attention to messages is heavily dependent on the audience's preexisting level of interest (involvement) for a specific topic.[58, 59] Much effort will be needed to gain the attention of audiences for topics or data that audiences do not have much immediate (or any) interest in. This may consist of attempting to increase the audiences' levels of emotion about the topic, such as through the use of narratives or pictures (Chapter 4), as well as using an active strategy to reach certain people.

## Audiences

One of the most important contributions from the field of communication is its emphasis on identifying and understanding audiences, with the goal of using the most appropriate sources, channels, and messages. Audience segmentation refers to categorizing and describing relatively homogeneous or similar subgroups among broader audiences, and has typically involved categorizing general public subgroups by certain common characteristics, such as by demographics, geography, beliefs, or psychological states.[59] Segmentation has also been used to categorize audiences by occupational groups and by media usage.[7, 60] Indeed, the authors of this book have segmented lay audiences into the general public, policy makers, and the press.

## General Audience Considerations

Although there are unique aspects of the three lay audiences we have selected, common features that influence communication, including communication about public health topics, are important factors for all of them. They are involvement and level of interest in health; education level; lay health beliefs and worldviews; and past experience, confirmation bias, and selective exposure.

### General Level of Interest in Health and Involvement with a Specific Health Issue

The level of interest in health issues among people varies widely.[25, 61, 62] For the majority of people in the United States, health issues are of moderate-to-low interest, especially on an ongoing basis. Women, people of older age, and those with self-reported good personal health show an increased interest in health topics, as do persons in the presence of individual or family health problems.[25] We are unaware of research on the general level of interest in health issues among policy makers or journalists; however, there is likely much self-selection based on preexisting level of interest, resulting in such persons becoming members of legislative committees that address health issues or becoming science or health reporters.[63–65]

A well-known characteristic that determines whether any audience member is likely to attend to messages about a specific health topic or issue is involvement.[58, 59] Involvement refers to personal relevance or interest in a specific topic or issue; involved individuals are likely to attend to messages on such issues or topics because they already find them salient to their interests, thus the method and type of message presentation may not be as critical for such individuals.[58]

Lay individuals who are personally involved with a topic are more likely to seek information about the topic than those without such involvement[4] and are likely to expect additional data and other types of information to be available to them along with material to support source credibility (Figure 2.2). Media stories or information about proposed legislative funding for services or new research on spinal cord injuries or autism, for example, will resonate strongly with individuals who are experiencing these conditions themselves or who have family members or friends with them. It is a well-established adage that some of the best legislative champions for a specific disease or health condition are personally familiar with individuals who have the disease or condition. Although there is limited research, involvement also extends to journalists, as the personal interests of reporters and editors influence their choice of stories and how they are framed for audiences.[66]

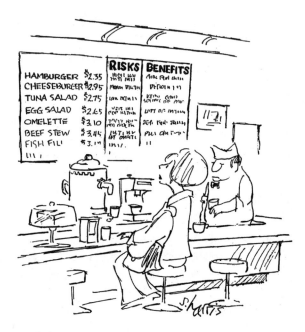

**Figure 2.2** Source: ScienceCartoonsPlus.com

Involved individuals not only are more likely to attend to communication messages, but based on the Elaboration Likelihood Model (Figure 2.3), they are also likely to use the central route to process (elaborate) messages.[58, 59] This means that involved individuals are much more likely than uninvolved persons to listen carefully to scientific findings and explanations, including those based on data,[58, 59] as well as to seek additional information on the topic.[4] Conversely, when involvement levels are low, the Elaboration Likelihood Model suggests that audiences use a peripheral pathway to process messages.[58] This means that message presentation is especially important and may require the use of certain formats (e.g., emotional appeals), well-known spokespeople, trusted organizations, or message tones[67] (Box 2.4).

*Education Level*

Education is strongly associated with use of books, magazines, and newspapers; computer use; and awareness of health topics covered by the news media.[4, 25] Well-educated persons tend to live within rich "health information fields" and networks.[4] They are proficient in seeking health information, especially through libraries and the Internet. When making health-related decisions, better-educated people are more likely to obtain information from multiple sources.[4]

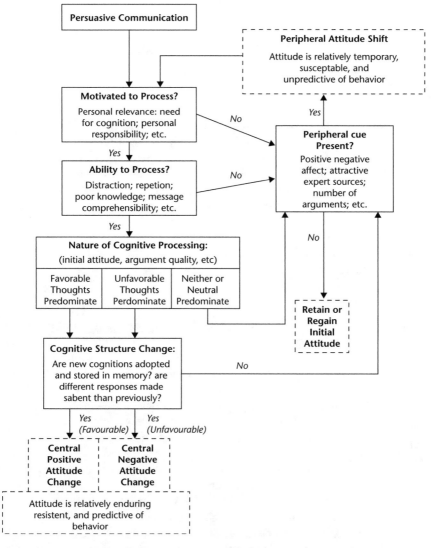

**Figure 2.3** Elaboration likelihood model. Note the critical importance of the "Motivated to Process?" box as to whether persons process messages through central or peripheral routes. (Source: Petty RE, Cacioppo JT. *Communication and Persuasion: Central and Peripheral Routes to Attitude Change.* New York, N.Y.: Springer-Verlag; 1986. With kind permission of Springer Science + Business Media.)

### Lay Health Beliefs and Worldviews

Public health practitioners and scientists may have little appreciation about the types of existing health beliefs or the extent of lay theorizing about health,[68–73] and many people are reluctant to share such beliefs with health professionals. Table 2.1 lists some common lay health beliefs in the United States and other Western countries.

**Box 2.4** Higher and lower levels of involvement: A tale of two audiences

### Highly involved

An audience's level of involvement with a specific health issue has a strong influence on how likely they are likely to pay attention to a topic. For example, an audience with higher involvement, such as antivaccine advocates who believe that childhood vaccinations cause autism, is likely to readily attend to new information about vaccines (especially reports of adverse effects) because this health topic is of great interest to them. Many persons opposed to vaccines may be parents of affected children or have relatives or friends with autistic children. They are likely to pay close attention to the details in news or other reports, including pro and con arguments about vaccine safety.

### Less involved

By comparison, it is much more difficult to gain the attention of parents or caregivers about preventing accidental poisoning of children. It is not that people do not want to prevent poisonings, but messages about poison control usually reach audiences when poisoning is not an immediate threat. Serious accidental poisonings are a relatively rare event; the intended audiences for messages are likely to have low levels of involvement with poison prevention because most parents and caregivers of young children are unlikely to have first-hand knowledge or experience with this problem.

This means that poison control advocates have to work hard to create memorable messages to which parents and caregivers of young children are likely to attend. For example, when the American Association of Poison Control Centers instituted its toll-free poison control hotline, the group publicized it with a large campaign that included radio and print public service announcements coupled with distributing stickers, magnets, brochures, and posters with a telephone number to call in the event of a suspected accidental poisoning.

Source: Centers for Disease Control and Prevention. *Injury Fact Book. 2001–2002. Poison Control: Campaign to Raise Awareness of Poison Control Services*; 2002. Centers for Disease Control and Prevention. *National Immunization Program: Leading the Way to Healthy Lives*; 2006. Centers for Disease Control and Prevention. *Vaccine Safety: Issues of Interest*; 2006.

**Table 2.1 Selected lay health beliefs in the United States**

| |
| --- |
| Exposure to cold temperatures or cold air causes upper respiratory infections |
| Natural foods are healthier |
| Stress plays the most important role in the development of, or recovery from, disease |
| Vaccines are harmful (e.g., autism is caused by childhood immunizations) |
| HIV is God's revenge on homosexuals |
| Antibiotics cure upper respiratory or other types of viral infections |
| An injury to the breast increases the chance of breast cancer |
| Sexually transmitted diseases can be transmitted from toilet seats |
| A positive attitude can prevent or cure many serious diseases |
| High doses of vitamins have restorative or curative powers |

Source: Furnham A. Explaining health and illness: Lay perceptions on current and future health, the causes of illness, and the nature of recovery. *Soc Sci Med.* 1994;39:715–725. Prior L. Belief, knowledge and expertise: The emergence of the lay expert in medical sociology. *Sociol Health Illn.* 2003;23:41–57.

Uncovering audiences' lay health beliefs is important for many communication efforts, as it may be necessary to acknowledge or address such beliefs before communicating intended messages. People filter and process new information based on knowledge they already have on a particular topic.[74] Failing to account for lay beliefs and making communication adjustments can result in lay audiences not attending to, or integrating, science-based messages into their knowledge base at all.[69, 74]

Not only are there specific lay health beliefs, but also broader societal beliefs. In the United States, people have great faith in science and technological fixes for most health problems, no matter how complex or multifactorial they are.[64, 71, 75] Not surprisingly, such beliefs can result in extensive coverage by reporters of potential new "breakthroughs" and "progress," which help to encourage support among the public and policy makers for "curative" research.[64, 69, 75] This is in marked contrast to most public health activities, which are more everyday, mundane, and aimed at prevention.

Worldviews are general viewpoints about life and society that influence people's judgment.[76] Common examples of worldviews include concepts such as fatalism, a certain level of trust in authorities or experts, individualism, egalitarianism, and technological enthusiasm. From a public health perspective, the concepts of individualism and egalitarianism may be the most important, especially concerning the level of support for broad societal or governmental interventions to address societal issues. These worldviews influence beliefs about the extent to which people control their own destinies, as well as beliefs about the appropriate distribution of power and wealth in society. People with a strongly individualistic worldview, for example, may not be persuaded by scientific research findings (no matter how strong) that demonstrate the positive impact on the public's health of a government policy or regulation.

*Past Experience, Confirmation Bias, and Selective Exposure*

An individual's past experiences with a particular issue have a strong influence on their understanding, judgment, and decision making when they are faced again with the same or a closely related issue.[77] Such experiences are used to create mental models, or schema, that people unconsciously use for similar situations.[53, 78] Specific schemas are used to understand, explain, or predict future events or outcomes. For example, an individual who previously received acupuncture for a musculoskeletal injury that resolved quickly may develop a schema that acupuncture would be helpful for many other types of health problems.

Confirmation bias and selective exposure are closely related. They can best be considered as people wanting to hear what they want to hear or see what they want to see. Confirmation bias refers to the tendency of people to see situations or to interpret messages in such a way as to confirm their preexisting beliefs or attitudes (e.g., worldviews), perceptions, or behaviors[79] (Box 2.5). Thus, a teen smoker who hears that one out of three adolescents who smoke will die from a tobacco-related disease may interpret this to confirm his or her belief that "smoking isn't as bad as they say."

---

**Box 2.5** Willy Wonka's revenge—Is chocolate good for you?

For many years chocolate was considered a dietary disaster, as chocolate products typically contain much fat and sugar. Although the widely touted connection between chocolate consumption and acne has long since been disproved, the presence of cocoa butter and high levels of stearic acid would hardly seem to make chocolate a candidate for being a "health food." Imagine the delight of chocolate lovers everywhere when researchers began publishing results of studies suggesting that, because of its health benefits, they can have their chocolate and eat it too.

Studies have shown that chocolate, particularly dark chocolate, contains antioxidant and flavonoid compounds similar to those found in red wine and tea, which are also reputed to have benefits. A few research studies with small numbers of participants suggest that, because of the presence of these compounds, chocolate potentially may have health benefits such as reducing blood pressure, improving glucose metabolism, and perhaps even anticarcinogenic effects, without raising blood cholesterol levels. Not surprisingly, these positive health findings have been widely publicized by the news media, with reporters using phrases such as "dark chocolate reduces blood pressure" or "doctors are recommending dark chocolate as part of a healthy diet." Chocolate manufacturers

*(continued)*

took notice of these findings; in fact, some research studies have been funded by manufacturers themselves.

Not as widely reported, however, are the caveats associated with these studies. Among them are that study populations have been extremely small (several had fewer than 15 participants), results do not apply to other types of chocolate, chocolate is high in calories and fat, and antioxidants and flavonoids are also present in other plant-based foods such as fruits, vegetables, and whole grains, all of which also contain fiber, vitamins, and minerals that chocolate lacks. Researchers have consistently cautioned that these findings do not mean that chocolate is a health food and have made no dietary recommendations about chocolate.

But the belief that chocolate is good for you will be difficult to change among many people. Chocolate lovers everywhere (including the authors of this book) found these research findings to be music to their ears, providing them with another reason besides taste to consume chocolate. Future studies about chocolate's presumed health benefits reported by the news media and elsewhere will be readily attended to because they confirm an existing bias for chocolate aficionados, with studies that show either no benefits or detrimental effects from chocolate likely to be resisted by these same individuals.

Source: Grassi D, Necozione S, Lippi C, et al. Cocoa reduces blood pressure and insulin resistance and improves endothelium-dependent vasodilation in hypertensives. *Hypertension.* 2005;46(2):398–405. Grassi D, Lippi C, Necozione S, Desideri G, Ferri C. Short-term administration of dark chocolate is followed by a significant increase in insulin sensitivity and a decrease in blood pressure in healthy persons. *Am J Clin Nutr.* 2005;81(3):611–614. Harder B. Can chocolate fight diabetes, too? *Science News Online;* 2005:7. Healthier Life. Chocolate and health: Is dark chocolate really good for you? *The Healthier Life;* 2003.

Selective exposure refers to people's tendency to rely on information sources likely to provide messages with which they will agree.[34] Thus, at the interpersonal level, people tend to befriend like-minded individuals with beliefs and opinions that are much like their own. Given today's array of information sources from the Internet, mass media, and elsewhere, the opportunity for people to selectively expose themselves to messages confirming their own views has never been greater.

## The Public as a Lay Audience

### Gender and Age

Besides education, gender and age are important demographic considerations when communicating data to the public. For example, women are much more likely than men to attend to health issues.[25] This probably occurs for several reasons, such as women's richer interpersonal communication networks, more frequent visits to health care providers, and greater family caretaking responsibilities.[4, 80, 81] Attention to health issues increases with age, as older individuals are more likely than younger persons to experience disease and health limitations.[25] They are also more likely than younger persons to have regular health care providers and visit them more frequently.[80]

### Social Networks and Culture

People live within social networks that influence health beliefs, attitudes, and behaviors.[82] Family members, friends, neighbors, work colleagues, faith communities, social organizations, and even online communities create social ties for individuals. In some instances, the influence of social networks can be positive to a person's health, such as two or more friends exercising together regularly; however, networks can also have negative influences, such as close friends or family members who misuse alcohol, use illegal drugs, or have unhealthy diets.

Scientific and mathematical reasoning and trust in science and scientists derives predominantly from Western cultural values.[64, 83] Persons from other cultures commonly have different understandings and views about disease and health. For example, some Latinos may believe in *susto*, which is illness that is believed to arise from fright.[84] Many persons from Asian and other cultures have strong beliefs about the close interrelationship between mind, body, and soul and may have a holistic approach to health.[83]

Some individuals may place more trust in a well-respected individual from their own culture rather than a U.S-trained scientist or health practitioner. People from some cultures may prefer explanations presented as narratives (stories) rather than explanations based on scientific data. Language barriers can present further challenges and increase the chance of misunderstanding (Box 2.6).[85–87]

Sociocultural historical experiences can also influence level of trust in science and scientists, such as the long history of discrimination against certain racial and ethnic groups in the United States.[82] This lack of trust is probably most evident among African Americans as a legacy of the Tuskegee experiments conducted by the U.S. Public Health Service (Box 2.7).[88]

### Structural Factors

Structural, or macro-level, factors in society have a strong influence on the public and on communicating health information. For example, persons in the United States without health insurance have more limited access to health care providers as information sources than do people with insurance.[80]

**Box 2.6** Failing to account for a lay audience member's knowledge base causes a medication error

A 45-year-old Hispanic immigrant, Mr. G., undergoes a job health screening and is told that his blood pressure is very high and he will not be allowed to continue work until his blood pressure is controlled. He visits a local hospital and receives prescriptions for beta-blocker and diuretic medications. The physician prescribed these medications because they are known to be effective, simple to use, and because they are supposed to be taken once a day.

Mr. G. presents to the emergency department 1 week later with dizziness. His blood pressure is very low, and Mr. G. says he has been taking the medicine just like it says to take it on the bottle. The puzzling case is discussed by multiple practitioners until one that speaks Spanish asks Mr. G. how many pills he took each day. "11," Mr. G. replies. The provider explains to his colleagues that "once" means "11" in Spanish.

Source: Institute of Medicine. *Health Literacy: A Prescription to End Confusion.* Washington, D.C.: National Academies Press; 2004:116.

**Box 2.7** An HIV prevention program for rural African Americans in Alabama

Incorporating the cultural beliefs and preferences of an audience is a common challenge in real-world prevention efforts. Community-based organizations (CBOs) in rural Alabama creating an HIV prevention campaign for African Americans faced a particularly difficult challenge. Alabama was the site of the decades-long Tuskegee study in which African American men with syphilis were left untreated so that public health officials could study the course of the disease. Given this decidedly negative history, the long-term legacy has been that many African Americans are suspicious about the intentions of government health efforts.

To effectively address African American beliefs and values as part of a broad-scale community campaign, CBO planning groups worked closely with rural Alabama community members to help design events to improve prevention through education and HIV testing. To create a successful program, the CBOs determined the needs of the community and incorporated African American cultural values into communication messages. The CBOs used preferred and credible information sources and channels for audiences

*(continued)*

47

**Box 2.7** (continued)

(i.e., community leaders, clergy, social networks, and family settings) to disseminate information and encourage discussion about HIV among community
members. They also brought HIV prevention messages directly to the community instead of asking people to seek information on their own.

In one event, for example, the target population consisted of disenfran-
chised African American women living in housing projects. An HIV prevention event was brought to them by holding it in an athletic field adjacent to
their homes. Tents were set up to display and distribute culturally tailored
educational materials, and the sponsoring organization offered free food,
beverages, and prizes while a popular African American disc jockey conducted a live broadcast on  a local radio station about the event's activities.

These various efforts ultimately paid off by helping to overcome
suspicions. The program was successful, as there were large turnouts at
community events, resulting in a substantial number of persons at high
risk for HIV receiving educational materials.

Source: Myrick R. In search of cultural sensitivity and inclusiveness:
Communication strategies used in rural HIV prevention campaigns designed for
African Americans. *Health Commun.* 1998;10:65–85.

But lack of insurance is only one factor. Persons with low socioeconomic
status (SES) and those living in medically underserved parts of the country
(e.g., rural areas, inner cities) also have less access to sources of health information. Low-income populations are less likely to have access to the Internet
because of cost and other issues.[89] Access to public libraries is highly variable but is generally lower in low-income areas.[4] In many low-income areas,
there are limited educational opportunities and poorer quality schools, both
of which contribute to reduced literacy levels. Furthermore, hopelessness,
anomie, and fatalism, which tend to be greater among persons with low SES,
provide additional barriers to seeking health-related information.[4, 53]

*Regular Sources of Health Information*

As mentioned earlier, people have differences in their access, preferences, and trust of health information sources. Although doctors are the
most trusted sources,[25, 28] one national survey found that television news was
named by more than half the public as their most important source of health
information.[90] Some members of the general public also have high levels of
trust in certain Internet Web sites as health information sources.[26, 32, 35, 37, 91]
Finally, much of the public's exposure to health messages from a variety of

sources is incidental or accidental and not the result of any active process on their part.[4, 92]

## Policy Makers as a Lay Audience

For policy makers, as with the general public, there is substantial heterogeneity. Nevertheless, there are similarities among them that can help improve the chances of communicating successfully with them about public health information, including data (Table 2.2).

## Individual Characteristics

There is variability among policy makers, depending on whether they work in the private or public sector, are elected or appointed, or work in for-profit or nonprofit organizations. Demographically, policy makers tend to be white men aged 40 years or older who are college graduates, although there is

**Table 2.2 Characteristics, occupational and institutional factors, and regular sources of information for policy makers**

**Individual characteristics**
  Usually older white men
  Ambitious, hard working, savvy
  Attuned to financial implications
  Intuitive decision making common
  Want certainty from experts

**Occupational and institutional factors**
  Public versus private systems; elected versus appointed individuals
  Formal and informal processes
  Public policy usually made by legislators, executives, or administrators
  Interpersonal relationships crucial
  Rely on gatekeepers
  Busy and subject to multiple communication efforts and requests

**Regular sources of information**
  Interpersonal sources important
  Attend to relevant news media coverage

Source: Arceneaux K. The "gender gap" in state legislative representation: New data to tackle an old question. *Polit Res Q.* 2001;54:143–160. Armor S. More women at the top. *USA Today.* June 25, 2003. Sect. 3. Bacharach S, Lawler E. *Power and Politics in Organizations.* San Francisco, Calif.: Jossey-Bass; 1980. Harris TE. *Applied Organizational Communication: Principles and Pragmatics for Future Practice.* Mahwah, N.J.: Lawrence Erlbaum; 2002. Morgan G. *Images of Organizations.* 2nd ed. Thousand Oaks, Calif.: Sage; 1997. Spasoff RA. *Epidemiologic Methods for Health Policy.* New York, N.Y.: Oxford University Press; 1999. Stone DA. *Policy Paradox: The Art of Political Decision Making.* Rev. ed. New York, N.Y.: Norton; 2002. Weissert CS, Weissert WG. State legislative staff influence in health policy making. *J Health Polit Policy Law.* 2000;25:1121–1148.

variability in educational status among state and local legislators.[93–97] Elected public officials, especially at the state and federal level, are usually businesspersons or lawyers.[98, 99] Most policy makers are ambitious, hardworking, savvy, and have limited amounts of free time.[100] They tend to be aware of, and pay careful attention to, the perceived wants and desires of superiors, constituents, and important people within their working environments before making decisions.[63, 100]

Although not usually well versed in science or advanced mathematics,[101] policy makers are likely to comprehend basic mathematics, especially those related to finances, given their common role of making resource allocation decisions.[63, 102] However, research among organizational leaders, especially in the private sector, demonstrates that they are much more likely to rely on their own intuition (gut feelings), rather than data when making major decisions.[100]

Because policy makers frequently make decisions in their jobs across several topic areas, they may have to rely on input from experts when facing unfamiliar issues. Scientists are comfortable with the concept of uncertainty across multiple dimensions, but uncertainty may be especially vexing for policy makers who desire definitive answers to inform their decision making.[103] During the 1970s, for example, Alexander Schmidt, the former commissioner of the Food and Drug Administration, was reported to have said, "I'm looking for a clear bill of health, not a wishy-washy iffy answer on cyclamates [a soft drink additive]" when referring to a report from a scientific panel that stated they were "95% certain" cyclamates do not cause cancer (see Ref. 103, p. 111). Similarly, former Maine senator Edmund Muskie wanted one-armed scientists who did not say on the "one hand or the other hand" when asked about the evidence that pollutants cause adverse health effects (see Ref. 104, p. 891).

### Occupational and Institutional Factors

Policy makers operate within systems that have formal and informal rules for getting things done.[102, 105, 106] For public administrators and elected policy makers, formal written processes are likely to exist, such as legislative or regulatory language for funding documents or ballot initiatives. Informal processes, however, are also important.[63, 105] Policy and other types of decision making by leaders in the private sector may be highly centralized, especially in extremely hierarchical organizations.[100, 102] Though often accountable to a board of directors or other type of advisory group, private policy makers may have great leeway in making decisions and implementing them rapidly without any type of appeals process. There may be one or a few individuals within public or private organizations who wield power and whose opinion is strongly influential (Box 2.8).[107]

**Box 2.8** Health insurance for low-income individuals in Massachusetts: Understanding the public policy-making process

The large number of persons who lack health insurance is an ongoing challenge in the United States. In the absence of recent action at the federal level, several states have enacted policies or begun programs to increase health insurance coverage, especially for lower income individuals. The Health Care for All (HCA) coalition in Massachusetts worked tirelessly for many years, with their efforts ultimately resulting in the enactment of a 1996 state law that expanded health care coverage for children and low-income residents. A key aspect of HCA's success was their decision to work closely with a prominent and powerful state senator who was intimately familiar with the occupational and institutional factors within the legislature.

Realizing the importance of having a political champion, the HCA coalition began to work in the late 1980s and early 1990s with a state senator, John McDonough, to reduce uninsurance in Massachusetts through the development of a Family Health Plan. Passing any piece of legislation requires more than lining up "yes" votes; an intimate knowledge and understanding of the legislative process are required for success. The state legislature had addressed health care cost issues for several years by regulating the rates hospitals could charge for services. McDonough, a member of the legislature's Health Care Committee, worked to add a section to a hospital deregulation bill that was eventually enacted that also expanded health insurance to children ("Healthy Kids").

In 1995, McDonough became chair of the Health Care Committee. When a committee report mentioned the state's number of uninsured persons in one of its reports (nearly 700,000 uninsured residents and 160,000 uninsured children), McDonough held a public hearing of the committee to publicize the extent of the problem. The HCA coalition and other advocates used the number of uninsured persons, especially uninsured children, widely in efforts to raise awareness about uninsurance. The coalition and McDonough worked closely to design a more comprehensive bill to expand health coverage for children and low-income adults. To gain further support, the bill included a repeal of a universal employer insurance mandate widely disliked by businesses and provided funding for the insurance expansion through a proposed 25-cent increase in the states' cigarette tax.

A statewide poll found that 77% of Massachusetts adults agreed with a proposal to raise cigarette taxes by 25 cents if the revenue was used to "fund health insurance for children who don't have it and help buy prescription drugs for elders who can't afford such coverage." The HCA coalition and other organizations used these poll findings to

*(continued)*

> **Box 2.8** (continued)
>
> demonstrate widespread support for the bill. The bill eventually passed in the Massachusetts House and the Senate in 1996 with strong bipartisan support, as evidenced by both legislative chambers voting to override a veto by the governor.
>
> Source: McDonough JE. *Experiencing Politics: A Legislator's Stories of Government and Health Care.* Berkeley, Calif.: University of California Press; 2000.

Interpersonal relationships between advocates and select elected officials or their gatekeepers can be very influential in determining the success or failure of efforts to influence elected policy makers.[63] Knowing both formal and informal processes is essential for those desiring to communicate effectively with private or public policy makers.[102, 108]

Gatekeepers, such as top aides or executive secretaries, play a key role in determining which people, and to what information, private or public policy makers are exposed.[102, 107, 109] Policy makers rely heavily on legislative or executive aides and on assistants to the executives or administrators who control information and access.[100, 108] These assistants may be inexperienced or not knowledgeable about public health issues, let alone science or mathematics.[109, 110]

Several types of policy making occur in the public sector and have different institutional factors.[63, 109, 111] In the United States, legislative policy making involves decisions by local, state, or federally elected members of legislative bodies (e.g., state senates or city councils). Legislators are subject to many influences, especially from well-financed groups.[63] Elected government executives, such as mayors, governors, or county managers, also can make or influence policies. They can be highly visible and dominate public and media perceptions about government.[63] Much of their influence involves their ability to lead and persuade others, for example, legislators or administrators.

Administrative public policy making involves rule making and adjudication of policies decided by legislators.[63, 109] It involves interpreting and implementing the language in legislative bills or administrative directives, such as promulgating rules or regulations. Administrative policy makers are typically civil servants, that is, "permanent" government employees within the executive branch of government.[109] Public administrative policy makers may be more cautious than their counterparts in the private sector, as they can face intensive scrutiny from other policy makers or organizations about controversial decisions.[108]

Private and public policy makers are often extremely busy people. As part of their jobs, they interact regularly with individuals and organizational representatives who want something from them, for example, resources, support, or personal assistance.[63, 100] They are often subject to a large number of communication attempts.[4, 100] Thus, in addition to understanding the formal and informal processes in policy-making environments, it is important to identify and develop good relationships with gatekeepers.[108] Ideally, this involves developing long-term relationships with key policy makers and their assistants, especially at times other than when key policy decisions are imminent.[63, 108] Furthermore, the messages provided need to be concise, communicate main points quickly, and require little reading.[100, 108, 112]

### Regular Sources of Health Information

Because of time pressure and extensive communication efforts from others, interpersonal sources of information are of paramount importance for private and public policy makers.[63, 100] Elected officials, for example, tend to pay close attention to communication (e.g., letters, personal visits, phone calls) from constituents, especially if they receive a substantial amount of communication attempts from citizens about a specific issue or subject.[63] As for communication channels, preferences will be highly variable, depending on personal preferences, organizational culture, and other factors; brevity in messages, however, is essential.[100, 108] Policy makers are probably the least likely of lay audiences to seek information from Web sites; this may not be true for gatekeepers, however, who may be of younger age and prefer to obtain information from Internet sources.

Elected or appointed public policy makers closely attend to news media coverage relevant to their area of interest or responsibility.[21, 63] Elected legislators usually attend to news stories and letters to the editor in local newspapers and on television shows in their districts.[63] Private organization policy makers are also likely to closely attend to news media reports or editorials that may be relevant to their organizations.[100]

## Journalists as a Lay Audience

Despite widespread changes occurring in news media field, fueled by the Internet, changing demographic preferences, and other factors,[113, 114] journalists have the potential to reach a large number of members of the general public, and policy makers attend to news stories relevant to them. Furthermore, news media representatives have an important role in agenda setting and framing of issues, that is, helping to define which issues are most important and how they are described and presented to lay audiences.[13, 115, 116] Earned media, that is, gaining news coverage for a public health topic or issue, can be a highly cost-effective way to reach lay audiences with messages. Thus, it is essential for those seeking to communicate public health information to the public or to policy makers to have a good understanding of journalists and their worlds (Table 2.3). As with other lay audiences, there are certain commonalities among journalists, and knowledge of these can improve the chances of communicating data and other public health information more effectively.

### Individual Characteristics

The demographics of journalists are well known: despite some changes, the majority of reporters in the different news media venues are white men, especially those who have more than 20 years of experience or are in senior editorial positions.[66, 117] Female editors are more likely to cover health and education topics than are male editors,[118] and many health reporters are women.[119]

**Table 2.3 Characteristics, occupational and institutional factors, and regular sources of information for journalists**

**Individual characteristics**
    Often white men, especially editors
    Progressive "mainstream" values and beliefs
    Concerned about individual freedom issues
    May be intimidated by scientists or health professionals
    General reporters, specialty reporters, and editorialists

**Occupational and institutional factors**
    Business considerations: attuned to topics of interest to the public
    Short deadlines common
    Differences between specific news media (e.g., newspapers, TV)
    Certain characteristics make stories more "newsworthy" (e.g., local tie-in)
    Prefer personal stories (narratives)
    Much competition for news space
    Follow news outlet "leaders," e.g., elite papers such as *The New York Times*

**Regular sources of information**
Preselected list of trusted experts

Source: Blum D, Knudson M, Henig RM, eds. *A Field Guide for Science Writers: The Official Guide of the National Association of Science Writers*. 2nd ed. New York, N.Y.: Oxford University Press; 2006. Brownson RC, Malone BR. Communicating public health information to policy makers. In: Nelson DE, Brownson RC, Remington PL, Parvanta C, eds. *Communicating Public Health Information Effectively: A Guide for Practitioners*. Washington, D.C.: American Public Health Association; 2002. p. 97–114. Friedman SM, Dunwoody S, Rogers CL, editor. *Scientists and Journalists: Reporting Science as News*. New York, N.Y.: Free Press; 1986. Gastel B. *Health Writer's Handbook*. Ames, IA: Iowa State University Press; 1998. Greenwell M. Communicating public health information to the news media. In: Nelson DE, Brownson RC, Remington PL, Parvanta C, eds. *Communicating Public Health Information Effectively: A Guide for Practitioners*. Washington, DC: American Public Health Association; 2002. p. 73–96. Manning P. *News and News Sources: A Critical Introduction*. Thousand Oaks, Calif.: Sage; 2001. Dumro R, Duke S. The Web and e-mail in science communication. *Science Communication* 2003;24:283–308.

The values, beliefs, and ideologies of journalists and editors are considered "progressive mainstream," that is, they generally believe in altruistic democracy, responsible capitalism, the preservation of the existing social order, and individual moderatism (i.e., they are antifanatic and antilawbreaking).[66] Journalists are attentive to individual freedom issues,[66] which may make them less supportive of certain public health policies, but tend to be proenvironment.[64, 118]

Full-time journalists can broadly be classified as general assignment reporters, specialty (or "beat") reporters, or editorialists[64, 66, 120]; there are relatively few full-time health journalists in the United States. Few journalists have training or expertise in health, science, or mathematics and may be intimidated by the expertise and credentials of the scientists and health professionals.[64, 69, 120, 121]

### Occupational and Institutional Factors

The news media can be envisioned as news factories that produce stories that fit within certain acceptable boundaries.[66] They are also businesses that need to make a profit, relying heavily on advertising revenue; thus, they try to avoid offending advertisers or other powerful interests.[66] Media organization leaders have a good understanding of the demographics and preferences of their audiences for news stories.[66, 120]

There are basically two types of news stories written by reporters: hard news or features.* Hard news is typically what is presented as headline news on television, radio, or within the first few pages of newspapers, and focuses on new, discrete events (i.e., new findings or "crises").[120] A key occupational component of most journalists who write hard news stories, particularly those who work for newspapers and television, is that they usually work on short deadlines from a few minutes to a few hours.[120, 122] Feature stories are more in-depth, typically longer and more explanatory than hard news stories, with timeliness not as important.

Although the news media are often referred to generically, there are differences among them. Despite consolidation and declining readership, there are several thousand newspapers in the United States,[22] which means most news stories are written by newspaper reporters. There are a few "elite" papers (e.g., *The New York Times, Wall Street Journal*), which are influential and tend to have some of their stories picked up by regional or local newspapers.[22, 120]

Television news has some distinctive features. It tends to reach audiences of a larger size than do other news media sources (especially local television

---

* Editorials and other types of opinion pieces (e.g., essays by regular columnists or opinion-editorials [op-ed pieces]) are also common in newspapers and some magazines. These types of articles are not covered here because they are not considered to be news stories and also because some are written by persons who are not journalists.

news),[123] and it is strongly dependent on good visual images.[120] Television news stories tend to be short, averaging about 60–100 s in length.[120, 124] Most magazines have highly specialized readerships, and magazine reporters are especially attuned to the potential salience of stories for their audiences. The use of the Internet for "streaming" news through Internet Service Providers such as America OnLine (AOL) is increasing, but they typically rely on news stories produced by newspaper, news wire, or television organizations for content.[125] With the exception of National Public Radio (NPR), radio journalism in the United States is rare, relying on brief stories from other news media.[120, 123]

Characteristics of news stories that gain audience interest have been well researched.[66, 122, 126] They include (a) information considered to be new (not previously reported or well known), (b) prominence or importance of the individuals involved or seriousness of the problem, (c) human interest, (d) conflict or controversy, (e) unusualness, (f) timeliness, (g) proximity (e.g., of local interest), (h) entertainment potential, (i) irony, or (j) seasonal aspect or anniversary.

A local tie or "angle" for most news media outlets is especially important for many local journalists. Personal stories (narratives) are commonly used by journalists to provide human interest or drama for audiences[64, 69, 120, 124, 127] (Box 2.9).

---

**Box 2.9 Journalists and health-related storytelling**

In a survey conducted by the National Cancer Institute, health and science journalists said that they select information and develop news stories based on their potential for public impact, the possibility of educating the public with accurate information, and self-help. Journalists strive to use the information they gather in order to tell a story. Storytelling about health topics is greatly enhanced by adding a human element to news articles, such as through interviews with sources or a more in-depth focus on people affected by a specific issue.

For example, federal data demonstrated that in 2000–2001, the rate of alcohol-related driving deaths in the United States increased from the rate observed during most of the 1990s. Because national data do not necessarily attract people's attention, an Austin, Texas, newspaper reporter highlighted the problem of drinking and driving by publishing a comprehensive news story about a local young woman who nearly died as a result of being struck by a drunk driver. Highlighting the injuries, rehabilitation, and future challenges faced by this young woman helped to put a human face on the problem.

*(continued)*

The practical or self-help implications of new research findings for individuals are a common focus of health studies. After a large mumps outbreak occurred in the Midwest in the spring of 2006, a Washington Post newspaper story described the extent of mumps in the Washington metropolitan area (which had no outbreak-related cases) and symptoms of the disease. Practical recommendations were included in conjunction with the news story through the use of a "mumps to-do list" with tips for young children, teens, young adults, and adults, and a question and answer (Q & A) sheet that addressed common questions about vaccinations, prevention, and activity restrictions.

Source: Edwards A. Mumps watch: Parents are urged to verify child immunizations as outbreak spreads. *The Washington Post*. 2006. Hafetz D. Jaqueline and Amadeo: Chasing hope. *Austin American-Statesman Special Report*. May 12, 2002.

Regardless of the medium, competition for space for news stories is high.[120, 123] This means that public health stories have to compete with other potential stories for the attention and interest of journalists and editors. Public health individuals or organizations interested in gaining news media coverage of their issue need to provide information and materials considered compelling to journalists to be successful. Finally, journalists closely attend to stories covered in other news media outlets. This can lead to pack reporting where journalists follow a particular story, often using similar news story frames and drawing similar conclusions.[64, 120]

### Regular Sources of Health Information

Journalists' sources for stories and editorials can be influential.[64, 66, 118] Health or science journalists, especially those with extensive experience, usually have a preselected list of trusted individual experts whom they routinely use based on their own past experience.[64] If a new research study or report is released, journalists often prefer to speak with the lead author of the study or report rather than a public relations staff member or other organization official.[64, 69] The selection of sources, not surprisingly, depends on their availability. In the past, journalists relied heavily on telephone contacts with sources but email has increasingly become an important communication channel.[128]

Reporters commonly rely on Web sites for two important functions: to rapidly obtain background and other information for stories, and to monitor news stories produced by other news media outlets,[128] hence the importance of making material available on Web sites and ensuring that it is current. News wire services, such as the Associated Press, also play an important role as a resource for stories, especially for newspapers.[22] Scientific journals are sometimes read and used as sources, depending on the time constraints and reporter initiative.[64]

Press releases and press conferences may be held in conjunction with major health meetings or scientific publications. Press releases from major health journals, such as the *New England Journal of Medicine, JAMA*, and *BMJ*, from major voluntary or other organizations (e.g., Institute of Medicine, Office of the Surgeon General, American Cancer Society), and from other sources considered trustworthy are also used, at times, as sources.[118, 128]

## Purpose, Strategy, and Context

### Purpose

There are four purposes for communicating public health information, including data, to lay audiences. These are to (a) increase knowledge, (b) instruct, (c) facilitate informed decision making, or (d) persuade. Increasing knowledge refers to providing audiences with factual information to increase understanding, which may not be of immediate or practical use. Instruction means to directly inform people what actions or steps they need to perform for a specific task, such as how to use a respirator. Data are rarely necessary for instruction.

Informed decision making consists of a source sharing information in an unbiased and understandable manner with intended audiences, allowing them to make decisions based on their own understanding of the information.[6] (In clinical settings, this is usually referred to as shared decision making.[129]) It is used when there is a lack of scientific consensus on a specific topic, when potentially serious side effects are possible, or when personal values are critical to a decision.

Persuasion means attempting to change beliefs, perceptions, attitudes, or behaviors, such as increasing immunizations or discouraging illicit drug use.[5, 27, 34, 50] The primary purpose for many, if not most, public health communication efforts involve some aspect of persuasion.[130, 131] As discussed in Chapter 1, it is important when engaging in persuasion to explicitly acknowledge the roles that values and ethics play. The desire to persuade may tempt public health practitioners to downplay, exaggerate, overinterpret, or imply greater certainty to scientific findings than is justifiable based on data.[130] The scientific basis for messages must be defensible and not presented in misleading ways that could potentially result in audience members making inappropriate or dangerous decisions.[132] If public health practitioners are found to have lied or exaggerated about the findings they present, they, as well as their institutions, will lose trust and credibility among lay audiences; unfortunately, once trust is lost it is difficult to regain.[76, 133, 134]

## Strategy

Related to purpose is the strategy that senders use in their attempts to reach intended audiences with messages. Strategy is passive, active, or some combination of the two.[4] Passive communication is the repository or "library" model in which senders place information in one or more places and rely on information-seeking audiences to find it. Releasing routine health agency reports, or placing information on Internet Web sites, are examples of passive strategies. The effectiveness of this approach depends on several factors, such as the audience's education level, preferred information sources, language proficiency, information seeking strategies, awareness, involvement, belief in source credibility, ease of access, and computer or electronic proficiency.[4]

An active communication strategy involves making some effort to gain audience attention. Active strategies to reach audiences involve the use of mass or small media, attempting to activate interpersonal social networks through the efforts of selected individuals (word of mouth), or some other means. Active strategies are usually much more expensive than passive strategies and may need to be used over a long period of time to maximize effectiveness.

There is overlap between passive and active communication strategies, as some combination of the two strategies is commonly used. This is sometimes referred to as the "push–pull" model (Box 2.10), that is, actively pushing messages toward audiences and making additional materials available to interested information seekers (e.g., paid advertising in print media or television ads that contain the name of a Web site with further information or encourage readers to call a specific phone number to reach their local health department).[135] Even the most passive of communication efforts are likely to require some effort to inform potential audiences about the availability of information repositories in order to succeed.

## Context

Contextual factors are outside influences on audiences that may change their receipt or interpretation of communication messages. Communication does not occur in a vacuum, and many factors, often beyond the control of senders, can play critical roles.[3] Public health communication efforts seemingly based on a topic highly salient to audiences, use credible sources, rely on accessible and preferred audience communication channels that reach people, and use

**Box 2.10** The Red Dress Campaign: Push and pull

Despite the fact that heart disease is far and away the most common cause of death among women, many women are unaware of this fact. In a major campaign led by the National Heart Lung and Blood Institute (NHLBI), the Push (sending information that has not been requested) and Pull (making information available on demand) approach to communication has been used effectively to help raise awareness among women about their risk of heart disease.

Calling their education campaign "The Heart Truth," using the tag line "Heart disease doesn't care what you wear—it's the #1 killer of women," and adopting the red dress as the national symbol for women and heart disease awareness, NHLBI and its partners implemented the following Push and Pull activities:

**Push** (Sending information)

- Directly providing educational materials to women to help them learn about heart disease and reduce their risks (including Spanish language materials).
- National public service media advertising (television, radio, and print).
- Compelling photos and stories of real women telling how heart disease changed their lives.
- Forming partnerships with corporate and nonprofit organizations, including nontraditional partners (e.g., Association of Black Cardiologists, National Association of Latina Leaders) and providing materials to them to distribute to women through their state and local networks.

**Pull** (Encouraging people to seek further information or materials)

- Providing and notifying partners about a speaker's kit and other promotional materials available to disseminate information.
- Developing an online Internet toolkit containing activity ideas and materials to help individuals and organizations interested in planning their own Heart Truth events.
- Sponsoring the Red Dress Single City Program in local communities nationwide, which involved local hospitals, community groups, and women's health organizations holding Red Dress–themed health fairs, free health screenings, luncheons, fashion shows, and other events that encouraged women to attend.

Follow-up surveys have demonstrated the positive impact of the Push and Pull efforts used by the Red Dress Campaign. Between 2001 and

*(continued)*

2005, the campaign helped increase the percentage of women who recognized that heart disease is their leading cause of death from 34% to 57%.

Source: National Heart, Lung, and Blood Institute. *The Heart Truth: A National Awareness Campaign for Women about Heart Disease*; 2005. National Coalition for Women with Heart Disease. One in four U.S. women recognize the red dress as the national symbol for women and heart disease awareness; nearly half say the symbol would prompt them to talk to or see their doctor; 2005.

well-designed and well-presented messages for intended audiences may still not be effective.

Many other sources besides public health practitioners provide health-related messages to lay audiences, such as friends or relatives, and commercial interests (e.g., businesses through marketing or lobbying), and some of these messages contradict those based on science. Individuals within intended audiences may be experiencing certain emotions that influence the communication experience (Chapters 3 and 6),[136–139] such as when there has been a community environmental health exposure or an unexpected problem with a consumer product or service.[140] People may feel fearful or outraged, which can influence their judgment about the credibility of sources and the information provided to them.[138]

Competing, short-term priorities may also arise among audiences, such as weather-related problems, budget crises, or deaths or illnesses within families. A celebrity may be involved in a scandal, resulting in minimal news media coverage for a public health story. Computer system or power failures may prevent individuals from delivering effective oral presentations.

### Rationale for Communicating Data to Lay Audiences

This chapter thus far has provided an overview of the many factors influencing communication with lay audiences. Given this myriad of factors and influences, it is legitimate to ask whether it is even worthwhile to communicate data to lay audiences.

As described elsewhere in this book, there are certain situations and audiences for which presenting data is not recommended, such as when the purpose for communication is instruction. But data have been shown to be influential in many instances with lay audiences. Using terms derived from the fields of debate and rhetoric, scientific data provide reasons that support a claim[51, 52]; that is, they are a form of evidence that lead to conclusions.[51, 141, 142]

Although some individuals rely almost solely on authority from family, community, national, or religious leaders, most people in Western cultures, when assessing the credibility of messages from scientists and health professionals, are likely expect some evidence to be proffered in support of statements or conclusions.[63, 64, 105] Quantitative data are the dominant form of evidence used in scientific fields to provide reasons that answer the question of "why"[105, 142] (e.g., Why should I use condoms? Because regular condom use substantially reduces the risk of contracting certain sexually transmitted diseases).

Research has shown that communicating data to lay audiences can have two types of effects: enhancing source credibility and increasing the believability of messages. As discussed, expertise and trust are the major dimensions of source credibility.[34–36] There is consistent research from the persuasion and related literatures showing that sources who use evidence, including statistical evidence, to support their claims are rated by audiences as having higher credibility.[34, 35, 141, 143, 144]

In Western societies such as the United States, data are commonly considered as cultural icons of objectivity,[105, 143, 145] with official or government data especially viewed in this light.[105] This makes a compelling case for sources to communicate data not only to support the major messages they present to lay audiences (see below), but also to demonstrate that they are knowledgeable about the current "state of the science." The opposite demonstrates this point: a scientist who relied solely on reasons other than data to support a claim (i.e., personal experience, case examples, or anecdotes) would likely be viewed by lay audiences as having lower credibility, particularly for complex issues or involved presentations.[35, 146–149]

Some research suggests that using data can increase lay audiences' knowledge and understanding, assist them with informed decision making, and increase the persuasiveness of arguments (e.g., for changing belief, attitudes, perceptions, or behaviors) in health and other settings.[34, 36, 143, 147, 149–154] Much of this research is based on comparing statistical evidence (numbers) with information provided in the form of narratives (i.e., case studies, personal testimonies, anecdotes).[149] However, research findings on the effectiveness of using messages with data are not consistent. For example, although several studies have shown statistics to be more persuasive than narratives, others have not.[34, 36, 143, 149, 155] Similarly, a review of research on cancer-treatment decision aids, many of which involved presenting data to patients, found limited support for their effectiveness.[156]

These inconsistent findings about communicating data to lay audiences are not really surprising, given the many factors influencing communication discussed previously.[34, 149, 152] Of particular importance when it comes to communicating data are (a) involvement, (b) level of emotion, (c) education level, (d) mathematical, science, and document literacy, (e) worldviews, (f) the initial attitude or belief about an issue, (g) the complexity of the issue or information, (h) audience familiarity with the topic or issue, (i) and how information is presented (Chapters 3 and 4).[76, 80, 141, 143, 147, 149, 157, 158] Furthermore, as discussed previously, lay audiences have a broader view of what they consider valid types of evidence for scientific, health, and other issues beyond what scientists have to offer.[159]

Accordingly, no blanket recommendations can be made about the effects of data, or whether to use or not use them in messages to lay audiences. In general, however, data-containing messages are most likely to be effective with audiences who have (a) higher levels of involvement, (b) lower levels of emotion (especially fear or anger), (c) higher levels of education, (d) higher levels of mathematic, scientific, and document literacy, (e) a rational orientation, and (f) an original opinion in favor of the position advocated that data support. Data messages are also more likely to be effective for topics or situations that are complex, or which are unfamiliar to audiences. Given the wide variation among audiences and situations, the general recommendation by Allen[160] to use data in combination with other approaches (e.g., words, visual modalities) has merit.

## Conclusion

At heart, communicating about data is first and foremost a communication activity. Providing a large amount of data and relying on the "numbers to speak for themselves" is wishful thinking: the selection and presentation of scientific data requires thought and consideration. Public health scientists, practitioners, and others desiring to communicate data with the public, policy makers, or the press will need to familiarize themselves with the communication process to communicate data effectively.

Of special note is the need to understand the characteristics of lay audiences, and the many factors that can influence or affect them, prior to considering whether or how to communicate public health data. Such knowledge is gained from careful audience analysis; in many instances, the use of formal or informal testing methods can provide invaluable input and guide communication efforts (Chapter 5).

**The bottom line**

Learning to communicate quantitative data effectively is part of becoming
expert at communication itself

Science-based storylines, that is, the major conclusions that communicators
would like audiences to understand, form the foundation on which
messages are developed

The purposes for communicating quantitative data to lay audiences are
to (a) increase knowledge, (b) instruct, (c) facilitate informed decision
making, and (d) persuade

Data messages are most likely to be effective with audiences who have (a)
higher levels of involvement, (b) lower levels of emotion (especially fear
or anger), (c) higher levels of education, (d) higher levels of mathematic,
scientific, and document literacy, (e) a rational orientation, and (f) an
original opinion in favor of the position advocated that data support

## Further Reading

### Communication Fundamentals

Albers, MJ. *Communication of Complex Information: User Goals and Information
Needs for Dynamic Web Information.* Mahwah, N.J.: Lawrence Erlbaum; 2004.

Littlejohn SW, Foss KA. *Theories of Human Communication.* 9th ed. Belmont, Calif.:
Wadsworth; 2007.

Nelson DE, Brownson RC, Remington PL, Parvanta C. eds. *Communicating Public
Health Information Effectively: A Guide for Practitioners.* Washington, D.C.:
American Public Health Association; 2002.

Schiavo R. *Health Communication: From Theory to Practice.* San Francisco, Calif.:
Jossey-Bass; 2007.

### Mass Media

Friedman SM, Dunwoody S, Rogers CL. eds. *Communicating Uncertainty: Media
Coverage of New and Controversial Science.* Mahwah, N.J.: Lawrence Erlbaum;
1999.

Hayes R, Grossman D. *A Scientist's Guide to Talking with the Media: Practical Advice
from the Union of Concerned Scientists.* New Brunswick, N.J.: Rutgers University
Press; 2006.

McQuail D. *McQuail's Mass Communication Theory.* 5th ed. London, UK: Sage; 2005.

Shoemaker PJ, Reese SD. *Mediating the Message: Theories of Influences on Mass Media
Control.* 2nd ed. White Plains, N.Y.: Longman; 1996.

## Public and Private Policy Makers

Longest BB. *Health Policymaking in the United States.* 4th ed. Ann Arbor, Mich.: Health Administration Press; 2005.

McDonough JE. *Experiencing Politics: A Legislator's Stories of Government and Health Care.* Berkeley, Calif.: University of California Press; 2000.

Sabatier PA. ed. *Theories of the Political Process.* 2nd ed. Boulder, Colo.: Westview Press; 2007.

Shockley-Zalabak PS. *Fundamentals of Organizational Communication.* 6th ed. Boston, Mass.: Allyn & Bacon; 2005.

## Persuasion and Behavior Change

Dillard JP, Pfau M. eds. *The Persuasion Handbook: Developments in Theory and Practice.* Thousand Oaks, Calif.: Sage; 2002.

Glanz K, Rimer BK, Lewis FM. eds. *Health Behavior and Health Education.* 3rd ed. San Francisco, Calif.: Jossey-Bass; 2002.

O'Keefe DJ. *Persuasion: Theory and Research.* Thousand Oaks, Calif.: Sage; 2002.

Perloff RM. *The Dynamics of Persuasion: Communication and Attitudes in the 21st Century.* 3rd ed. Mahwah, N.J.: Erlbaum, 2007.

## References

1. Lum M, Parvanta C, Maibach E, Arkin E, Nelson DE. General public: Communicating to inform. In: Nelson DE, Brownson RC, Remington PL, Parvanta C, eds. *Communicating Public Health Information Effectively: A Guide for Practitioners.* Washington, D.C.: American Public Health Association; 2002:47–57.

2. Littlejohn SW, Foss KA. *Theories of Human Communication.* 9th ed. Belmont, Calif.: Wadsworth; 2007.

3. McQuail D. *McQuail's Mass Communication Theory.* 5th ed. London, UK: Sage; 2005.

4. Johnson JD. *Cancer-Related Information Seeking.* Cresskill, N.J.: Hampton Press; 1997.

5. McGuire WJ. Theoretical foundations of campaigns. In: Rice RE, Atkin CK, eds. *Public Communication Campaigns.* 2nd ed. Beverly Hills, Calif.: Sage; 1989:43–65.

6. Parvanta C, Maibach E, Arkin E, Nelson DE, Woodward J. Public health communication: A planning framework. In: Nelson DE, Brownson RC, Remington PL, Parvanta C, eds. *Communicating Public Health Information Effectively: A Guide for Practitioners.* Washington, D.C.: American Public Health Association; 2002:11–32.

7. National Cancer Institute. *Making Health Communication Programs Work.* Washington, D.C.: US Department of Health and Human Services, National Institutes of Health, National Cancer Institute; 2002. NIH Pub. No. 02–5145.

8. Perse EM. *Media Effects and Society.* Mahwah, N.J.: Lawrence Erlbaum; 2001.

9. Kreuter MW, Farrell D, Olevitch L, Breman L. *Tailoring Health Messages: Customizing Communication Using Computer Technology.* Mahwah, N.J.: Lawrence Erlbaum; 1999.

10. Rimer BK, Halabi S, Sugg SC, et al. The short term impact of tailored mammography decision-making interventions. *Patient Educ Couns.* 2001;43:269–285.

11. Rimer BK, Kreuter MW. Advancing tailored health communication: A persuasion and message effects perspective. *J Commun.* 2006;56:S184–S201.

12. Rogers EM. *Diffusion of Innovations.* 4th ed. New York, N.Y.: Free Press; 1995.

13. Dearing JW, Rogers EM. *Agenda-Setting.* Thousand Oaks, Calif.: Sage; 1996.

14. Southwell BG, Torres A. Connecting interpersonal and mass communication: Science news exposure, perceived ability to understand science, and conversation. *Commun Monogr.* 2006;73:334–350.

15. Niederdeppe J, Frosch DL, Hornik RC. Cancer news coverage and information seeking. *J Health Commun.* 2008;13:181–199.

16. DeFleur ML, Ball-Rokeach S. *Theories of Mass Communications.* 5th ed. White Plains, N.Y.: Longman; 1989.

17. Suggs LS. A 10-year retrospective of research in new technologies for health communication. *J Health Commun.* 2006;11(1):61–74.

18. Hesse BW, Shneiderman B. eHealth research from the user's perspective. *Am J Prev Med.* 2007;32(5 Suppl):S97–S103.

19. Burke W, Psaty BM. Personalized medicine in the era of genomics. *JAMA.* 2007;298(14):1682–1684.

20. Shneiderman B. *Leonardo's Laptop: Human Needs and the New Computing Technologies.* Cambridge, Mass.: MIT Press; 2002.

21. Croteau D, Hoynes W. *Media/Society.* 3rd ed. Thousand Oaks, Calif.: Sage; 2003.

22. Alexander A, Owers J, Carveth R, Hollifield CA, Greco AN. *Media Economics: Theory and Practice.* Mahwah, N.J.: Lawrence Erlbaum; 2004.

23. Brailer D. Action through collaboration: A conversation with David Brailer. The national coordinator of HIT believes that facilitation, not mandates, are the way to move the agenda forward. Interview by Robert Cunningham. *Health Aff (Millwood).* 2005;24(5):1150–1157.

24. Vivian J. *The Media of Mass Communication.* 9th ed. Boston, Mass.: Allyn & Bacon; 2008.

25. Miller JD, Kimmel LG. *Biomedical Communications: Purposes, Methods, and Strategies.* San Diego, Calif.: Academic Press; 2001.

26. Rutten LJF, Squiers L, Hesse B. Cancer-related information seeking: Hints from the 2003 Health Information National Trends Survey (HINTS). *J Health Commun.* 2006;11:147–156.

27. Rice RE, Atkin CK, eds. *Public Communication Campaigns.* 3rd ed. Thousand Oaks, Calif.: Sage; 2001.

28. Science Panel on Interactive Communication and Health. *Wired for Health and Well-Being: The Emergence of Interactive Health Communication.* Washington, D.C.: U.S. Department of Health and Human Services; 1999.

29. Wood AF, Smith MJ. *Online Communication: Linking Technology, Identity, and Culture.* 2nd ed. Mahwah, N.J.: Lawrence Erlbaum; 2005.

30. Institute of Medicine. *Speaking of Health: Assessing Health Communication Strategies for Diverse Populations.* Washington, D.C.: National Academies Press; 2002.

31. Rains SA. Perceptions of traditional information sources and use of the World Wide Web to seek health information: Findings from the Health Information National Trends Survey. *J Health Commun.* 2007;12:667–680.

32. Hong T. Contributing factors to the use of health-related websites. *J Health Commun.* 2006;11:149–165.

33. Hastie R, Dawes RM. *Rational Choice in an Uncertain World: The Psychology of Judgment and Decision Making.* Thousand Oaks, Calif.: Sage; 2001.
34. O'Keefe DJ. *Persuasion: Theory and Research.* Thousand Oaks, Calif.: Sage; 2002.
35. Pornpitakpan C. The persuasiveness of source credibility: A critical review of five decades' experience. *J Appl Psychol.* 2004;34:243–281.
36. Stiff JB, Mongeau PA. *Persuasive Communication.* New York, N.Y.: Guilford; 2003.
37. Hesse BW, Nelson DE, Kreps GL, et al. Trust and sources of health information: The impact of the Internet and its implications for health care providers: Findings from the first Health Information National Trends Survey. *Arch Intern Med.* 2005;165(22):2618–2624.
38. McComas KA, Trumbo CW. Source credibility in environmental health-risk controversies: Application of Meyer's credibility index. *Risk Anal.* 2001;21:467–480.
39. Treise D, Walsh-Childers K, Weigold MF, Friedman M. Cultivating the science internet audience: Impact of brand and domain on source credibility for science information. *Sci Commun.* 2003;24:309–332.
40. Bates BR, Romina S, Ahmed R, Hopson D. The effect of source credibility on consumers' perceptions of the quality of health information on the Internet. *Med Inform Internet Med.* 2006;31(1):45–52.
41. Warnick B. Online ethos: Source credibility in an "authorless" environment. *Am Behav Scientist.* 2004;48:256–265.
42. Rains SA. The anonymity effect: The influence of anonymity on perceptions of sources and information on health websites. *J Appl Commun Res.* 2007;35:197–214.
43. Zaza S, Briss PA, Harris KW, eds. *The Guide to Community Preventive Services: What Works to Promote Health?* New York, N.Y.: Oxford University Press; 2005.
44. U.S. Preventive Services Task Force. *Guide to Clinical Preventive Services.* Rockville, Md.: Agency for Healthcare Research and Quality; 2008.
45. The Cochrane Collaboration. *Cochrane Reviews.* Oxford, UK: The Cochrane Collection; 2008.
46. Green EC, Witte K. Can fear arousal in public health campaigns contribute to the decline of HIV prevalence? *J Health Commun.* 2006;11:245–259.
47. Witte K, Meyer G, Martell D. *Effective Health Risk Messages: A Step-by-Step Guide.* Thousand Oaks, Calif.: Sage; 2001.
48. Tufte ER. *The Visual Display of Quantitative Information.* 2nd ed. Cheshire, Conn.: Graphics Press; 2001.
49. Albers MJ. *Communication of Complex Information: User Goals and Information Needs for Dynamic Web Information.* Mahwah, N.J.: Lawrence Erlbaum; 2004.
50. Dillard JP, Pfau M, eds. *The Persuasion Handbook: Developments in Theory and Practice.* Thousand Oaks, Calif.: Sage; 2002.
51. Ramage JD, Bean JC, Johnson J. *Writing Arguments: A Rhetoric with Readings.* 6th ed. New York, N.Y.: Pearson/Longman; 2003.
52. Weston A. *A Rulebook for Arguments.* 3rd ed. Indianapolis: Hackett; 2000.
53. Glanz K, Rimer BK, Lewis FM. *Health Behavior and Health Education: Theory, Research, and Practice.* 3rd ed. San Francisco, Calif.: Jossey-Bass; 2002.
54. Kotler P, Lee N. *Social Marketing: Influencing Behaviors for Good.* 3rd ed. Thousand Oaks, Calif.: Sage; 2007.
55. Hastings G. *Social Marketing: Why Should the Devil Have All the Best Tunes?* Oxford, UK: Butterworth-Heinemann; 2007.

56. Siegel M, Doner L. *Marketing Public Health: Strategies to Promote Social Change.* 2nd ed. Sudbury, Mass.: Jones and Bartlett; 2007.

57. Hornik RC, ed. *Public Health Communication: Evidence for Behavior Change.* Mahwah, N.J.: L. Erlbaum Associates; 2002.

58. Petty RE, Cacioppo JT. *Communication and Persuasion: Central and Peripheral Routes to Attitude Change.* New York, N.Y.: Springer-Verlag; 1986.

59. Slater MD. Persuasion processes across receiver goals and message genres. *Commun Theory.* 1997;7:125–148.

60. Rodgers S, Chen Q, Duffy M, Fleming K. Media usage as a health segmentation variable. *J Health Commun.* 2007;12:105–119.

61. Brodie M, Hamet EC, Altman DE, Blendon RJ, Benson JM. Health news and the American public, 1996–2002. *J Health Polit Policy Law.* 2003;26:927–950.

62. Maibach EW, Weber D, Massett H, Hancock GR, Price S. Understanding consumers' health information preferences: Development and validation of a brief screening instrument. *J Health Commun.* 2006;11:717–736.

63. McDonough JE. *Experiencing Politics: A Legislator's Stories of Government and Health Care.* Berkeley, Calif.: University of California Press; 2000.

64. Nelkin D. *Selling Science: How the Press Covers Science and Technology.* New York, N.Y.: W. H. Freeman; 1995.

65. Weigold ME. Communicating science: a review of the Literature. *Science Commun.* 2001;23:164–193.

66. Shoemaker PJ, Reese SD. *Mediating the Message: Theories of Influences on Mass Media Control.* 2nd ed. White Plains, N.Y.: Longman; 1996.

67. Maibach E, Parrott RL, ed. *Designing Health Messages: Approaches from Communication Theory and Public Health Practice.* Thousand Oaks, Calif.: Sage; 1995.

68. Angermeyer MC, Dietrich S. Public beliefs about and attitudes towards people with mental illness: A review of population studies. *Acta Psychiatr Scand.* 2005;113:163–179.

69. Friedman SM, Dunwoody S, Rogers CL, eds. *Communicating Uncertainty: Media Coverage of New and Controversial Science.* Mahwah, N.J.: Lawrence Erlbaum; 1999.

70. Gwyn R. *Communicating Health and Illness.* London, UK: Sage; 2002.

71. Hughner R, Kleine SS. Views of health in the lay sector: A compilation and review of how individuals think about health. *Health.* 2004;8:395–422.

72. Schlomann P, Schmitke J. Lay beliefs about hypertension: An interpretive synthesis of the qualitative research. *J Am Acad Nurse Pract.* 2007;19(7):358–367.

73. Silk KJ, Bigbsy E, Volkman J, et al. Formative research on adolescent and adult perceptions of risk factors for breast cancer. *Soc Sci Med.* 2006;63:3124–3136.

74. Morgan MG, Florig HK, Nair I, et al. Lay understanding of low-frequency electric and magnetic fields. *Bioelectromagnetics.* 1990;11:313–335.

75. Harter LM, Japp PM. Technology as the representative anecdote in popular discourses of health and medicine. *Health Commun.* 2001;13:409–425.

76. Slovic P, ed. *The Perception of Risk.* Sterling, Va.: Earthscan; 2000.

77. Kahneman D, Tversky A, eds. *Choices, Values, and Frames.* Cambridge, UK: Cambridge University Press; 2000.

78. Morgan MG, Fischhoff B, Bostrom A, Atman CJ. *Risk Communication: A Mental Models Approach.* Cambridge, UK: Cambridge University Press; 2002.

79. Plous S. *The Psychology of Judgment and Decision-Making.* New York, N.Y.: McGraw-Hill; 1993.

80. National Center for Health Statistics. *Health, United States, 2007 with Chartbook on Trends in the Health of Americans.* Hyattsville, Md.: Centers for Disease Control and Prevention, National Center for Health Statistics; 2007.

81. Institute of Medicine. *Crossing the Quality Chasm: A New Health System for the 21st Century.* Washington, D.C.: National Academies of Science; 2001.

82. Institute of Medicine. *Health and Behavior: The Interplay of Biological, Behavioral, and Societal Influences.* Washington, D.C.: National Academy Press; 2001.

83. Thompson TL. *Handbook of Health Communication.* Mahwah, N.J.: Lawrence Erlbaum; 2003.

84. Rigoglioso RL. Multiculturalism in practice. *Picker Rep.* 1995;3(1):12–13.

85. Jandt FE. *Intercultural Communication: An Introduction.* 3rd ed. Thousand Oaks, Calif.: Sage; 2001.

86. Samovar LA, Porter RE, McDaniel ER. *Communication between Cultures.* Belmont, Calif.: Wadsworth; 2006.

87. Gudykunst WB, Mody B. *Handbook of International and Intercultural Communication.* 2nd ed. Thousand Oaks, Calif.: Sage; 2001.

88. Jones JH. *Bad Blood: The Tuskegee Syphilis Experiment: A Tragedy of Race and Medicine.* New York, N.Y.: Collier, Macmillan, Free Press; 1981.

89. Horrigan JB. *A Typology of Information and Technology Communication Users.* Washington, D.C.: Pew Internet and American Life Project; 2007.

90. Kaiser Family Foundation/Harvard School of Public Health. *September/October 2001 Health News Index.* Menlo Park, Calif.: Kaiser Family Foundation; 2001.

91. Baker L, Wagner TH, Singer S, Bundorf MK. Use of the Internet and e-mail for health care information: Results from a national survey. *JAMA.* 2003;289(18):2400–2406.

92. McLeod JM, Bybee CR, Durall JA. Evaluating media performance by gratifications sought and received. *Journal Q.* 1982;59:3–12.

93. Arceneaux K. The "gender gap" in state legislative representation: New data to tackle an old question. *Polit Res Q.* 2001;54:143–160.

94. Armor S. More women at the top. *USA Today.* June 25, 2003:3B.

95. Kenworthy L, Malami M. Gender inequality in political representation: A worldwide comparative analysis. *Soc Forces.* 1999;78:235–268.

96. U.S. Census Bureau. *Statistical Abstract of the United States: 2008.* Washington, D.C.: U.S. Census Bureau; 2007.

97. Waldrop J. The demographics of decision makers. *Am Demographics.* 1993;15(6):26–32.

98. National Conference of State Legislatures. *Legislator Demographics 2008.* Washington, D.C.: National Conference of State Legislatures; 2008.

99. Amer M. *Congressional Research Service Report for Congress. Membership of the 109th Congress: A Profile.* Washington, D.C.: Congressional Research Service; 2006.

100. Harris TE. *Applied Organizational Communication: Principles and Pragmatics for Future Practice.* Mahwah, N.J.: Lawrence Erlbaum; 2002.

101. Bier VM. On the state of the art: Risk communication to decision-makers. *Reliab Eng Syst Saf.* 2001;71:151–157.

102. Morgan G. *Images of Organizations.* 2nd ed. Thousand Oaks, Calif.: Sage; 1997.

103. Slovic P. *The Perception of Risk.* London; Sterling, Va.: Earthscan; 2000.

104. David EE. One-armed scientists? *Science.* 1975;189:891.

105. Stone DA. *Policy Paradox: The Art of Political Decision Making*. Rev. ed. New York, N.Y.: Norton; 2002.
106. Novick LF, Morrow CB, Mays GP, eds. *Public Health Administration: Principles for Population-Based Management*. 2nd ed. Sudbury, Mass.: Jones and Bartlett; 2007.
107. Bacharach S, Lawler E. *Power and Politics in Organizations*. San Francisco, Calif.: Jossey-Bass; 1980.
108. Brownson RC, Malone BR. Communicating public health information to policy makers. In: Nelson DE, Brownson RC, Remington PL, Parvanta C, eds. *Communicating Public Health Information*. Washington, D.C.: American Public Health Association; 2002:97–114.
109. Spasoff RA. *Epidemiologic Methods for Health Policy*. New York, N.Y.: Oxford University Press; 1999.
110. Weissert CS, Weissert WG. State legislative staff influence in health policy making. *J Health Polit Policy Law*. 2000;25:1121–1148.
111. Van Horn C, Baumer D, Gormley W. *Politics and Public Policy*. Washington, D.C.: Congressional Quarterly Press; 1992.
112. Konheim CS. Risk communication in the real world. *Risk Anal*. 1988;8:367–373.
113. Croteau D. The growth of self-produced media content and the challenge to media studies. *Crit Stud Media Commun*. 2006;23:340–344.
114. Alterman E. Out of print: The death and life of the American newspaper. *The New Yorker*. New York, N.Y.; 2008:48–59.
115. Reese SD, Gandy OH, Grant AE, eds. *Framing Public Life: Perspectives on Our Understanding of the Social World*. Mahwah, N.J.: Lawrence Erlbaum; 2001.
116. Scheufele DATD. Framing, agenda setting, and priming: The evolution of three media effects models. *J Commun*. 2007;57:9–20.
117. Pein C. White space in the newsroom. *Columbia J Rev*. 2004;43(3):19.
118. Manning P. *News and News Sources: A Critical Introduction*. Thousand Oaks, Calif.: Sage; 2001.
119. Nelson DE. Reducing information pollution in the Internet age. *Prev Chronic Dis*. 2007;4(1):A03.
120. Friedman SM, Dunwoody S, Rogers CL, eds. *Scientists and Journalists: Reporting Science as News*. New York, N.Y.: Free Press; 1986.
121. Cohn V, Cope L. *News and Numbers: A Guide to Reporting Statistical Claims and Controversies in Health and Other Fields*. 2nd ed. Ames, Iowa: Iowa State Press; 2001.
122. Greenwell M. Communicating public health information to the news media. In: Nelson DE, Brownson RC, Remington PL, Parvanta C, eds. *Communicating Public Health Information Effectively: A Guide for Practitioners*. Washington, D.C.: American Public Health Association; 2002:73–96.
123. Ball-Rokeach SJ, Loges WE. Ally or adversary? Using media systems for public health. *Prehosp Disast Med*. 2000;15:188–194.
124. Blum D, Knudson M, Henig RM, eds. *A Field Guide for Science Writers*. 2nd ed. Oxford [England]; New York, N.Y.: Oxford University Press; 2006.
125. Fallows D, Rainie L. *Millions Go Online for News and Images not Covered in the Mainstream Press*. Washington, D.C.: Pew Internet and American Life Project; 2004.
126. Easton G. Reporting risk—that's entertainment. *BMJ*. 2003;327:756.
127. Gastel B. *Health Writer's Handbook*. Ames, Iowa: Iowa State University Press; 1998.

128. Dumro R, Duke S. The Web and e-mail in science communication. *Sci Commun.* 2003;24:283–308.

129. Briss P, Rimer B, Reilley B, et al. Promoting informed decisions about cancer screening in communities and healthcare systems. *Am J Prev Med.* 2004;26(1):67–80.

130. Nelson DE, Brownson RC, Remington PL, Parvanta C, eds. *Communicating Public Health Information Effectively: A Guide for Practitioners.* Washington, D.C.: American Public Health Association; 2002.

131. Witte K. The manipulative nature of health communication research: Ethical issues and guidelines. *Am Behav Sci.* 1994;38(2):285–293.

132. Higginson J, Chu F. Ethical consideration and responsibilities in communicating health risk information. *J Clin Epidemiol.* 1991;44(Suppl 1):S51–S56.

133. McComas KA, Trumbo CW, Besley JC. Public meetings about suspected cancer clusters: The impact of voice, interactional justice, and risk perception on attendees' attitudes in six communities. *J Health Commun.* 2007;12:527–549.

134. Meredith LS, Eisenman DP, Rhodes H, Ryan G, Long A. Trust influences response to public health messages during a bioterrorist event. *J Health Commun.* 2007;12:217–232.

135. Perreault WD, McCarthy EJ, Cannon JP. *Basic Marketing: A Market Planning Strategy Approach.* 16th ed. Columbus, Ohio: McGraw-Hill/Irwin; 2006.

136. Allen MPR, Gayle BG, Burrell N, ed. *Interpersonal Communication Research: Advances through Meta-Analysis.* Mahwah, N.J.: Lawrence Erlbaum; 2002.

137. Dillard JP, Pfau M, eds. *The Persuasion Handbook: Developments in Theory and Practice.* Thousand Oaks, Calif.: Sage; 2002.

138. Sandman PM. *Responding to Community Outrage: Strategies for Effective Risk Communication.* Fairfax, Va.: American Industrial Hygiene Association; 1993.

139. Dillard JP, Nabi RL. The persuasive influence of emotion in cancer prevention and detection messages. *J Commun.* 2006;56:S123-S139.

140. Bennett P, Calman K, eds. *Risk Communication and Public Health.* New York, N.Y.: Oxford University Press; 1999.

141. Dennis MR, Babrow AS. Effects of narrative and paradigmatic judgmental orientations on the use of qualitative and quantitative evidence in health-related inference. *J Appl Commun Res.* 2005;33:328–347.

142. Parrott R, Silk K, Dorgan K, Condit C, Harris T. Risk communication and judgments of statistical evidentiary appeals. When a picture is not worth a thousand words. *Hum Commun Res.* 2005;32:423–452.

143. Reinard JC. The persuasive effects of testimonial assertion evidence. In: Allen M, Preiss RW, eds. *Persuasion: Advances through Meta-Analysis.* Cresskill, N.J.: Hampton Press; 1988.

144. Reynolds RA, Reynolds JL. Evidence. In: Dillard JP, Pfau M, eds. *The Persuasion Handbook: Developments in Theory and Practice.* Thousand Oaks, Calif.: Sage; 2002:427–444.

145. Alonso W, Starr P, National Committee for Research on the 1980 Census. *The Politics of Numbers.* New York, N.Y.: Russell Sage Foundation; 1987.

146. Brownson RC, Malone BR. Communicating public health information to policy makers. In: Nelson DE, Brownson RC, Remington PL, Parvanta C, eds. *Communicating Public Health Information Effectively: A Guide for Practitioners.* Washington, D.C.: American Public Health Association; 2002:97–114.

147. Cooper J, Bennett EA, Sukey HL. Complex scientific testimony: How do jurors make decisions? *Law Hum Behav.* 1996;20:379–394.

148. Kadous K, Koonce L, Towry KL. Quantification and persuasion in managerial judgment. *Contemp Acc Res.* 2005;22:643–686.
149. Reynolds RA, Reynolds JL. Evidence. In: Dillard JP, Pfau M, eds. *The Persuasion Handbook: Developments in Theory and Practice.* Thousand Oaks, Calif.: Sage; 2002:427–444.
150. Ancker JS, Senathirajah Y, Kukafka R, Starren JB. Design features of graphs in health risk communication: A systematic review. *J Am Med Inform Assoc.* 2006;13(6):608–618.
151. Edwards A, Hood K, Matthews E, et al. The effectiveness of one-to-one risk communication interventions in health care: A systematic review. *Med Decis Making.* 2000;20:290–297.
152. Hibbard JH, Peters, E. Supporting informed consumer health care decisions: Data presentation approaches that facilitate the use of information in choice. *Annu Rev Public Health.* 2003;24:413–433.
153. Schapira MM, Nattinger AB, McHorney CA. Frequency or probability? A qualitative study of risk communication formats used in health care. *Med Decis Making.* 2001;21(6):459–467.
154. Woloshin S, Schwartz LM, Byram SJ, et al. Women's understanding of the mammography screening debate. *Arch Intern Med.* 2000;160(10):1434–1440.
155. Greene K, Brin LS. Messages influencing college women's tanning bed use: Statistical versus narrative evidence format and a self-assessment to increase perceived susceptibility. *J Health Commun.* 2003;8:443–461.
156. Whelan TM, O'Brien MA, Villasis-Keever M, et al. *Impact of Cancer-Related Decision Aids: Evidence Report/Technology Assessment No. 46.* Rockville, Md.: Agency for Healthcare Research and Quality; 2002.
157. Pratkanis AR, Aronson E. *Age of Propaganda: The Everyday Use and Abuse of Persuasion.* Rev. ed. New York, N.Y.: W.H. Freeman; 2001.
158. Rothman AJ, Kiviniemi MT. Treating people with information: An analysis and review of approaches to communicating health risk information. *J Natl Cancer Inst Monogr.* 1999(25):44–51.
159. Garvin T. Analytical paradigms: The epistemological distances between scientists, policy makers, and the public. *Risk Anal.* 2001;21(3):443–455.
160. Allen M, Bruflat R, Fucilla R, et al. Testing the persuasiveness of evidence: Combining narrative and statistical forms. *Commun Res Rep.* 2000;17:331–336.

# 3

## Overcoming General Audience Tendencies and Biases to Enhance Lay Understanding of Data

> I hate these studies. Millions of American women feel exactly the same way. Despite those very precise statistics ("seven more heart attacks per 10,000 women"), last week's announcement [about increased health risks associated with hormone therapy from a July 2002 study published in JAMA] did not suggest any specific alternative treatments.
>
> Health information consumer Sammy Stevens commenting on a 2002 announcement from the National Institutes of Health[1]

### Introduction

In Chapter 2, we pointed out the broad factors involved in communicating public health information to lay audiences effectively. Messages, and the purposes for communicating them, can vary from highly directed persuasive arguments,[2–4] to assisting information seekers in readily locating and comprehending the quantitative information they need to increase their knowledge or make crucial decisions.[5, 6] Regardless of the context in which communication occurs, the basic process remains the same: information about scientific health findings must be converted from technical language into communications that lay audiences can more easily understand.

To complicate matters, lay audiences of all types interact with health-related data in environments that can be information intensive, highly fragmented, and infused with input from multiple sources and channels. In this chapter, we examine what happens when lay audiences are exposed to information presented in a quantitative format. First, we examine national assessment findings on adult literacy to understand how well lay audiences comprehend the basics of numbers and mathematical operations underlying statistical presentations. Next, we examine general comprehension tendencies of people when faced with technical or complex information, along with the specific heuristics—or mental shortcuts—they use when dealing with numbers. Finally, we synthesize this research and its implications to provide recommendations for data selection and presentation.

## Public Understanding of Quantitative Findings

As introduced in Chapter 1, quantitative data refers to numbers, mathematical operations, statistical or scientific calculations, or mathematical terms commonly used in public health research or surveillance. Before considering how audiences of all types interact with quantitative data, it is worthwhile to consider how well prepared the general public is for dealing with the specifics of mathematical operations or statistical reasoning. How comfortable are lay audiences in interpreting statistical statements? Do they understand basic statistical concepts such as probability or measures of central tendency, and can they navigate their way through the tables and graphs that are the mainstay in some types of quantitative presentations? How well has the educational system done in familiarizing public audiences with quantitative concepts? Might we expect differences based on levels of education? Answers to questions such as these, we believe, could assist communication planners in the organization phase (see Chapter 5) of their planned data communications.

### The National Assessment of Adult Literacy (NAAL)

An important source of data on this topic is the NAAL, which is conducted periodically by the U.S. Department of Education to assess progress in achieving national literacy goals. This survey, conducted in 1992 and most recently again in 2003 using a large and nationally representative sample of adults, provides a glimpse at how well literacy skills are distributed among U.S. adults.

Three basic types of literacy skills relevant to communicating data were assessed in the survey: prose literacy, document literacy, and quantitative literacy[7, 8]:

- *Prose literacy* was defined as maintaining the "knowledge and skills needed to search, comprehend, and use information from continuous texts." This concept corresponds most directly to classic definitions for English reading skills and is relevant to the degree that the gist of a scientific finding may be presented in a text format.
- *Document literacy* was defined functionally as being able to "search, comprehend, and use information from noncontinuous texts." Performance on the document literacy scale is relevant to the degree that quantitative

information may be presented to the public in the form of a table or chart, or across a series of pages in a Web site. It is also relevant to the use of data in printouts designed to support informed decision making, as is becoming the norm within many health care and insurance contexts.

- *Quantitative literacy* was defined as being able to demonstrate "the knowledge and skills required to apply arithmetic operations, either alone or sequentially," and is most directly related to the task of communicating numeric information to audiences. Assessing quantitative literacy involved performance on such tasks as calculating the amount of life insurance coverage offered by an employer's health plan, or determining the time at which medications could be taken given numeric instructions on a prescription bottle.

For purposes of reporting, the National Research Council's Board on Testing and Assessment recommended that the scores on each of these scales be translated into one of four overall reporting categories. The lowest category of competence was labeled *below basic*, succeeded next by ratings of *basic*, *intermediate*, and at the highest level, *proficient*. Weighted population estimates along with their accompanying standard errors across multiple sub-populations were prepared and included on the Department of Education's Web site as a report to the nation.[9]

In Figure 3.1, we provide an excerpt of the NAAL report to summarize proficiency ratings (*below basic, basic, intermediate,* and *proficient*) across levels of educational attainment. What is striking from the graph is the contribution that education makes to adult proficiency in the quantitative area. Almost two-thirds (65% in 1992 and 64% in 2003) of those who had not graduated from high school performed at a *below* basic level of proficiency in mathematical tasks. Roughly a quarter (26% in 1992 and 24% in 2003) of high school graduates performed at a *below basic* level, while that number shrunk to about 5% (5% in 1992, 4% in 2003) for those with at least a bachelor's degree. At the high end of the rating scale, a little less than a third of bachelor's degree recipients (31% in both years) and considerably more than a third of graduate degree recipients (39% in 1992 and 36% in 2003) scored at a *proficient* level of quantitative performance.

One implication of these results is that persons who are communicators of health information should think twice before relying on written materials to convey data, or other health findings, to audiences who have less than a high school education. Oral presentations, or perhaps even pictorial presentations through video imagery (see Box 3.1), are much more compelling as a way of communicating numeric concepts to audiences who are not quantitatively literate. Another implication is that for even the most educated

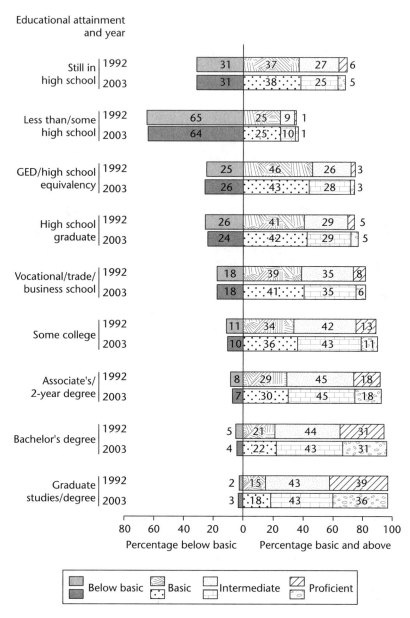

**Figure 3.1** Percentage of adults in each quantitative literacy level by highest educational attainment: 1992 and 2003. (Source: Institute of Education Sciences. *National Assessment of Adult Literacy.* Washington, D.C.: U.S. Department of Education; 2007.)

audiences, the majority of audience members maintain only a basic or intermediate level of familiarity with mathematical concepts. Care should always be taken to explain the meaning of numeric representations and to remind the audience of how to put data into context. Even the most common public

**Box 3.1** Communicating quantities without using numbers: The Truth Campaign

One of the challenges public health practitioners and parents jointly face is in reaching the hearts and minds of adolescents. A fight between two opposing forces broke out with disturbing—but from the context of this book, predictable—results.

The fight had to do with hooking teenagers into the addictive habit of smoking. The big tobacco companies had long been criticized for subtly marketing their products to young audiences. Responding to pressure, the tobacco companies agreed to sponsor "antismoking" resources for children and their parents, with the Philip Morris company developing its "Think: Don't Smoke" advertisements. The Philip Morris campaign, a seemingly innocuous set of antismoking resources, emphasized to parents that they talk to their teenagers, that they reason with them, and that they encourage teens to "think on their feet." Brochures and a Web site were prepared to support the campaign, all with text-heavy presentations of logical arguments and statistics.

The American Legacy Foundation, a not-for-profit organization focused on reducing tobacco use, launched a different type of campaign. Labeled the "Truth Campaign," their public service announcements used engaging visual images to get the point across that smoking is deadly. In its most compelling television spot, hundreds of body bags were piled in the street outside of a fictional tobacco company's headquarters. Images, not graphs, were used to illustrate the numbers.

Researchers evaluating the effectiveness of these two campaigns soon discovered a concerning finding: the Philip Morris–sponsored advertisements resulted in a "reactionary effect" among adolescents, with adolescents reporting an increased interest in smoking *after reviewing the materials* than before. The Legacy Campaign, on the other hand, had the desired effect: the campaign messages resulted in a decreased likelihood of teens beginning to smoke. Public advocacy groups soon lobbied for Philip Morris to pull their ads.

Source: Nicholson C. Framing science: Advances in theory and technology are fueling a new era in the science of persuasion. *APS Observer*. 2007;20(1). Farrelly MC, Healton CG, Davis KC, Messeri P, Hersey JC, Haviland ML. Getting to the truth: Evaluating national tobacco countermarketing campaigns. *Am J Public Health*. 2002;92(6):901–907.

health statistics such as percentages or ratios may be misunderstood without supporting explanation.

## Health Literacy

Another facet of literacy explored by the 2003 NAAL was health literacy or "the degree to which individuals have the capacity to obtain, process, and understand basic health information and services needed to make appropriate health decisions."[10] The inclusion of a health literacy scale in the 2003 NAAL is notable; it points to an acknowledged trend that the public's comprehension of words, documents, and numbers contributes to personal and public health outcomes.[11–15] To assess health literacy, 12 of the prose items, 12 of the document items, and 4 of the quantitative items were couched in terms of preventing disease, interacting with clinical services, and navigating the health care system.

Results suggested that a slight majority of adults in the United States was operating at an intermediate level of health literacy. Again, the effects of education were evident throughout the survey. Some 45% of those who had never attended high school or who had never obtained a GED equivalent demonstrated a below basic level of health competence. Level of competence increased with each year of education attained. Other findings reflected trends obtained from other sources. Women demonstrated higher levels of competence in health-related skills than men, reflecting the general finding that women are more engaged health information users than men.[16] Those who were under 65 responded with higher levels of competence than those over 65. This finding may reflect a generational gap not only in education but also in predispositions to be proactive about health care, as uncovered in other national surveys.[17] Those who were not fluent in English scored at lower levels of health literacy than those who had spoken English before starting school, illustrating the repeated observation that non-English speakers are at high risk for missing crucial communications necessary for health.[10, 18]

Health literacy as a concept is especially important because of its relationship to health communication[12] and its documented connection to health outcomes, including mortality. In cross-sectional studies, those with low levels of health literacy have been shown to maintain less health knowledge generally, to engage in poorer self-management for chronic disease, to show lower use of preventive services, and to exhibit worse health than those with higher levels of literacy.[11, 12, 14, 15, 19, 20] In a prospective cohort study of 3,260 Medicare-managed enrollees in four U.S. metropolitan areas, elderly patients who had scored low on a validated measure of health literacy experienced a 50% higher mortality rate over the 5 years of the study when compared to their more health-literate counterparts.[11]

If negative health outcomes are so prominent with those who are not facile with words, charts, or numbers then—paraphrasing an Institute of Medicine report[21]—what can be done to keep the public healthy? For health care providers in a face-to-face situation, the goal is to present health-related findings in a clear, jargon-free way and then to ask questions to be sure the person listening understands the main points.[6] Some health care professionals have used a "teach back" technique in clinical settings to positive effect.[15, 22] Using the technique, the professional will ask a patient to reiterate crucial instructions—for example, what quantities of medication to take, or what levels of blood cholesterol are risky—in their own words.

Usability and health experts advocate designing communication materials to be as useful to as many different types of audiences and users as possible, a concept referred to as "universal design." Designing government pamphlets with a language that is understandable to citizens with an eighth grade education is one example of universal design, as is creating public health information portals on the Web that can be read by Spanish speakers or citizens with visual limitations. Using icons on traffic signs and in hospital corridors can help visitors from foreign countries navigate the unfamiliar environs of a new city, regardless of the language spoken. The goal of universal design is to make products and information as usable across as many different levels of literacy as possible.

The main point to consider here is that numbers and health data are part of the conversation that will keep people healthy, but by creating communications without considering issues of literacy, we may put lay audiences at risk. Fortunately, in an age of expanding consumer involvement in health decisions,[23] applied communication scientists are beginning to take the challenge seriously. Even something as ubiquitous as the quantity-focused instructions on a pill bottle have undergone reinvention to make the communication of numbers universally clear (see Box 3.2).[24–26]

## Common Mistakes

Regardless of how proficient an audience might be, there are some mistakes that most people routinely make when interpreting numbers. For example, studies have suggested that many audiences have difficulty comprehending numbers that are very small or very large.[27–30] Small ratios present difficulties, and the magnitude of difference between 100,000 and 1 million, or parts per million versus parts per trillion, is likely to be lost on many lay audiences.

Similarly, many people do not understand that probability estimates with larger denominator values indicate a smaller likelihood of occurrence (e.g.,

---

**Box 3.2 Making a better pill bottle**

The National Council on Patient Information and Education has estimated that the global costs of medication nonadherence can be as high
as $177 billion worldwide; the human costs of making mistakes from
not understanding directions on prescription labels can be astronom-
ical. The labels on pill bottles often contribute to mistakes, according
to health communication researchers, because the labels are riddled
with abbreviations, Latin terminology, imprecise measures, and legalis-
tic obfuscations.

With the recent popularization of "consumer-oriented medicine,"
some commercial firms have set out to improve adherence to prescriptions by remaking the pill bottle. In the August 18, 2005, issue of *New
York Magazine*, writer Sarah Bernard reports about one company, Target
Corporation, that used graphic design and health literacy principles to
improve consumer understanding of pharmacy labels.

Up until the pill bottle redesign, wrote Ms. Bernard, the industry standard was plagued by inconsistent labeling, an excessive use of branding
for pharmaceutical names, confusing numbers, poor color combinations,
a curved shape that was hard to read, and tiny type. By the time usability
experts finished working on the pill bottle all that had changed, at least as
a standard within the company. Among some of the improvements made:

- Color was used to convey information. The red bottle symbolized caution; different colored rings were used to differentiate family members.
- The shape of the bottle was flattened to allow for easy reading.
- References to quantities were tested and made clearer to a broader
  audience, following principles of universal design. The words "take
  daily" were used as instruction instead of "take once a day," as "once"
  means 11 in Spanish (Chapter 2).
- Information was organized hierarchically on the label, with the most
  important information (drug name, dosage) put into the primary
  positions and less important information placed below.
- The warnings used on the label (e.g., take on an empty stomach) were
  made clearer and more obvious based on results of user testing.

Source: Bernard S. The perfect prescription: How the pill bottle was remade—
sensibly and beautifully. *New York Magazine*. April 18, 2005.

---

a risk of 1 in 200 is believed to be greater than a risk of 1 in 25).[29, 31, 32]
In one study, participants consistently rated the risk of cancer, HIV, heart
disease, homicide, and other health problems as higher when the risk was
reported as killing 1,286 out of 10,000 (12.86%) people compared with

24.14 out of 100 people (24.14%). The differences in the two denominators created an illusory perception of greater risk in the first statistic over the latter.[33]

With the exception of very small numbers, most people have a basic understanding of percentage, although this varies considerably by education level.[34, 35] People are likely to understand, for example, that 70% represents 7 out 10 and vice versa. The limitation is that they may interpret "7 out of 10" as being a lower percentage or ratio than "70 out of 100."

The other limitation audiences generally have is converting proportions to percentages and percentages into probabilities. In studies assessing quantitative literacy in health, participants were asked to convert percentages to proportions and vice versa (e.g., 0.1% to 1 in 1,000; 1 in 1,000 to 0.1%), and to report accurately how many times out of 1,000 coin flips a fair coin would be expected to land as heads (i.e., 500 times).[5] Only 16% and 38% of the participants, respectively, answered all three questions correctly in these studies, with the larger percentage of correct answers being given by better educated persons.[36, 37] This finding is not only an issue in the United States, but similar findings involving misunderstanding of probability have also been found in other countries, such as among adults in Germany.[38] Other studies conducted among international audiences suggest that the class of events represented by the probability (e.g., that a 20% chance of rain means that out of 100 days with similar conditions rain occurred on 20 of those days) is not intuitively understood unless explicitly stated.[39]

## General Tendencies of Lay Audiences

Before providing specifics about how people process and consider data, we review some general tendencies, which, though not specific to data or public health–related topics, can be strongly influential (Table 3.1). These general tendencies provide important insights as to how people are likely to process, and respond to, data presentations.

### Cognitive Processing Limits

The cognitive capacity of individuals to process large amounts of information at one time is quite limited, and people make every effort to simplify the information to which they are exposed. The reason for this is that the human brain, when processing information, operates within preset tolerances for optimal functioning.[40] For example, studies suggest that people can optimally retain only 7 ($\pm$2) discretely new pieces of information at a time.[41, 42] Systems engineers applied those data to design telephone numbering

**Table 3.1 General tendencies and other considerations of lay audiences concerning information**

Cognitive processing limits
Satisficing
Expectations of experts
Challenge of uncertainty
Processing of risk information
Information framing effects
Scanning
Use of contextual cues
Resistance to persuasion
Role of emotion

systems with seven digits so as not to exceed human capacity. Other work on memory suggested that capacity could be expanded if sub-elements could be grouped, or "chunked," into larger units of meaning. Adding an area code to the prefix of a telephone number is often not a difficult memory task because the familiar three numbers contained in parentheses is remembered as a single "chunk" of information.

What this means is that simply presenting people with more information, especially if it is complex (which is often the case with scientific data), will likely to lead to cognitive (or "information") overload.[43] When this occurs, people are likely to ignore new information or to compensate by using fairly simple approaches, such as remembering only the first thing that they heard or saw. Research on persuasion is fully consistent with the need to be cautious about the amount of data presented to lay audiences: there is clear evidence that simply using more data does not increase argument strength.[44] For persuasive purposes, in general no more than one or two data points should be used to support arguments.[44]

## Satisficing

Satisficing refers to people's tendency to expend limited amounts of mental energy or effort to obtain information until they believe they have "enough" for any particular purpose. In other words, when it comes to processing new data, people tend to be cognitive misers.[45, 46] This is most evident in people who are time-pressured, such as policy makers or journalists, who often desire information on a topic for a specific, immediate task or activity. Quite simply, when busy people look for information to make a decision they often cannot afford to expend the mental energy needed to process data in deep, expansive ways. They look for the bottom line, the gist of what the information is telling them.[47, 48]

Professional Web site designers have come to understand the limitations of a "satisficing" audience. Analyses of Web traffic indicate that if new users do not find the information they need in a large Web site within 15 minutes or less, they are likely to leave the site perhaps never to return.[49, 50] Thus, ready accessibility of useful information for users is critical as people may not seek the most appropriate source if another is available.[51]

Satisficing is common among journalists. Given the time constraints they face, it is not surprising that reporters tend to satisfice by using a handful of available sources they trust.[52, 53] Increases in media consolidation have led to reductions in staff within news organizations, more work for those remaining, and a continued business pressure on cost reduction and savings. Investigating how to tap into these existing channels, perhaps by working closely with a press office or a news bureau service, should pay dividends by providing journalists with the information they need in a way that is usable.[54] Summarizing findings in ways that reflect the current state of the science,[43] and not just a single-study finding,[55, 56] should help journalists set the agenda[4, 57–59] for public health discourse by helping them focus on major health themes[43] and science-based health communication[54, 60–63] (see Chapters 2 and 5).

## Audience Expectations of Experts and the Challenge of Uncertainty

The concept of uncertainty is well understood and accepted by scientists, mathematicians, economists, and others in similar fields that rely heavily on statistical analyses. However, most lay audiences want experts with experience and credentials, including health experts, to provide them with definitive, prescriptive information.[64] To take a nonhealth example, persons who experience mechanical problems with their automobiles expect mechanics to tell them what the problem is and then recommend a solution for resolving it, as opposed to saying something such as "there's a 30% chance that the problem is the alternator," or "only about 1 in 1,000 cars like yours have defective gas lines."

There are two facets to the problem. One is that audiences do not have the time or training to understand the nuances of a statistically uncertain finding. As a result, they tend to force probabilistic answers into discrete categories.[45, 65–67] Using the terminology of cognitive information processing discussed earlier, they "chunk" the information into easily remembered notions. A 60% chance of rain is reduced to "it will probably rain, I better take an umbrella." A headline declaring that "scientists disagree on the link between overweight and adverse health outcomes" can be interpreted as "the jury is still out, no need to change my habits."

One of the reasons it is so important for health scientists to deal with the issue of tentativeness of findings is that many industry groups have been known to use the concept of uncertainty to undo the exhortations of public health professionals. In Figure 3.2, we offer a photocopy of a document prepared by the Brown and Williamson tobacco company proposing to use scientific "doubt" as their advertising product in a campaign to discredit the public health community. In many ways, this document was the "smoking gun" in litigation against the tobacco industry.[68] In a 2005 *Scientific American* article, epidemiologist David Michaels recounts several more recent attempts by industry groups in a number of different sectors—from chemical product manufacturing groups to the oil industry to pharmaceutical companies—to forestall government regulation by casting uncertainty on accepted scientific claims.[69]

The other facet of the problem has to do with the reason the public will turn to health experts in the first place: they are looking for advice on how

"Doubt is our product since it is the best means of competing with the 'body of fact' that exists in the mind of the general public. It is also the means of establishing a controversy. Within the business we recognize that a controversy exists. However, with the general public the consensus is that cigarettes are in some way harmful to the health. If we are successful in establishing a controversy at the public level, then there is an opportunity to put across the real facts about smoking and health."

**Figure 3.2** Excerpt from the infamous "Doubt is our product" document prepared in 1969 by Brown and Williamson that uses scientific uncertainty as the crux of a defensive advertising campaign. (Source: University of California, San Francisco. "Doubt is our product." San Francisco, Calif.: University of California Legacy Tobacco Documents Library; 1969. Available at http://legacy.library.ucsf.edu/tid/rgy93f00.)

to live their lives in healthy ways. Simply presenting data to audiences is not enough; audiences need to know what the data mean for purposes of decision making. One lesson to learn from the health communication literature is that presenting risk data will likely create emotional tension; indeed, many public service efforts are designed to create a sense of fear as a motivational state for change.[70] Once the emotional state is aroused, people are motivated to restore their emotional equilibrium. From a public health perspective, they look to health experts to provide clear "safety messages"[71, 72] for how to reduce the risk through clear prescriptions for action.[28, 70, 71, 73, 74] Without providing a clear course for preventive or recuperative action, the individual is left with a sense of paralysis and will be forced to cope with the emotional tension solely through psychological means. That could mean denying the relevance of the finding[72] or creating an unrealistic sense of personal optimism or invulnerability in the face of new information.[75, 76]

Unfortunately, the news media often exacerbate the public's sense of confusion by publicizing disagreement rather than agreement and publishing controversy rather than consensus. In a content analysis of news copy from samples of national print media in the United States, researchers found an inverse relationship between the amount of news coverage given to a particular cause of death and its prevalence as a leading cause of death in the population.[77] Put simply, rare causes of death (accidents, illicit drug use, toxic agents) garnered a lot of coverage whereas common causes of death (heart disease, tobacco use) received comparatively little coverage. The result of this publicized controversy can lead to a natural sense of confusion in the public's mind about what to do to prevent disease.

Scientists can help address the problem by thinking through the public health implications of health findings before talking to journalists. If a finding is preliminary, as is often the case when presenting at journalist-covered conferences, the scientist can exercise caution by putting the preliminary finding within the context of what is already known about a health issue. If new data point to important changes in what individual behaviors or policies can do to prevent disease or improve health, some would argue that it is the ethical obligation of the scientific community to disseminate the new knowledge to the public, policy makers, and journalists.[3, 78, 79]

The expectation that scientists will have definitive answers, and the desire for certainty, are especially great challenges in acute public health situations in which there can be high levels of fear and anger and a great desire for certainty (see Chapter 6). This, unfortunately, can present a dilemma, especially in situations such as suspected disease clusters in which the epidemiologic data are not yet clear on causation. For some audiences, especially well-educated audiences who understand the nature of uncertainty, having scientists admit that the data are not yet clear can increase trust ("they are leveling with us, admitting that they do not know for sure"). For others, especially those with a cultural history of disenfranchisement, admissions of uncertainty may increase fear and reduce trust ("even the scientists don't know for sure—maybe they are hiding something").[80–82] Tailoring messages to the tolerances of the intended audiences, while paying close attention to audience reactions, can help scientists negotiate the delicate balance between full disclosure and directive communications.

### Processing Risk Information

One of the more common ways in which data are presented to the public is in the form of information about risk, or its counterpart, benefit. Note that the term risk will generally be used throughout this book, but depending upon how data are presented, risks and benefits can be the inverse of each other. The term risk, in epidemiologic and statistical terminology, refers to probability in an associative sense (e.g., "based on a comprehensive study, persons exposed to the chemical groundwater contaminants had no increased risk of developing liver cancer," or "implementing the state vaccination policy for pertussis was associated with a 90% decreased risk of experiencing this disease").

Health data can either be presented as a relative risk (e.g., odds ratios indicating a 2.5 greater risk for behavior X versus behavior Y) or an absolute risk (1 in 500 showed complications). Because of their compelling language, relative risks are often used when the purpose of the communication is to persuade (e.g., the risk of lung cancer is 20 times greater for smokers than nonsmokers). The problem with relative risk, however, is that it may not tell a complete story. Data from a pharmaceutical trial may show that drug X is twice as effective as a placebo, but the underlying data may show only a slight improvement from 1 in 1,000 to 2 in 1,000 cases. For this reason, some have argued that direct-to-consumer advertising be made more honest by insisting on the inclusion of absolute risk statistics when communicating with lay audiences, either in conjunction with the relative risk statement or in lieu of it.[83–86]

Hundreds of studies in the risk perception and risk communication literature show that lay audiences understand risk in multifaceted ways involving far more than statistical probability. Most lay audiences understand risk as "hazard or peril."[66] For example, depending on the specific situation, perception and understanding of risk data can be strongly influenced by whether the risk factor is incurred voluntarily (e.g., smoking) or involuntarily (e.g., contaminants in the environment), by how emotions (especially anger or outrage) color perceptions, and by how optimistic or pessimistic the person is generally.[29, 30, 66, 67, 87–89] As would be expected, audiences prefer to live in a world without risk, especially when it pertains to involuntary risk (see Chapter 6 for further discussion of risk).

There is much misunderstanding among lay audiences about the epidemiologic concept of absolute risk, especially lifetime and cumulative risk.[29, 88, 90] Most people do not recognize that people repeatedly engaging in a low risk behavior at each occasion, such as failing to wear a safety belt each time they are in a car, increases their cumulative risk of adverse health outcome over time. Lifetime risk implies to some people that their risk is sometime in the distant future.[91] The commonly cited statistic that 1 in 8 women will develop breast cancer in their lifetime is understood by many women to mean that they have a 1 in 8 chance of developing this cancer each year, rather than the notion that over the course of her lifetime 1 woman in 8 will develop breast cancer.[90, 92, 93] Given these differences in lay audiences' and scientists' use and understanding of the concept of risk, care must be taken in creating definitions and descriptions.

## Framing

Cognitive scientists have demonstrated that individuals can interpret the same factual data in different ways depending on the mental model, or schema, through which they perceive the data.[66] Communication researchers have demonstrated that it is possible to influence health behavior by presenting data in a way that is consistent with common public frames.[94] The technique is referred to as "framing" the public health message.[2, 95]

One very productive way of framing public health data, especially in the area of prevention, is in terms of benefits (gains) versus risks (losses). When people make health decisions, they usually do so with an eye toward future prospects. Consider what happens when a person thinks about getting a colonoscopy. More than likely, the person's attention will be focused on the immediate prospects of setting up the appointment, preparing for the test, and undergoing a physically uncomfortable procedure. Those prospects are laden with costs, a dissuading influence on choosing to undertake the screening procedure. The task of the health communicator is to elevate the losses (colon cancer, colostomy, death) of *not getting* a screening test to a level of importance higher than that of the more immediate inconvenience. From this perspective, the minor discomforts associated with the colonoscopy are a trivial price to pay for peace of mind in avoiding the bigger loss associated with the disease. This type of communication is referred to as a "loss frame."

Now consider what happens when someone considers the prospect of losing weight or exercising. Many immediate benefits come to mind from engaging in these healthy behaviors, from looking more fit and attractive to feeling better physically and psychologically. The health communicator's role in these instances is to increase the relevance of these benefits even more as a way of making those rewards salient and tangible. This type of communication is referred to as a "gain frame."

Knowing that these types of frames exist and the ways they affect people's processing of health information can be helpful in selecting the types of data to present to the public, and choosing the context in which they should be presented. If data are related to primary prevention (engaging in behaviors to avoid the onset of a disease altogether), then data about the positive benefits of the preventive behavior (e.g., 67 out of 107 people reported feeling better after moderate exercise) should provide an impetus for engaging in the behavior—a gain frame. If the data concern secondary prevention (detecting the onset of disease early, usually through a screening test) then data about long-term losses for those not engaging in the behavior (e.g., 4 out of 10 in the nonscreening group were diagnosed with colon cancer at 5-year follow-ups) will be more effective—a loss frame (see Box 3.3).[29, 96, 97]

For some the notion of "framing science" has a negative ring to it; it sounds too much like political "spin" or communication with an ulterior motive.[98–101] In many respects these criticisms miss the point, suggests political communication scientist Matthew Nisbett.[95] All communication conveys a message, whether it be haphazardly constructed or carefully refined (see Chapter 2). When scientists talk only among themselves and eschew a conversation with the public or policy makers, those findings that do trickle down into public awareness will get framed for them, often with some very negative effects (sowing doubt for commercial gain as in Figure 3.2). The role of the public health scientist and practitioner is to be proactive in understanding how communications occur in the real world and then use that knowledge in combination with a strict sense of professional ethics to communicate health data to the public in ways that are understandable and engaging. In fact, there is evidence to suggest that being proactive in describing both the strength and weakness of data up front can be effective in "stealing thunder" from would-be detractors later on, effectively disarming them.[102]

## Scanning and Use of Contextual Cues

In scientific studies and reports, authors organize information so that it builds upon material presented earlier in the text and ends with a conclusion or conclusions. This approach works well for people interested in the subject

**Box 3.3** A matter of perspective: Choosing "gain" or "loss" frames

Psychologists have long been interested in the choices that people make in situations of risk. One of the empirical observations from that body of research is that people tend to organize information about their choices in terms of either potential benefits (gains) or potential costs (losses). Their willingness to engage in a risky action varied as a function of whether the gains or losses were emphasized.

When losses are emphasized, people are more inclined to take risks or engage in costly actions in order to prevent the loss. When gains are stressed, people are more inclined to behave in more predictable or risk-averse ways. For example, think of a game show where the contestant is likely to place a larger bet when told he or she might lose it all, but is likely to place a smaller bet when told that he or she will only be adding to their current winnings. This line of research generated a framework for studying decisions referred to as Prospect Theory.

Social psychologist Peter Salovey and his colleagues recognized that many of the health decisions people make are similar to the ways in which people make decisions in situations of risk. Two examples from their long line of research illustrate the point.

In one set of studies, he and his colleagues were interested in encouraging women to participate in routine mammography as a recommended screening tool for early stage breast cancer. The problem, they observed, is there are no immediate benefits to going in for a routine mammography. The test takes time, is uncomfortable, and highlights the risky thought that a positive finding might signal the onset of the disease. Applying the tenets of Prospect Theory, they hypothesized that by presenting data in a loss-framed message (i.e., explaining what bad things might happen if mammography were neglected) they could encourage people to take the risk. That is exactly what happened. In a 12-month follow-up, significantly more women (66%) had obtained a mammogram after watching a loss-framed video than after watching a gain-framed video (52%).

In another set of studies, the scientists were interested in the problem of encouraging the use of sun block to prevent skin cancer. Applying an effective sun block has relatively little cost to most people and would not be considered a risky behavior. Under these assumptions, the scientists hypothesized that a gain frame message would work better in persuading people to engage in the healthy behavior. In one experiment, 79% of women who had read a gain-framed brochure (explaining what the immediate benefits were) requested sun block for personal use. That compared to only 45% of those who read a loss-framed brochure.

*(continued)*

**Box 3.3** (continued)

Health behavior, from these studies, appeared to be a matter of perspective. Emphasizing gains was best for nonrisky behaviors, whereas emphasizing losses seemed to work well in cases in which a risky action (e.g., disease screening) was required.

Source: Salovey P, Williams-Piehota. Field experiments in social psychology: Message framing and the promotion of health protective behaviors. *Am Behav Sci.* 2004(47):488–505.

matter and for those who are willing to take the time to read, listen, or view a paper, report, or presentation from start to finish. However, many lay audiences, particularly those with low levels of involvement in the topic area being presented, do not use this approach; instead, they tend to scan written or visual material rapidly to see if it interests them, to determine what the major points might be, and to find the bottom line.[103, 104]

When people are exposed to data or other types of scientific information that are complex or detailed, or which are presented in less familiar formats, they tend to look for cues to help them to better process and understand the information.[105] Many text documents with scientific information and visual data presentations fit both these descriptions for lay audiences. This tendency to scan for cues explains why it is helpful to include contextual information to assist audiences.

Contextual cues can be provided for lay audiences in several ways. Including information about sources is an important cue, given the tendency of audiences to rely heavily on the expert heuristic and because including source information increases the credibility of communicators (see Chapter 2). Having base rate or some other type of comparison data (e.g., a national estimate to facilitate comprehension of the magnitude of a state or local estimate; time trend data) is another means of providing contextual cues, as are several techniques used to highlight key data points or findings in text, such as arrows, bolding of data, or short text messages (e.g., cases of disease Y declined 50% since the Z policy began) (see Chapter 4).

The tendency to scan is particularly noted among Internet users, who may be searching for a few specific pieces of information quickly but find themselves faced with hundreds or thousands of potential web sites.[50, 105] One consequence of browsing and scanning, especially on the Internet, is that users may happen upon a relevant piece of data without knowing where it came from or what the numbers mean. The problem is exacerbated by frequent use of common search engines (Google, Yahoo), the results from which may be linked deep within the information architecture of the located site. If individual Web pages are not contextualized, the person doing the scanning will quickly become disoriented and lost.[50]

One way to provide context cues in a document that may be photocopied or printed out is to make purposive use of headers, footers, and other identifiers. Professional journals in most scientific disciplines do this by clearly labeling each article with citable reference information: the author, the journal, date of publication, and issue number. Most *.pdf (portable document format) files will preserve the placement of such attribution information when they are made available as printable articles on the Web, whereas articles created using HTML (Hypertext Markup Language) may not. Successful Web site designers will usually insist on using templates to be sure that the sourcing organization, update information, URL (Uniform Resource Locator), and other identifying data are routinely included on each page.[50, 106, 107] Templates can also be used to ensure that data charts can be read by voice synthesis applications for persons with vision impairments in accordance with Section 508 of the Americans with Disabilities Act.[108]

## Resistance to Persuasion

As discussed in Chapters 1 and 2, much of public health communication involves persuasion. Getting people to attend to multiple public health messages is one challenge, but persuading people to change beliefs, attitudes, or behaviors, particularly if they are well established, is difficult because people use a variety of psychological means, or defensive processing, to blunt dissonant messages. Dissonant or threatening messages are those that are inconsistent with a person's current behavior, and thus encourage the person to change beliefs or actions away from ways that are normal for them (e.g., messages emphasizing that smoking is bad are inconsistent with, or dissonant with, a smoker's attitudes toward tobacco use).

Defensive processing of threatening messages can occur in several ways. Denial is one approach: people may simply deny that the message is true, regardless of the credibility of the source or the strength of the arguments ("I don't care what you say—I believe that I am correct").[72] People may have an optimistic bias, believing themselves to be at lower or no risk than others (invulnerable), particularly for behaviors that are under voluntary control,[67] such as recreational drug use. Optimistic bias is particularly evident among adolescents but is by no means restricted to persons in this age group.[76] This bias may cause people to agree with public health messages about health risks or recommended actions but to maintain belief that the messages don't really apply to themselves.

Yet another type of defensive processing is to develop counterarguments to minimize internal (cognitive) dissonance in order to maintain the status quo.[109] Probably the most common counterarguments are questioning the validity of the data or research itself, challenging the motivation behind the research, or questioning the credibility of the researchers or their institutions (attack ad hominem). Such approaches are not limited to individuals. Organizations, businesses, and other institutions use the same type of counterarguments to blunt messages perceived as threatening.

## The Role of Emotion

One theme that should be apparent from these discussions is that emotion can play an influential role in the ways in which people perceive, and respond to, health data. From the persuasion literature, we know that the use of statistics (e.g., 440,000 Americans will die from cigarette smoking this year) can have an evocative effect on audiences receiving a health message.[44, 110, 111] In fact, persuasive messages are often designed to provoke a personal sense of concern or fear.[112–114] Fear and other emotions can then exert a motivating influence for behavior change by heightening arousal, orienting attention, and spurring self-reflection.[111, 113, 114]

Provocation of an emotional response by itself, though, is usually not enough to effect a change in behavior. From the health communication literature, we know that fear on its own can be paralyzing and that a clear safety message is needed to provide individuals with a plan for coping (e.g., go to the Health Center to receive a flu shot).[71, 72, 115] Pragmatically, the person will also need to have access to resources (insurance, a car, a subsidized flu shot) and must have a sense that any response to the persuasive health message would be accepted by peers (e.g., that it is socially okay not to smoke).[116] Support from significant others (family, friends) is also valuable for helping people interpret their feelings[117] and in seeking instrumental assistance[118] (e.g., making a doctor's appointment or following through with a personal goal).

If the person hearing about the risk data is able to adopt a suitable coping strategy for reducing risk, the sense of fear can often go away. If not, the person is left with a sense of emotional tension that may spur psychological attempts at coping through rationalization or blunting.[72, 75] Audiences may discount their own sense of personal vulnerability to the risk, or they might discredit the source of the risk information, or they may simply "turn off" when hearing more data.[72, 117] Even having made an initial wrong decision can create a type of emotional tension, as people fear being perceived as "wishy washy," clinging to their first decisions in spite of new data to the contrary.[119] When coping means learning new skills—which can often be the case in medicine—people can often overestimate their own personal abilities to cope. Unfortunately, their lack of knowledge about the deficit can prevent them from seeking help.[120]

One particular type of emotional bias that has proven especially challenging in the area of health communication is what happens when people are forced to confront data relevant to their own possibility of dying. For most people, thinking about their own mortality is a terrifying experience and can motivate people to behave emotionally or irrationally.[121, 122] For example, in a study of possible campaign materials against binge drinking, researchers varied the degree to which the focus of the communications were on the mortality consequences of heavy drinking. Participants exposed to high mortality salience messages, both those with a history of binge drinking and those without, expressed a greater willingness to binge drink in the future than those who were exposed to other types of materials—a rebound effect.[123] Other researchers have found that a focus on mortality information can precipitate engagement in irrational phobic behaviors,[121] create a sense of social "distancing" from those who are sick,[124] spur reckless actions,[125] promote blind adherence to authority, foment aggressiveness,[126] and precipitate reactionary decision making.

In clinical settings, counselors suggest that it may be important to attend to these emotional effects first before dealing directly with threatening evidence or complicated treatment alternatives. One way to do this is to help patients focus on a sense of "bigger meaning" to their lives,[122] while promoting self-esteem[127] and a sense of connectedness to others.[128, 129] This can be done, for example, by asking people to describe their fears and hopes, working with them to help them recognize their strengths, and encouraging them to consider taking specific steps or actions. Once a person is able to put things back into perspective, it should be possible to resume communication about probabilities and risk.

## Specific Numeric Biases

In addition to the general lay audience tendencies described in the previous section, there are several specific biases that people bring to bear when faced with numbers that can influence their understanding of data, particularly if they have had little or no training in statistical methods. Such biases and resulting interpretation errors occur because people—novices and experts alike—process statistical information using highly automatic, intuitive processes,[45, 65, 130] with only selected information processed by a more effortful focus.[131]

These automatic patterns can become highly ingrained, running effortlessly below the surface of conscious awareness, and are used to accommodate incoming information in rapid and efficient ways; these shortcuts are sometimes referred to as heuristics, or schema.[65] Unfortunately, these shortcuts can lead to systematic error[76, 132] and illogical reasoning.[133, 134] Paralleling these automatic patterns of cognition, a more volitional system exists that allows for conscious analysis and attention.[130] This allows people to more effectively apply learned rules and deliberative judgment; educational efforts in statistical reasoning, however, are usually needed in order for people to use this system.

## Representativeness Heuristic

One common shortcut people use to make judgments is to base their estimations on implicit knowledge and stereotypes about the category to which an object belongs.[46, 135] For example, research about public perceptions of cancer demonstrate that people generally hold a strongly negative, visceral perception of cancer as a highly aggressive, lethal disease.[136] A communication challenge is to explain to people that cancer (a category) is actually a broad set of diseases; many types of cancer (the specific objects) are slow growing and easily detectable at a treatable stage, and an early diagnosis for some cancers may not be a death sentence but a life-saving discovery.

From a data perspective, the representativeness heuristic can result in people making inferences about a broad class of objects based on limited experiences. This tendency is referred to as the "law of small numbers" to show its dissimilarity to the "law of large numbers" that forms the foundation of statistical reasoning.[137] In a classic illustration, people were asked whether the number of days in which 60% of births turned out to be males would be more common at hospitals with 15 births a day, with 45 births a day, or be equally common. Most people chose the "equally common" answer, but for an equally distributed (50%) characteristic within a population such as sex at birth, the distribution of a sample will more closely approximate the population as the sample size is increased. This means that the hospital with a smaller number of births per day would be more likely to vary from the population average. In other words, there would be a greater probability of a

60% male birth rate in a hospital with 15 births a day than there would at a hospital with 45 births a day.

The representativeness heuristic is at play anytime someone infers population characteristics from a small set of salient, but statistically misrepresentative, observations. It is the reason why politicians can be so compelling when describing an individual case in great detail, even if that case contradicts broader trends. The individual case story is a natural draw for people because it is vivid, descriptive, salient, and engaging.[138] Individual case reasoning can also serve as a distracter for people looking to rationalize their risky behavior. When safety (seat) belt laws were first being proposed in the 1980s, it was common to hear people sharing anecdotes about how they "had heard of someone who had been thrown from a crash and lived precisely because he or she was not wearing his or her safety belt." Regardless of whether these urban myths were true, people put a lot of stock in the compelling single case (i.e., $n = 1$) story.

Data can serve to reorient people back to a statistical mind set. See, for example, the excerpt from a public service Web page hosted by the National Broadcasting Company meant to encourage safety belt usage. Although the page begins with a folksy quip from a familiar celebrity, it quickly moves to a recitation of data on how many lives are saved from the simple act of "buckling up." This more accurate depiction of true base rate information for deaths attributable to not wearing a safety belt focuses the reader back into a statistical mind set. Given the magnitude of the numbers cited, the data also make for a compelling story (Figure 3.3).

Another place in which the representativeness heuristic may be playing a role is when single studies, rather than evidence reviews, are popularized by the media. Journalists and their editors are naturally attracted to the "late-breaking story" for news coverage, which means they are inclined to pick up the latest—and often contradictory—finding. Scientists and professional journal editors can play into the problem by only publishing statistically significant contrasts[139] or by overestimating the critical contributions of a distinct finding to the overall knowledge base.[86] The result is that the popular news media give more attention to rare events and rare diseases than to more common and relevant risks threatening life and health on a daily basis.[55, 140] With such a mismatch in frequency of reporting, it is no wonder that people overestimate their risks of dying from gunshot wounds, bird flu, and airplane crashes while underestimating their vulnerability to heart disease, cancer, or automobile crashes.[45, 46] One way of addressing the problem is by giving a greater priority to evidence reviews and meta-analyses in academic journals and in the popular press.[43]

**Did You Know?**

- Over 40,000 people die each year in motor vehicle crashes, the leading cause of death for every age from 3 through 33.
- Research has found that lap/shoulder seat belts, when used, reduce the risk of fatal injury to front-seat passenger car occupants by 45 percent and the risk of moderate-to-critical injury by 50 percent.
- In 2005, 55 percent of those killed in passenger vehicles were not wearing seat belts.
- From 1975 through 2005, safety belts saved about 211,128 lives, including 15,632 lives saved in 2005. If all passenger vehicle occupants over age 4 wore safety belts, an additional 5,328 lives could have been saved in 2005."

**Figure 3.3** Excerpts from a public service announcement about seat belt use. Notice the use of data to break people away from nonstatistical thinking. (Source: "The More You Know," National Broadcasting Company, 2006, http://www.themoreyouknow.com/Seat_Belts/)

## Anchoring and Adjustment Bias

Anchoring and adjustment bias refer to the tendency of people to be anchored by the first number they have in mind; any adjustments they make are strongly influenced by that initial value (anchor). In an often-cited experiment, participants were randomly assigned a starting value of 10 or 65 and were then asked the relatively obscure question of whether the percentage of African countries in the United Nations exceeds or falls below the starting value. Universally, participants who were given a starting value of 10 indicated that the percentage must be higher and those who were given a starting value of 65 indicated that it must be lower. Participants were then asked to indicate what they estimated the true percentage to be. The median estimate for those with the starting value of 10 was 25; the median for those with the starting value of 65 was 45.[46]

The anchoring and adjustment bias accounts for the influence of first impressions in influencing subsequent judgments. It is one of the reasons why a data communicator should be careful about releasing preliminary findings.[56] If the wrong numbers enter into the public discussion, and then subsequent investigation yields new information, many in the public may still be anchored on the earlier estimates. The public may make adjustments once they find out the first numbers were wrong, but the adjustments will likely be constrained by first impressions.

Even professionals are subject to error from the anchoring and adjustment heuristic. Diagnosticians who consistently overestimate the base rate probability for a disease and are then told that the base rate was "less than" than the diagnostician thought will likely adjust the numbers as only a slight deviation from the original guess. Physicians and their patients who underestimate the chances of side effects from an inherently risky procedure, and who learn that their predictions have been wrong, may only adjust their guesses slightly. The erroneous number will influence subsequent guesses, unless data are used to dispel the erroneous adjustment.

## Correlation Equals Causation

People have a strong tendency to believe that if two types of data are correlated, then one causes the other.[45, 46] Demographers note that as the number of churches in a given geographic area increases so does violent crime. Lest anyone be concerned that churches cause crime, demographers are also quick to point out that there is a third variable—population density—that accounts for both trends simultaneously. Correlation in this instance does not imply causation, but the general public is bombarded by advertising and folk wisdom meant to suggest otherwise. It is no accident that models chosen for cigarette advertisements are those who appear as healthy as possible. It is also not a surprise that the homeopathic medicine and nutritional supplement industries are thriving, usually with very little true experimental data supporting claims for efficacy.

This is not to say that correlated events are unrelated to each other causally; in fact, they often are. But it takes rigorous study based on sound theoretical frameworks to rule out competing hypotheses and to determine the nature and direction of causal influences. Scientists who communicate correlated findings are ethically bound to restrain from implying (passively or actively) a strong causal link between variables that are associated through correlation only.[141] Integrating the findings into the broader scientific base can be helpful here.

### Failure to Consider Randomness

Related to the correlation/causation issue is the tendency of lay audiences not to consider chance or randomness as explanations for sequences, events, or occurrences. Many studies have shown that people tend to see patterns in data or results (or other types of information presented to them), even when data are generated at random.[45, 46] This leads them to develop explanations or attributions that may have no basis in reality, for example, elaborate explanations for how winners in games of chance (e.g., lotteries) correctly selected winning numbers.

The most common situation in public health where the tendency to attribute meaning to randomness occurs involves disease clusters, such as cases of cancer or birth defects.[142] Alleged community clusters of diseases or health conditions commonly lead to rapid public speculation and attempts to attribute them to one specific cause, which often is assumed to be environmental in nature (e.g., a nearby industry, recent receipt of a vaccine).

This does not imply that a specific and identifiable cause does not exist, especially when rare diseases or health conditions occur; however, disease cluster evaluations rarely uncover environmental etiologies.[25] Public health and many other examples demonstrate that people rarely consider randomness or chance as the most likely (or even a possible) explanation, even when extensive investigations conclude otherwise.

## Practical Suggestions

The range of specific situations, topics, and other variations in which public health data or other types of information can be provided is great (i.e., from developing a one-line statement with a single summary message for the press to face-to-face lengthy communication sessions in clinical settings, or community meetings to discuss uncertainty about environmental chemical exposure levels). Obviously in the latter types of situations, because of the high levels of involvement among lay audiences, there is much greater need to, and opportunity for, providing explanations about the science and mathematics involved in the creation of public health data.

As discussed in the first two chapters, there are also differences based on the purpose for the communication, audiences, and context. Nevertheless, based on the material presented in Chapter 2, an audience's quantitative literacy, and the general and specific tendencies and biases of lay audiences in interpreting material discussed in this chapter, there are several practical suggestions that can improve communication about public health data across a wide spectrum of situations.

## Determine Whether Data Should Be Presented

Most health messages will be considered by lay audiences in terms of their functionality.[143] Fundamentally, lay audiences expect health experts to describe what is going on, what it means, and what needs to be done about it (e.g., personal actions by members of the public, funding decisions for programs, policy decisions).[3]

As introduced in Chapters 1 and 2 and discussed in subsequent chapters, public health practitioners and researchers desiring to communicate scientific information to lay audiences need to develop a science-based storyline from which they will create messages to communicate with lay audiences. A storyline may be as simple as a "do this or don't do that" behavior or something as complex as facilitating a decision on treatment options based on comparisons of predictive risk of complications.

Regardless, a critical step is to decide whether data (a) can be used to support the storyline and (b) should be presented to intended audiences. The decision of "data or no data," and the selection of which data to present if data are to be used is highly dependent upon the communication purpose, audience, and context. As mentioned in Chapter 2, in some situations (e.g., instruction, acute situations requiring urgent action), there is little or no need to communicate data to lay audiences as data are not needed to support the storyline (Figure 3.4; note that for personal action to reduce health risks, a

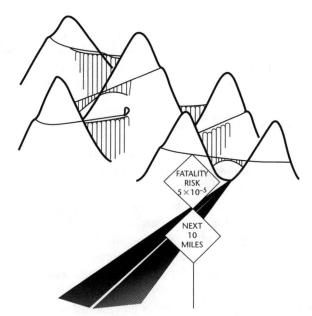

**Figure 3.4** Source: National Research Council. *Improving Risk Communication.* Washington, D.C.: National Academy Press; 1989.

simple warning message, such as "slow" or "dangerous curves ahead" would be sufficient than this data message).

As discussed earlier, whether because of low mathematical and scientific literacy, cultural preferences, reliance upon authority, or personal dislike or distrust of numbers, some audiences do not want to receive information in the form of data. These preferences need to be taken into account, and data should be used with such audiences only when necessary. Formal or informal research on audiences and their preferences (e.g., formative research on materials and messages[144]), is essential to help uncover such preferences or tendencies and is discussed in more detail in Chapter 5. It may appear that naïve audiences would never have the sophistication to comprehend statistical concepts. Persons with low levels of quantitative literacy, however, when they are motivated to comprehend and presented with materials of high quality, can learn some of the basic skills needed to understand medical statistics (such as treatment risk when making an informed medical decision).[145]

Another consideration is whether audiences are likely to be potential opponents to communicators' messages and have strongly held beliefs or opinions on the issue or topic under consideration. Public health data and scientific reasoning are unlikely to change the viewpoints of opponents: such communicated evidence will probably be ignored; the credibility of the data, proponent, or institution questioned; or opponents will generate counterarguments.[84, 146, 147] In such situations, public health proponents should consider not using data at all or at least supplementing data with narrative in the form of personal testimony (Chapter 7).[148, 149] Research on persuasion suggests that such direct personal stories may be the only approach that may reach those with strongly held opposition opinions, as it is more difficult for opponents to develop counterarguments to discount someone's personal experience.[2, 44, 148, 150]

## Select the Type of Statistics to Portray

As introduced in Chapter 1 and discussed in greater detail in the remaining chapters, if data are used, the selection or omission of data, along with the choice of words, can be highly influential and reflect the communicator's purpose, values, and ethics. The choice of whether to rely on relative risk estimates to convey a finding or absolute risk estimates is a case in point. Relative risk probability estimates (e.g., odds ratios), because they tend to be larger in magnitude than absolute risk estimates, are likely to be more effective for raising or maintaining awareness or persuading people. Just as exemplars (individual case studies or stories) can be used to make the point when underlying data support the illustrated conclusion, a compelling relative risk statement can be used to give succinct, straightforward messages when the public health science is clear and settled.

Some entities can use the power of relative risk information unethically. Product manufacturers frequently use relativistic statements to make claims for their products stronger. Some have argued that in these cases it is not appropriate to present relative statistics alone. Proposals have been made to include absolute risk information in all direct-to-consumer claims made by pharmaceutical companies, for example, given that the for-profit motive underlying advertising creates an inherent conflict of interest. It is better (the argument goes) to err on the side of full disclosure in these cases than to permit exaggerated claims.[5, 85, 151]

A general rule of thumb is to lead off with the more compelling statistic if the purpose of the communication is to persuade (remember the anchoring heuristic). Even if the purpose of the communication is to be persuasive and relative risk is used for impact, it is still generally a good idea to present the rest of the story in terms of absolute risk numbers, when feasible. The ethical obligation here is to be complete and transparent while not overburdening the audience with unnecessary details. Notice how the risk chart presented in Figure 3.5 can still present a compelling case against smoking, particularly in clinical settings, while relying solely on data estimates based on absolute risk.

### Identify and Counter Mistaken Health-Related Lay Audience Beliefs

Lay health beliefs and worldviews were discussed in Chapter 2. Before considering communicating data to lay audiences on a public health topic, it is useful to have a good understanding of audience beliefs that may bear on the issue, as certain myths or other mistaken beliefs may be present. Published surveys routinely include questions about the public's knowledge and beliefs about disease etiology and treatment, and can serve as a good starting point.[152] Formative testing, audience surveys, and personal interviews are another way of assessing public beliefs before launching a public health campaign or other major population-based effort (see Chapter 5).

It is important to uncover potential misconceptions or inaccurate intuitions lay audiences may have that clash with scientific evidence, and then attempt to correct them; otherwise, audiences are likely to have defensive reactions to messages. The tendency to equate correlation with causation and the failure to consider randomness represent common types of lay audience misunderstandings about science and statistics.

Countering inaccurate beliefs can often be done by using messages that acknowledge that an audience's misconception or explanation appears plausible, diplomatically stating why it is not accurate or complete, and presenting an alternate (and scientifically accurate) explanation that demonstrates the problems to the audience's understanding (see Box 3.4).

**Risk chart for men who currently smoke***

Find the line with your age. The numbers next to your age tell how many of 1,000 men will die in the next 10 years from each cause of death.

| Age, y | Vascular disease | | Cancer | | | Infection | | | Accidents | Any causes |
|---|---|---|---|---|---|---|---|---|---|---|
| | Heart attack | Stroke | Lung | Colon | Prostate | Pneumonia | Influenza | AIDS | | |
| 20 | | | | | | | | | 5 | 23 |
| 25 | | | | | | | | | 5 | 26 |
| 30 | 1 | 1 | 1 | | | | | | 4 | 30 |
| 35 | 2 | 1 | 2 | | | 1 | | 1 | 5 | 43 |
| 40 | 4 | 1 | 6 | 1 | | 1 | | 2 | 5 | 64 |
| 45 | 17 | 3 | 13 | 1 | | 1 | | 2 | 5 | 91 |
| 50 | 32 | 5 | 33 | 2 | 1 | 2 | | 2 | 4 | 145 |
| 55 | 51 | 8 | 55 | 4 | 2 | 3 | | 1 | 4 | 217 |
| 60 | 84 | 14 | 98 | 6 | 4 | 6 | | 1 | 5 | 341 |
| 65 | 91 | 18 | 152 | 9 | 8 | 11 | | 1 | 6 | 516 |
| 70 | 140 | 31 | 249 | 11 | 14 | 23 | | | 7 | 786 |
| 75 | 213 | 54 | 330 | 14 | 23 | 44 | 1 | | 11 | >950 |
| 80 | 295 | 80 | 275 | 16 | 32 | 76 | 1 | | 15 | >950 |
| 85 | 361 | 100 | 211 | 16 | 37 | 113 | 2 | | 19 | >950 |
| 90 | 335 | 109 | 133 | 14 | 36 | 147 | 2 | | 21 | >950 |

*Fewer than 1 death* (shaded cells)

*Calculations for this chart are based on data that use the standard Centers for Disease Control and Prevention (CDC) definition of a smoker: someone who has smoked at least 100 cigarettes in his lifetime and smokes any amount now. The numbers in each row do not add up to the chance of dying from any reason because there are many other causes of death in addition to the ones listed here. AIDS = acquired immunodeficiency syndrome.

**Figure 3.5** An illustration of a "risk chart" offering a comparison of risks in context using mortality rates in frequency format across several diseases. (Source: Woloshin S, Schwartz LM, Welch HG. Risk charts: Putting cancer in context. *J Natl Cancer Inst.* 2002;94(11):799–804.)

**Box 3.4** Addressing and countering lay audience misconceptions or inaccurate beliefs

Lay audiences may have strongly held, yet inaccurate, conceptions or beliefs (lay theories) about science, including many related to public health issues. Such lay theories can have substantial negative impacts on an audience's understanding of public health messages from credible scientific sources and subsequent negative impacts on individual and population-based health.

Simply providing audiences with more information, or using more clearly worded explanations or arguments, without acknowledging inaccurate lay theories and attempting to counteract them, is unlikely to result in effective communication. Fortunately, research from fields such as instructional design, science education, educational design, applied linguistics, and educational psychology can be used to help address such challenges. The following approach to address inaccurate lay theories has been shown to be effective based on multiple research studies:

- State the lay belief obstructing lay understanding
- Acknowledge its apparent plausibility
- Demonstrate its inadequacy
- State the (counterintuitive) orthodox scientific theory
- Establish its greater adequacy

A critical first step is to state the lay belief to get audiences to explicitly recognize that this, indeed, is their belief. (*Note*: Given that such lay theories or beliefs may not be readily "volunteered" by people underscores the importance of conducting formative research to undercover them.) Rather than stating that such beliefs are wrong, it is much better to acknowledge good, but mistaken, reasons as to why they may have these beliefs. Next, it is necessary to demonstrate why their belief is incorrect in order for them to potentially become dissatisfied with it. This then sets the stage for stating and explaining the current scientific consensus about the issue at hand.

Encouraging the use of child motor vehicle safety seats provides a good example of the process of countering a mistaken lay belief. One reason some people give for not using child safety seats is their belief that they can adequately protect their baby if a crash occurred by holding him or her in their arms. To counteract this belief, the first step would be simply to state that many parents believe they can adequately protect their infants in case of a motor vehicle crash by holding them. It is then necessary to acknowledge that for many of the activities of childrearing,

*(continued)*

**Box 3.4** (continued)

parents can protect their infants by holding them (acknowledging the apparent plausibility of this belief).

To demonstrate the inadequacy of this belief and to educate them about the current scientific consensus (especially for those not familiar with physics), it is helpful to compare the force of impact in a car crash with something that the parent is familiar with to provide context, that is, a crash occurring at 30 mph would be the equivalent of driving off a three-story building, and state that no parents' arms or laps could prevent their infants from sustaining serious, if not fatal, injuries.

Source: Rowan KE. When simple language fails: Presenting difficult science to the public. *J Tech Writ Commun.* 1991;21:369–382.

## Use Familiar Types of Data and Explain Key Scientific or Mathematical Concepts

When selecting data to present to lay audiences, choose those data most likely to be familiar to those audiences, if at all possible. When numbers themselves are used, frequencies and percentages are likely to be good choices and understood by most audiences. However, fractional percentages, such as 0.4% or 0.001% should be avoided, as they are very likely to be misunderstood.

Rounding numbers (e.g., 25,000 rather than 24,961) and avoiding unnecessary levels of precision (60% rather than 59.7%) are recommended. If proportions must be used, such as to explain probability or as an alternative to percentages, use the smallest denominator possible, for example, 4 out of 10 rather than 40 out of 100, given the challenges many lay audiences have understanding large denominators. Further recommendations on data presentation, particularly in visual formats, are described in Chapter 4.

A common mistake of many communicators of public health data is that they become so enamored with numbers that they forget to paint the rest of the picture, forgetting the low quantitative and scientific literacy of lay audiences. Seemingly straightforward concepts such as relative risk reduction, statistical significance, or probability are unfamiliar and likely to be poorly understood by lay audiences, most of whom would benefit from a careful explanation or provision of materials that clearly define and describe basic concepts and approaches.[3, 144, 153–157]

In addition to explaining details through interpersonal communications, additional written materials can also be made available to provide more details. This may be done through the use of glossaries, Question and Answer (Q & A) documents, Frequently Asked Questions (FAQs) sheets, multiple-page "backgrounders," or longer white papers about technical matters. Fortunately, Web sites provide an especially useful means for making such material available to lay audiences; journalists in particular may appreciate additional materials if they are readily accessible and well written.

Under certain circumstances, particularly those involving teaching, training, or perhaps in an extended acute public health situation (see Chapter 6), lay audiences are capable of correctly applying statistical reasoning principles and overcoming heuristics and other biases and tendencies. In a series of studies, people who were sensitized to the role of chance, particularly when dealing with a small number of cases, improved their ability to make correct probability inferences.[158] Studies have shown that providing learners with even a brief amount of training and orientation to statistical reasoning (e.g., as little as 20 min) can help them perform better on quantitative literacy tasks afterward. These and other studies suggest that people are capable of taking advantage of "teachable moments" to learn more about the quantitative skills they need to interpret health-related data.[85, 145, 157, 159]

When taking advantage of teachable moments, it is always useful to draw on analogies from familiar activities to help increase understanding. For example, a lot of people have direct experience with probability whenever they visit a gaming casino, or they can be extremely facile in tracking ranges and means when analyzing sports statistics.[158] Helping people to understand probabilities or odds in terms of a gambling metaphor (you've got a 50% chance; those are even odds—almost like flipping a coin). Even when *Las Vegas* television show star James Lesure warned young viewers that riding in a car without a safety belt was like "gambling with your life," he made an implicit appeal to a familiar metaphor in explaining how the odds would be stacked against them if they didn't buckle up. Sports metaphors can even be used to explain such complex statistical concepts as regression toward the mean ("once you've bowled a near perfect game, the chances are your next score will be lower no matter how good you are—there's no way to go but down").

## Directly Address Uncertainty

For many reasons, science is filled with uncertainty, either because of incomplete knowledge, differing interpretations, statistical imprecision in estimates, or changing recommendations based on new findings. As discussed earlier in this chapter, uncertainty among scientists can cause distress among many members of the public and policy makers, who expect clear and definitive comments and recommendations from experts.[64] Scientific uncertainty becomes especially troubling for lay audiences with high levels of involvement, when people need to make decisions about personal health care (e.g., health care treatments, screening), or in acute public health situations such as environmental exposures (Chapter 6).

Scientists need to be up front about uncertainty with lay audiences. In face-to-face encounters, such as for personal care decision making in clinical settings; in community or similar settings involving such things as unsolved disease outbreaks, environmental exposures, or issues with medical products; or in policy-maker deliberation situations, the best advice is to be honest about the tentative nature of the science and then to work with people to answer their questions about what the uncertainty means for them.[6] This usually will involve emphasizing why scientists cannot make a definitive explanation by carefully explaining the limitations of scientific and statistical methods, and by helping people understand what the trade-offs are in their own decision making.[6, 34, 52, 160]

Health education tools can help people better understand uncertainty. Some brochures and decision support software have shown promise in assisting people with the uncertainties inherent in choosing between health care treatments.[161] Health guidelines documents may be helpful, such as the Guide to Clinical Preventive Services[162] or the Guide to Community Preventive Services,[163] as they illustrate which findings have made their way into the standard of care and which findings are still tentative.[164] For further information on addressing the challenge of uncertainty, see Chapter 6.

### Reduce Cognitive Burden by Ensuring Usability

Because of the many reasons outlined in this book, lay audiences are likely to perceive science, numbers, and other types of technical information as complex. Presenting data, particularly a large amount of data, places a cognitive burden on most lay audiences. When data are presented in formats that are difficult to understand, human performance falters.[6, 161, 165, 166] In contrast, selecting "user friendly" formats that reduce cognitive burden can increase the accuracy and efficiency by which audiences process information[3, 40, 167–170]; in a nutshell, "usability matters—a lot"[171] (see Chapter 4).

Cognitive burden is reduced when audiences are not presented with too much data and can easily locate key points of information; hence the value to communicators of highlighting key points, using aesthetically pleasing layouts, and providing summaries or key points upfront.[49, 154, 165, 171–173] Highlighting key points within the materials can be done in several ways: adding short text messages that state the key points or conclusions, bolding certain text, adding arrows to show key points or relationships, and using effective labeling or legends. Consistent use of certain approaches to written document layouts are increasingly recognized as essential, particularly for Web sites. These include such techniques as paying attention to the amounts of white (open) space to avoid crowding, font size, color, consistency, location of information, and navigational ease (see http://usability.gov/ as a resource). Finally, whenever possible it is best to include summaries or to use the inverted pyramid approach to write documents by stating the main points or conclusions at the beginning.

Being inclusive and clear on all the critical information someone needs to interpret a number, a map, or a graph is also an important part of ensuring usability. Labels should be clear and located in close proximity to the data they are intended to describe (Chapter 4). Plain, jargon-free language should be used throughout and abbreviations should not be used unless spelled out first. It is also worth the effort to be sure that the underlying concepts the data describe are clear. Box 3.5 gives an example of what can happen when descriptions of the reference class are unclear when describing single point probabilities (probability of *what*).

---

**Box 3.5** Explaining the reference class for single-point probabilities

A psychiatrist who prescribed Prozac to depressed patients used to inform them that they had a 30% to 50% chance of developing a sexual problem, such as impotence or loss of sexual interest. On hearing this, many patients became concerned and anxious. Eventually, the psychiatrist changed his method of communicating risks, telling patients that out of every 10 people to whom he prescribes Prozac, 3 to 5 of those people experienced sexual problems.

This way of communicating the risk of side effects seemed to put patients more at ease, and it occurred to the psychiatrist that he had never checked how his patients understood what "a 30–50% chance of developing a sexual problem" means. It turned out that many patients thought that something would go awry in 30% to 50% of their sexual encounters.

The psychiatrist's original approach to risk communication left the reference class unclear: "Does the percentage refer to a class of people (patients who take Prozac) to a class of events (a given person's sexual encounters), or to some other class?"

Source: Gigerenzer G., Hertwig R., Van den Broek E., Fasolo B, Katsikopoulos KV. "A 30% chance of rain tomorrow": How does the public understand probabilistic weather forecasts? *Risk Anal.* 2005;25(3):623–629.

## Provide Contextual Information

A central theme of this chapter is that when people interact with health data they are often doing so with an eye toward understanding how the findings are relevant to themselves or to their loved ones. Specifically, people want to understand what they can do to maintain a healthy lifestyle, avoid risky situations, or make their disease conditions better. That is, people are oriented toward action: "what can be done now, if anything, to reduce a risk?"

For this reason, it is important to provide a clear context for what people can do with the information being given them in their own circumstances. That may mean offering clear instructions for how to reduce the risk, perhaps by offering a helpline number or giving instructions on where to go for follow-up information. It might even mean working with journalists to tailor findings to the needs of their expected audience. Research conducted jointly between the Columbia School of Journalism and Saint Louis University has demonstrated how it is possible to tailor national press releases to fit into the local context, making the information more relevant to the local community and offering places to go for further assistance (see Figure 3.6).

Another way of providing contextual information is to be sure to embed any individual finding within the overall context of existing public health recommendations. The public may not care if there was a slight recalculation in cost/benefit modeling for the use of one type of dormant flu strain versus

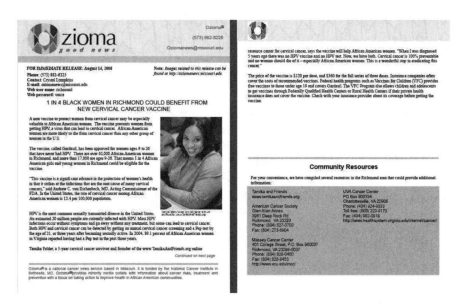

**Figure 3.6** Illustration of how a press release can be tailored for local context. (Courtesy of the Saint Louis Center of Excellence in Cancer Communication Research, 2006.)

another in an overarching epidemiological model. What they really want to know is what the gist of the findings means for them—whether they should be asking their physician for a flu shot in the upcoming winter season. As we see in Chapter 5, integrating individual findings within the larger perspective of public health recommendations is an important part of *making data talk*.

## Conclusion

Lay audiences have, at best, a fairly rudimentary understanding of quantitative findings. Their understanding is rooted in their level of education, but any person who does not use mathematical concepts or numeric representations regularly will find many data presentations difficult to understand. This means that it is not appropriate to assume that lay audiences will grasp the meaning of public health data without communicators filling in gaps with explanations about what the data mean along the way.

Lay audiences have certain expectations of health and other experts, typically expecting that these experts will have concrete answers to their questions about risk and uncertainty. Even though these answers are not likely to exist, lay audiences remain fairly resistant to persuasion.

The limits that lay audiences have in their ability to process information are universally human and easily overwhelmed. Faced with too much data, people commonly rely on cognitive shortcuts (heuristics) and other approaches to deal with information presented to them (e.g., scanning and reliance on contextual cues), and have well-known biases when faced with certain forms of data, especially probability data. Often such approaches work well enough to handle the information demands of daily life, but they can lead to bias and error when interpreting scientific data.

It is essential to understand the general tendencies of audiences and how they understand data. The concepts and key points of this chapter form the basis for the recommendations and case examples described in Chapters 4–7, as they help communicators better decide whether to present data, what data to select, how much data to present, and what additional information to include to promote lay audience understanding.

---

**The bottom line**

For prose, document, and quantitative literacy, audiences without a high
  school education were most challenged by quantitative literacy, highlighting the need to explain data included in public health messages

Lay audiences expect definitive answers from scientists and public
  health practitioners; because science allows for uncertainty, it may be
  necessary to explain parts of the scientific process to lay audiences so
  they understand why an answer may not seem clear

Use a gain frame for messages about primary prevention; use a loss frame
  for messages about secondary prevention

Effectively communicating data to lay audiences means understanding
  and overcoming the normal shortcuts (heuristics) our brains use to deal
  with more information than we can readily comprehend

Care should be taken to reduce "cognitive burden" in a world of
  proliferating information and "data smog"

The use of data in messages can help orient readers to "statistical
  thinking"; that is, getting away from anecdotes and thinking about
  quantitative findings

---

## Further Reading

### Quantitative Literacy and Biases

Koehler DK, Harvey N. eds. *Blackwell Handbook of Judgment and Decision Making*.
  Boston, Mass.: Wiley-Blackwell, 2007.

Nielsen-Bohlman L, Panzer AM, Kindig DA. eds. *Health Literacy: A Prescription to
  End Confusion*. Washington, D.C.: National Academy Press, 2004.

Sox H, Blatt MA, Higgins MC, Marton KI. *Medical Decision Making*. Philadelphia, Pa.:
  The American College of Physicians, 2006.

Zaˋacadoolas C, Pleasant A, Greer DS. *Advancing Health Literacy: A Framework for
  Understanding and Action*. San Francisco, Calif.: Jossey-Bass, 2006.

### Psychological Aspects of Health Communication

Cameron LD, Leventhal H. *The Self-Regulation of Health and Illness Behaviour*.
  London; New York, N.Y.: Routledge, 2003.

Berry D. *Risk, Communication and Health Psychology*. Berkshire, UK: Open University
  Press, 2004.

Heath RL, O'Hair, HD. *Handbook of Risk and Crisis Communication*. New York, N.Y.:
  Routledge; 2008.

Lundgren RE, McMakin AH. *Risk Communication: A Handbook for Communicating
  Environmental, Safety, and Health Risks*. 3rd ed. Columbus, Ohio: Battelle Press; 2004.

## References

1. Kalb C, Rosenberg D, Springen K, Gossard MH. What's a woman to do? *Newsweek.* July 22, 2002;42.
2. O'Keefe DJ. *Persuasion: Theory and Research.* Thousand Oaks, Calif.: Sage; 2002.
3. Nelson DE, Brownson RC, Remington PL, Parvanta C, eds. *Communicating Public Health Information Effectively: A Guide for Practitioners.* Washington, D.C.: American Public Health Association; 2002.
4. Maibach E, Parrott RL, eds. *Designing Health Messages: Approaches from Communication Theory and Public Health Practice.* Thousand Oaks, Calif.: Sage; 1995.
5. Schwartz LM, Woloshin S. The case for letting information speak for itself. *Eff Clin Pract.* 2001;4(2):76–79.
6. Epstein RM, Alper BS, Quill TE. Communicating evidence for participatory decision making. *JAMA.* 2004;291(19):2359–2366.
7. Kirsch IS, Jungeblut A, Jenkins L, Kolstad A. *Adult Literacy in America: A First Look at the Findings for the National Adult Literacy Survey.* 3rd ed. Report No.: NCES 1993–275. Washington, D.C.: U.S. Department of Education; 2003.
8. Kutner M, Greenberg E, Jin Y, et al. *Literacy in Everyday Life: Results from the 2003 National Assessment of Adult Literacy.* Report No.: NCES 2007–480. Washington, D.C.: U.S. Department of Education; 2007.
9. Institute of Education Sciences. *National Assessment of Adult Literacy.* Washington, D.C.: U.S. Department of Education; 2007.
10. Nielsen-Bohlman L, Institute of Medicine (U.S.). *Committee on Health Literacy. Health Literacy: A Prescription to End Confusion.* Washington, D.C.: National Academies Press; 2004.
11. Baker DW, Wolf MS, Feinglass J, et al. Health literacy and mortality among elderly persons. *Arch Intern Med.* 2007;167(14):1503–1509.
12. Parker RM, Gazmararian JA. Health literacy: Essential for health communication. *J Health Commun.* 2003;8(Suppl 1):116–118.
13. Parker RM, Baker DW, Williams MV, Nurss JR. The test of functional health literacy in adults: A new instrument for measuring patients' literacy skills. *J Gen Intern Med.* 1995;10(10):537–541.
14. Davis TC, Wolf MS, Bass PF, 3rd, et al. Literacy and misunderstanding prescription drug labels. *Ann Intern Med.* 2006;145(12):887–894.
15. Villaire M, Mayer G. Low health literacy: The impact on chronic illness management. *Prof Case Manag.* 2007;12(4):213–216; quiz 217–218.
16. Hesse BW, Nelson DE, Kreps GL, et al. Trust and sources of health information: The impact of the Internet and its implications for health care providers: Findings from the first Health Information National Trends Survey. *Arch Intern Med.* 2005;165(22):2618–2624.
17. Jung HP, Baerveldt C, Olesen F, Grol R, Wensing M. Patient characteristics as predictors of primary health care preferences: A systematic literature analysis. *Health Expect.* 2003;6(2):160–181.
18. Viswanath K, Breen N, Meissner H, et al. Cancer knowledge and disparities in the information age. *J Health Commun.* 2006;11(Suppl 1):1–17.
19. Rudd RE, Comings JP, Hyde JN. Leave no one behind: Improving health and risk communication through attention to literacy. *J Health Commun.* 2003;8(Suppl 1):104–115.

20. Parker RM, Jacobson TA. The role of health literacy in narrowing the treatment gap for hypercholesterolemia. *Am J Manag Care.* 2000;6(12):1340–1342.

21. Gebbie KM, Rosenstock L, Hernandez LM, Institute of Medicine (United States). *Committee on Educating Public Health Professionals for the 21st Century. Who Will Keep the Public Healthy? Educating Public Health Professionals for the 21st Century.* Washington, D.C.: National Academy Press; 2003.

22. Flowers L. Teach-back improves informed consent. *OR Manager.* 2006;22(3):25–26.

23. Cayton H. The flat-pack patient? Creating health together. *Patient Educ Couns.* 2006;62(3):288–290.

24. Hardie NR, Gagnon JP, Eckel FM. Feasibility of symbolic directions on prescription labels. *Drug Intell Clin Pharm.* 1979;13(10):588–595.

25. Brownson RC, Baker EA, Leet TL, Gillespie KN. *Evidence-Based Public Health.* New York, N.Y.: Oxford University Press; 2003.

26. National Council on Patient Information and Education. *Educate Before You Medicate.* Bethesda, Md.: National Council on Patient Information and Education; 2007.

27. Edwards A, Elwyn G. Understanding risk and lessons for clinical risk communication about treatment preferences. *Qual Health Care.* 2001;10(Suppl 1):i9–i13.

28. National Research Council. *Improving Risk Communication.* Washington, D.C.: National Academy Press; 1989.

29. Rothman AJ, Kiviniemi MT. Treating people with information: An analysis and review of approaches to communicating health risk information. *J Natl Cancer Inst Monogr.* 1999(25):44–51.

30. Redelmeier DA, Rozin P, Kahneman D. Understanding patients' decisions: Cognitive and emotional perspectives. *JAMA.* 1993;270(1):72–76.

31. Paling J. Strategies to help patients understand risks. *BMJ.* 2003;327(7417):745–748.

32. Sandman PM, Weinstein ND, Hallman WK. Communications to reduce risk underestimation and overestimation. *Risk Decis Policy.* 1998;3:93–108.

33. Yamagishi K. When a 12.86% mortality is more dangerous than 24.14%: Implications for risk communications. *Appl Cognit Psychol.* 1997;11:495–506.

34. Bottorff JL, Ratner PA, Johnson JL, Lovato CY, Joab SA. Communicating cancer risk information: The challenges of uncertainty. *Patient Educ Couns.* 1998;33(1):67–81.

35. Lipkus IM, Samsa G, Rimer BK. General performance on a numeracy scale among highly educated samples. *Med Decis Making.* 2001;21(1):37–44.

36. Schwartz LM, Woloshin S, Black WC, Welch HG. The role of numeracy in understanding the benefit of screening mammography. *Ann Intern Med.* 1997;127(11):966–972.

37. Woloshin S, Schwartz LM, Moncur M, Gabriel S, Tosteson AN. Assessing values for health: Numeracy matters. *Med Decis Making.* 2001;21(5):382–390.

38. Gigerenzer G. *Calculated Risks: How to Know When Numbers Deceive You.* New York, N.Y.: Simon & Schuster; 2002.

39. Gigerenzer G, Hertwig R, Van den Broek E, Fasolo B, Katsikopoulos KV. "A 30% chance of rain tomorrow": How does the public understand probabilistic weather forecasts? *Risk Anal.* 2005;25(3):623–629.

40. Norman DA. *The Design of Everyday Things.* 1st Basic paperback ed. New York, N.Y.: Basic Books; 2002.

41. Engle RW, Tuholski SW, Laughlin JE, Conway ARA. Working memory, short-term memory, and general fluid intelligence: A latent-variable approach. *J Exp Psychol Gen.* 1999;128(3):309–331.

42. Miller GA. The magical number seven, plus or minus two: Some limits on our capacity for processing information. *Psychol Rev.* 1956;63:81–97.

43. Shenk D. *Data smog: Surviving the information glut.* New York, N.Y.: Bantam; 1997.

44. Reynolds RA, Reynolds JL. Evidence. In: Dillard JP, Pfau M, eds. *The Persuasion Handbook: Developments in Theory and Practice.* Thousand Oaks, Calif.: Sage; 2002;427–444.

45. Hastie R, Dawes RM. *Rational Choice in an Uncertain World: The Psychology of Judgment and Decision Making.* Thousand Oaks, Calif.: Sage; 2001.

46. Plous S. *The Psychology of Judgment and Decision Making.* Philadelphia, Pa.: Temple University Press; 1993.

47. Reyna VF, Adam MB. Fuzzy-trace theory, risk communication, and product labeling in sexually transmitted diseases. *Risk Anal.* 2003;23(2):325–342.

48. Reyna VF, Hamilton AJ. The importance of memory in informed consent for surgical risk. *Med Decis Making.* 2001;21(2):152–155.

49. Eveland W, Cortese J, Park J, Dunwoody S. How Web site organization influences free recall, factual knowledge, and knowledge structure. *Hum Commun Res.* 2004;30(2):208–233.

50. Nielsen J. *Designing Web Usability.* Indianapolis, Ind.: New Riders; 2000.

51. Grama LM, Beckwith M, Bittinger W, et al. The role of user input in shaping online information from the National Cancer Institute. *J Med Internet Res.* 2005;7(3):e25.

52. Friedman SM, Dunwoody S, Rogers CL, eds. *Communicating Uncertainty: Media Coverage of New and Controversial Science.* Mahwah, N.J.: Lawrence Erlbaum; 1999.

53. Manning P. *News and News Sources: A Critical Introduction.* Thousand Oaks, Calif.: Sage; 2001.

54. Gregory J, Miller S. *Science in Public: Communication, Culture, and Credibility.* New York, N.Y.: Plenum Trade; 1998.

55. The Royal Institution of Great Britain. *Guidelines on Science and Health Communication.* London, England: The Royal Institution of Great Britain; 2001.

56. Woloshin S, Schwartz LM. What's the rush? The dissemination and adoption of preliminary research results. *J Natl Cancer Inst.* 2006;98(6):372–373.

57. Dearing JW, Rogers EM. *Agenda-Setting.* Thousand Oaks, Calif.: Sage; 1996.

58. Curtin PA. Reevaluating public relations information subsidies: Market driven journalism and agenda-building theory and practice. *J Public Relat Res* 1999;11:53–90.

59. Curtin PA, Rhodenbaugh E. Building the news media agenda on the environment. A comparison of public relations and journalistic sources. *Public Relat Rev.* 2001;27:179–195.

60. Greenwell M. Communicating public health information to the news media. In: Nelson DE, Brownson RC, Remington PL, Parvanta C, eds. *Communicating Public Health Information Effectively.* Washington, D.C.: American Public Health Association; 2002:73–96.

61. Klein T, Danzig F. *Publicity: How to Make the Media Work for You.* New York, N.Y.: Scribner; 1985.

62. Wright KB, Moore SD. *Applied Health Communication.* Cresskill, N.J.: Hampton Press; 2007.

63. Wright KB, Sparks L, O'Hair D. *Health Communication in the 21st Century.* Malden, Mass.: Blackwell; 2008.

64. Johnson BB. Further notes on public response to uncertainty in risks and science. *Risk Anal* 2003;23(4):781–789.

65. Kahneman D, Slovic P, Tversky A, eds. *Judgment under Uncertainty: Heuristics and Biases.* Cambridge, UK: Cambridge University Press; 1982.
66. Morgan MG, Fischhoff B, Bostrom A, Atman CJ. *Risk Communication: A Mental Models Approach.* Cambridge, UK: Cambridge University Press; 2002.
67. Slovic P. *The Perception of Risk.* London; Sterling, Va.: Earthscan; 2000.
68. Moore MC, Mikhail CJ. A new attack on smoking using an old-time remedy. *Public Health Rep.* 1996;111(3):192–203.
69. Michaels D. Doubt is their product. *Sci Am.* 2005;292(6):96–101.
70. Witte K, Meyer G, Martell D. *Effective Health Risk Messages: A Step-by-Step Guide.* Thousand Oaks, Calif.: Sage; 2001.
71. Leventhal H, Brissette I, Leventhal EA. The common-sense model of self-regulation of health and illness. In: Cameron LD, Leventhal H, eds. *The Self-Regulation of Health and Illness Behaviour.* New York, N.Y.: Routledge; 2003:42–65.
72. Cameron LD, Leventhal H. *The Self-Regulation of Health and Illness Behaviour.* New York, N.Y.: Routledge; 2003.
73. Garvin T. Analytical paradigms: The epistemiological differences between scientists, policy makers, and the public. *Risk Anal.* 2001;21(3):443–455.
74. Merskin D. Media dependency theory: Origins and directions. In: Demers D, Viswanath K, eds. *Mass Media, Social Control and Social Change: A Macrosocial Perspective.* Ames, Iowa: Iowa State University Press; 1999:77–98.
75. Croyle RT, ed. *Psychosocial Effects of Screening for Disease Prevention and Detection.* New York, N.Y.: Oxford University Press; 1995.
76. Croyle RT, Loftus EF, Barger SD, et al. How well do people recall risk factor test results? Accuracy and bias among cholesterol screening participants. *Health Psychol* 2006;25(3):425–432.
77. Frost K, Frank E, Maibach E. Relative risk in the news media: A quantification of misrepresentation. *Am J Public Health* 1997;87(5):842–845.
78. Nelkin D. *Selling Science: How the Press Covers Science and Technology.* New York, N.Y.: W. H. Freeman 1995.
79. Brownson RC, Malone BR. Communicating public health information to policy makers. In: Nelson DE, Brownson RC, Remington PL, Parvanta C, eds. *Communicating Public Health Information Effectively: A Guide for Practitioners.* Washington, D.C.: American Public Health Association; 2002:97–114.
80. Bier VM. On the state of the art: Risk communication to decision-makers. *Reliab Eng Syst Saf.* 2001;71:151–157.
81. Bier VM. On the state of the art: Risk communication to the public. *Reliab Eng Syst Saf.* 2001;71:139–150.
82. Frewer L. The public and effective risk communication. *Toxicol Lett.* 2004;149(1–3):391–397.
83. Naylor CD, Chen E, Strauss B. Measured enthusiasm: Does the method of reporting trial results alter perceptions of therapeutic effectiveness? *Ann Intern Med.* 1992;117(11):916–921.
84. Stone ER, Yates JF, Parker AM. Risk communication: Absolute versus relative expressions of low-probability risks. *Org Behav Hum Decis Process.* 1994;60:387–408.
85. Woloshin S, Schwartz LM. Reducing the risk that patients get it wrong. *Gastroenterology* 2005;129(2):748–750.
86. Schwartz LM, Woloshin S. On the prevention and treatment of exaggeration. *J Gen Intern Med* 2003;18(2):153–154.

87. Fischhoff B. Risk perception and communication unplugged: Twenty years of process. *Risk Anal* 1995;15(2):137–145.
88. Fischhoff B, Bostrom A, Quadrel MJ. Risk perception and communication. *Annu Rev Public Health* 1993;14(14):183–203.
89. Slovic P. Perception of risk. *Science* 1987;236(4799):280–285.
90. Hopwood P. Breast cancer risk perception: What do we know and understand? *Breast Cancer Res.* 2000;2(6):387–391.
91. National Cancer Institute. *How the Public Perceives, Processes, and Interprets Risk Information: Findings from Focus Group Research with the General Public.* Report No. POS-T086. Bethesda, Md.: National Cancer Institute; 1998.
92. Morris CR, Wright WE, Schlag RD. The risk of developing breast cancer within the next 5, 10, or 20 years of a woman's life. *Am J Prev Med.* 2001;20(3):214–218.
93. Fagerlin A, Zikmund-Fisher BJ, Ubel PA. How making a risk estimate can change the feel of that risk: Shifting attitudes toward breast cancer risk in a general public survey. *Patient Educ Couns.* 2005;57(3):294–299.
94. Salovey P, Williams-Piehota. Field experiments in social psychology: Message framing and the promotion of health protective behaviors. *Am Behav Sci.* 2004;(47):488–505.
95. Nisbet MC, Mooney C. Science and society. Framing science. *Science.* 2007;316(5821):56.
96. Rothman AJ, Salovey P. Shaping perceptions to motivate healthy behavior: The role of message framing. *Psychol Bull.* 1997;121(1):3–19.
97. Salovey P, Rothman AJ, Detweiler JB, Steward WT. Emotional states and physical health. *Am Psychol.* 2000;55(1):110–121.
98. Gerst R. The risks and advantages of framing science. *Science* 2007;317(5842):1168–1170; author reply 1168–1170.
99. Holland EM. The risks and advantages of framing science. *Science* 2007;317(5842):1168–1170; author reply 1168–1170.
100. Pleasant A. The risks and advantages of framing science. *Science* 2007;317 (5842):1168–1170; author reply 1168–1170.
101. Quatrano S. The risks and advantages of framing science. *Science* 2007;317(5842): 1168–1170; author reply 1168–1170.
102. Williams KD, Bourgeois MJ, Croyle RT. The effects of stealing thunder in criminal and civil trials. *Law Hum Behav.* 1993;17:597–609.
103. Niederdeppe J, Hornik RC, Kelly BJ, et al. Examining the dimensions of cancer-related information seeking and scanning behavior. *Health Commun.* 2007;22(2):153–167.
104. Shim M, Kelly B, Hornik R. Cancer information scanning and seeking behavior is associated with knowledge, lifestyle choices, and screening. *J Health Commun.* 2006;11(Suppl 1):157–172.
105. Albers MJ. *Communication of Complex Information: User Goals and Information Needs for Dynamic Web Information.* Mahwah, N.J.: Lawrence Erlbaum; 2004.
106. Sherman P. *Usability Success Stories: How Organizations Improve by Making Easier-to-Use Software and Web Sites.* Aldershot, England; Burlington, Vt.: Gower; 2006.
107. Pearrow M, Pearrow M. *Web Usability Handbook.* 2nd ed. Boston, Mass.: Charles River Media; 2007.
108. Horton S. *Access by Design: A Guide to Universal Usability for Web Designers.* Berkeley, Calif.: New Riders; 2006.
109. Cooper J. *Cognitive Dissonance: Fifty Years of a Classic Theory.* Los Angeles, Calif.: Sage; 2007.

110. Reynolds BA, Galdo JH, Sokler L. *Crisis and Emergency Risk Communication.* Atlanta, Ga.: Centers for Disease Control and Prevention; 2002.

111. Thompson TL. *Handbook of Health Communication.* Mahwah, N.J.: Lawrence Erlbaum; 2003.

112. DeJong W. The role of mass media campaigns in reducing high-risk drinking among college students. *J Stud Alcohol.* 2002;14(Suppl):182–192.

113. Ruiter RA, Kok G, Verplanken B, Brug J. Evoked fear and effects of appeals on attitudes to performing breast self-examination: An information-processing perspective. *Health Educ Res.* 2001;16(3):307–319.

114. Ruiter RA, Kok G, Verplanken B, van Eersel G. Strengthening the persuasive impact of fear appeals: The role of action framing. *J Soc Psychol.* 2003;143(3):397–400.

115. Glanz K, Rimer BK, Lewis FM. *Health Behavior and Health Education: Theory, Research, and Practice.* 3rd ed. San Francisco, Calif.: Jossey-Bass; 2002.

116. Fishbein M. A theory of reasoned action: Some applications and implications. *Nebr Symp Motiv.* 1980;27:65–116.

117. Croyle RT, Hunt JR. Coping with health threat: Social influence processes in reactions to medical test results. *J Pers Soc Psychol.* 1991;60(3):382–389.

118. Taylor SE, Falke RL, Shoptaw SJ, Lichtman RR. Social support, support groups, and the cancer patient. *J Consult Clin Psychol.* 1986;54(5):608–615.

119. Kruger J, Wirtz D, Miller DT. Counterfactual thinking and the first instinct fallacy. *J Pers Soc Psychol.* 2005;88(5):725–735.

120. Kruger J, Dunning D. Unskilled and unaware of it: How difficulties in recognizing one's own incompetence lead to inflated self-assessments. *J Pers Soc Psychol.* 1999;77(6):1121–1134.

121. Strachan E, Schimel J, Arndt J, et al. Terror mismanagement: Evidence that mortality salience exacerbates phobic and compulsive behaviors. *Pers Soc Psychol Bull.* 2007;33(8):1137–1151.

122. Arndt J, Greenberg J, Cook A. Mortality salience and the spreading activation of worldview-relevant constructs: Exploring the cognitive architecture of terror management. *J Exp Psychol Gen.* 2002;131(3):307–324.

123. Jessop DC, Wade J. Fear appeals and binge drinking: A terror management theory perspective. *Br J Health Psychol.* 2008, Jan. 21; PMID: 18208639.

124. Schimel J, Simon L, Greenberg J, et al. Stereotypes and terror management: Evidence that mortality salience enhances stereotypic thinking and preferences. *J Pers Soc Psychol.* 1999;77(5):905–926.

125. Ben-Ari OT, Florian V, Mikulincer M. The impact of mortality salience on reckless driving: A test of terror management mechanisms. *J Pers Soc Psychol.* 1999;76(1):35–45.

126. McGregor HA, Lieberman JD, Greenberg J, et al. Terror management and aggression: Evidence that mortality salience motivates aggression against worldview-threatening others. *J Pers Soc Psychol.* 1998;74(3):590–605.

127. Harmon-Jones E, Simon L, Greenberg J, et al. Terror management theory and self-esteem: Evidence that increased self-esteem reduces mortality salience effects. *J Pers Soc Psychol.* 1997;72(1):24–36.

128. Simon L, Arndt J, Greenberg J, Pyszczynski T, Solomon S. Terror management and meaning: Evidence that the opportunity to defend the worldview in response to mortality salience increases the meaningfulness of life in the mildly depressed. *J Pers* 1998;66(3):359–382.

129. Florian V, Mikulincer M, Hirschberger G. The anxiety-buffering function of close relationships: Evidence that relationship commitment acts as a terror management mechanism. *J Pers Soc Psychol.* 2002;82(4):527–542.

130. Kahneman D. A perspective on judgment and choice: Mapping bounded rationality. *Am Psychol.* 2003;58(9):697–720.

131. McClelland JL, Rumelhart DE, Hinton GE. Parallel distributed processing: Explorations in the microstructure of cognition. In: Munger MP, ed. *The History of Psychology: Fundamental Questions.* New York, N.Y.: Oxford University Press; 2003:478–492.

132. National Advisory Mental Health Council. Basic behavioral science research for mental health: Thought and communication. *Am Psychol.* 1996;51(3):181–189.

133. Gilovich T, Griffin DW, Kahneman D. *Heuristics and Biases: The Psychology of Intuitive Judgement.* Cambridge, UK; New York, N.Y.: Cambridge University Press; 2002.

134. Gilovich T, Savitsky K. Like goes with like: The role of representativeness in erroneous and pseudo-scientific beliefs. In: Gilovich T, Griffin D, Kahneman D, eds. *Heuristics and Biases: The Psychology of Intuitive Judgment.* New York, N.Y.: Cambridge University Press; 2002:617–624.

135. Kahneman D, Frederick S. Representativeness revisited: Attribute substitution in intuitive judgment. In: Gilovich T, Griffin D, Kahneman D, eds. *Heuristics and Biases: The Psychology of Intuitive Judgment.* New York, N.Y.: Cambridge University Press; 2002:49–81.

136. Freimuth VS, Stein JA, Kean TJ. *Searching for Health Information: The Cancer Information Service Model.* Philadelphia, Pa.: University of Pennsylvania Press; 1989.

137. Tversky A, Kahneman D. Belief in small numbers. *Psychol Bull.* 1971;76:31–48.

138. Griffin D, Buehler R. Frequency, probability, and prediction: Easy solutions to cognitive illusions? *Cognit Psychol.* 1999;38(1):48–78.

139. Greenwald AG, Kazdin AE. Consequences of prejudice against the null hypothesis. In: Kazdin AE, ed. *Methodological Issues and Strategies in Clinical Research.* Washington, D.C.: American Psychological Association; 1992:407–438.

140. Brodie M, Hamet EC, Altman DE, Blendon RJ, Benson JM. Health news and the American public, 1996–2002. *J Health Polit Policy Law.* 2003;26:927–950.

141. Huff D. *How to Lie with Statistics* (paperback reissue). New York, N.Y.: Norton; 1993.

142. Kulldorff M, Feuer EJ, Miller BA, Freedman LS. Breast cancer clusters in the northeast United States: A geographic analysis. *Am J Epidemiol.* 1997;146(2):161–170.

143. Nielsen-Bohlman L, Panzer AM, Kindig DA, eds. *Health Literacy: A Prescription to End Confusion.* Washington, D.C.: National Academy Press; 2004.

144. National Cancer Institute. *Making Health Communication Programs Work.* Washington, D.C.: U.S. Department of Health and Human Services, National Institutes of Health, National Cancer Institute; 2002. NIH Pub. No. 02–5145.

145. Woloshin S, Schwartz LM, Welch HG. Patients and medical statistics. Interest, confidence, and ability. *J Gen Intern Med.* 2005;20(11):996–1000.

146. Tesh S. *Hidden Arguments: Political Ideology and Disease Prevention Policy.* New Brunswick, N.J.: Rutgers University Press; 1988.

147. Pratkanis AR, Aronson E. *Age of Propaganda: The Everyday Use and Abuse of Persuasion.* Rev. ed. New York, N.Y.: W.H. Freeman; 2001.

148. Green MC, Strange JJ, Brock TC, eds. *Narrative Impact: Social and Cognitive Foundations.* Mahwah, N.J.: Erlbaum; 2002.

149. O'Keefe DJ. *Persuasion: Theory and Research.* Thousand Oaks, Calif.: Sage; 2002.

150. Sopory P, Dillard JP. Figurative language and persuasion. In: Dillard JP, Pfau M, eds. *The Persuasion Handbook: Developments in Theory and Practice.* Thousand Oaks, Calif.: Sage; 2002:407–426.

151. Schwartz LM, Woloshin S. Marketing medicine to the public: A reader's guide. *JAMA* 2002;287(6):774–775.

152. Gansler T, Henley SJ, Stein K, et al. Sociodemographic determinants of cancer treatment health literacy. *Cancer* 2005;104(3):653–660.

153. Schwartz LM, Woloshin S. Patient decision making: In search of good decisions. *Eff Clin Pract.* 1999;2(4):184.

154. Aldridge MD. Writing and designing readable patient education materials. *Nephrol Nurs J.* 2004;31(4):373–377.

155. Miller JD, Kimmel LG. *Biomedical Communications: Purposes, Methods, and Strategies.* San Diego, Calif.: Academic Press; 2001.

156. Lipkus IM, Klein WM, Rimer BK. Communicating breast cancer risks to women using different formats. *Cancer Epidemiol Biomark Prev.* 2001;10(8):895–898.

157. Woloshin S, Schwartz LM. How can we help people make sense of medical data? *Eff Clin Pract.* 1999;2(4):176–183.

158. Nisbett RE, Krantz DH, Jepson C, et al. The use of statistical heuristics in everyday inductive reasoning. In: Gilovich T, Griffin DW, Kahneman D, eds. *Heuristics and Biases: The Psychology of Intuitive Judgment.* New York, N.Y.: Cambridge University Press; 2002:510–533.

159. McBride CM, Emmons KM, Lipkus IM. Understanding the potential of teachable moments: The case of smoking cessation. *Health Educ Res.* 2003;18(2):156–170.

160. Rowan KE. Effective explanation of uncertain and complex science. In: Friedman SM, Dunwoody S, Rogers CL, eds. *Communicating Uncertainty: Media Coverage of New and Controversial Science.* Mahwah, N.J.: Lawrence Erlbaum; 1999:201–223.

161. Trevena LJ, Davey HM, Barratt A, Butow P, Caldwell P. A systematic review on communicating with patients about evidence. *J Eval Clin Pract.* 2006;12(1):13–23.

162. U.S. Preventive Services Task Force. *The Guide to Clinical Preventive Services: Recommendations of the U.S. Preventive Services Task Force.* [Washington, D.C.]: Agency for Healthcare Research and Quality; 2006.

163. Zaza S, Briss PA, Harris KW, Task Force on Community Preventive Services (United States). *The Guide to Community Preventive Services: What Works to Promote Health?* New York, N.Y.: Oxford University Press; 2005.

164. James B. Implementing practice guidelines through clinical quality improvement. *Front Health Serv Manag.* 1993;10(1):3–37; discussion 54–56.

165. Waters EA, Weinstein ND, Colditz GA, Emmons K. Formats for improving risk communication in medical tradeoff decisions. *J Health Commun.* 2006;11(2): 167–182.

166. Weinstein ND, Atwood K, Puleo E, et al. Colon cancer: Risk perceptions and risk communication. *J Health Commun.* 2004;9(1):53–65.

167. Gigerenzer G. The psychology of good judgment: Frequency formats and simple algorithms. *Med Decis Making.* 1996;16(3):273–280.

168. Gigerenzer G. Why does framing influence judgment? *J Gen Intern Med.* 2003;18(11):960–961.

169. Hoffrage U, Gigerenzer G. Using natural frequencies to improve diagnostic inferences. *Acad Med.* 1998;73(5):538–540.
170. Kohn LT, Corrigan J, Donaldson MS. *To err is human: Building a safer health system.* Washington, D.C.: National Academy Press; 2000.
171. Bates DW, Kuperman GJ, Wang S, et al. Ten commandments for effective clinical decision support: Making the practice of evidence-based medicine a reality. *J Am Med Inform Assoc.* 2003;10(6):523–530.
172. Dillman DA, Christian L. *The Influence of Words, Symbols, Numbers, and Graphics on Answers to Self-Administered Questionnaires: Results from 18 Experimental Comparisons.* Washington, D.C.: U.S. Census Bureau; 2002.
173. Zwaga HJG, Boersema T, Hoonhout H. By way of introduction: Guidelines and design specifications in information design. In: Zwaga HJG, Boersema T, Hoonhout HCM, eds. *Visual Information for Everyday Use: Design and Research Perspectives.* London, UK: Taylor & Francis; 1998:xvii–xxxiv.

# 4

## Presenting Data

> If you can't explain something simply, you don't understand it well. Most of the fundamental ideas of science are essentially simple, and may, as a rule, be expressed in a language comprehensible to everyone.
>
> Everything should be as simple as it can be, yet no simpler.
>
> Albert Einstein, *The Expanded Quotable Einstein*[1]

### Introduction

In communication, the way in which information is presented matters. Just as the appropriate choice of words in a sentence can make the difference between a literary masterpiece and gibberish, the choice of numbers, symbols, and explanations used to present health data can make the difference between public understanding and confusion. A large body of research about how people process information demonstrates that data selection and presentation influence comprehension, decision making, and behavior in health and other areas.[2-8] Conversely, poor data selection and presentation can lead to audience confusion,[9-12] medical errors,[13-15] flawed policy making,[10, 16, 17] and impaired organizational functioning.[18, 19]

### A Real-World Example

Figure 4.1 demonstrates just how powerful a role presentation can play in audiences' understanding and use of health data. The two charts in this figure were used in a series of studies on decision making by Hibbard and Peters.[20] Both charts include identical information for a task that is familiar to many people: choosing a health care plan by comparing features.

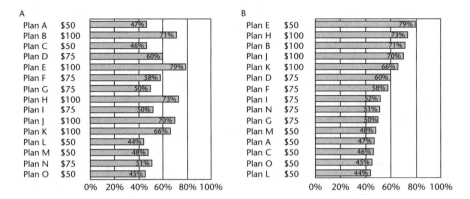

**Figure 4.1** Presentations of health care plans from the Hibbard and Peters research indicating percentage of members endorsing plan. The same data are arranged differently in the two charts: (a) The figure on the left lists plans in alphabetical order and (b) the figure on the right lists plans in descending order of member endorsement. Note that the dollar amounts refer to the monthly premium associated with the health plan. (Source: Hibbard JH, Peters E. Supporting informed consumer health care decisions: Data presentation approaches that facilitate the use of information in choice. *Annu Rev Public Health*. 2003;24:413–433. Reprinted with permission from the Annual Review of Public Health, Volume 24 ©2003 by Annual Reviews, http://www.annualreviews.org.)

Figure 4.1(a) and (b) contain identical information presented in two very different ways. Both contain the names of the plans, costs, and horizontal bars representing the percentage of people with each plan who have rated it satisfactory. Figure 4.1(a) has been organized alphabetically, with "Plan A" listed at the top of the chart and "Plan O" listed at the bottom. Figure 4.1(b) has been organized numerically by member satisfaction rating, with the most highly endorsed plan (79%) at the top of the chart and the least endorsed plan (44%) at the bottom. In these studies, persons who were presented with the data organized by member endorsement (as in Figure 4.1(b)) tended to select plans that were more highly rated, even if those plans were more expensive. The salience of member endorsement as a cue overrode concerns about cost.

This study illustrates an important point introduced in Chapter 3. Information processing is a constructive process that relies on cues in the environment that are interpreted in light of existing cognitive structures (referred to as schema[21] or mental models[22]) to create meaning. From a public health perspective, the task of the health communicator is to use the tools of scientific communication—words, symbols, and numbers—to support that constructive process in accurate and ethical ways (see Ref. 20, p. 415).

We should mention at the outset that no research has shown a clear superiority of one single data presentation format over another across all situations—much depends on the audience, the purpose of the communication, and the context of each situation (Chapter 2).[23–26] Still, research provides suggestions as to the perceptual rules that govern comprehension[4, 23, 27–32] and the types of formats that are more supportive of perceptual processes than others. Knowing these rules gives communicators options when developing presentations that are compelling and, more importantly, useful to audiences. Regardless of the individual format chosen for any presentation, the overarching goal is the same: to portray data accurately, clearly, and ethically so that audiences can update their own knowledge base.[7, 33]

This chapter covers the broad subject of presenting quantitative information once data have been selected and the purposes of communication determined. Chapter 3 presented a review of general audience tendencies with an eye toward improving understanding. This chapter describes the "palette" of data presentation formats, ranging from words only to advanced three-dimensional, computer-designed visual displays. It is not meant to be a cookbook of possibilities from which to pick and choose. (*Note*: See Further Reading recommendations at the end of this chapter, many of which contain extensive examples of data presentation.) Instead, a review of the research on data presentation principles, and on presentation formats, is combined with guidance and several examples about when and how to use each format to improve audience comprehension. Health communicators who can skillfully integrate the words, numbers, and symbols comprising all health communications will optimize the effectiveness of data presentation and reduce the chance that data will be misused or misunderstood.

## Background

As discussed in Chapter 1, scientists and others who are familiar with data and mathematics often make an implicit assumption that the "numbers will speak for themselves" and that worrying about the presentation of data or objective fact should not matter in a world that values rational decision making. Chapters 2 and 3 demonstrate the fallacy of this way of thinking. Presenting health data is essentially a communication activity, and as such should be given the same concern and meticulous attention to understanding audiences as in other types of important communication activities. It is not always a given that audiences will have the background needed to interpret data once they are presented to them, nor will they necessarily have the context needed to integrate abstract numerical concepts.

Perhaps one of the major reasons why scientists and other "data-philes" sometimes struggle when crafting a storyline around quantitative findings is that there has been a historical separation between educational courses that emphasize language, word use, and writing structure (e.g., English composition, rhetoric), courses involving the more abstract language of numbers and symbols (e.g., mathematics and, the sciences), and courses in more visually oriented curricula (e.g., graphic design, art, architecture). The emphasis of each set of coursework had its own strengths: composition and rhetoric reinforced an awareness of audiences and the choices available for crafting a compelling storyline to fit the situation. Mathematics (including statistics) and the sciences focus on the algorithmic nature of deriving a single right answer with advanced statistical courses emphasizing technological competence and computational accuracy. The skills taught in graphic design, art, and architecture provide students with a keen understanding of human perception.[34]

What is emerging today is a new transdisciplinary science that is breaking down the barriers separating these complementary skill sets. The good news is that the transition is being enabled by the emergence of a powerful new set of information technologies that allow health scientists to bring together the textual, numeric, and graphical elements of data presentations in new ways. Mainstream information technology companies (e.g., Microsoft and Google) are beginning to experiment with powerful new ways for scientists to extract and communicate trends from real-time health data.[35] The U.S.-based National Science Foundation is predicting that the next generation of "cyber infrastructure" tools will promulgate a whole new era of innovation and discovery in science.[36]

Paradoxically, this same expansion in capacity is also muddying the waters. Powerful new software programs come preloaded with a dizzying array of easy-to-use presentation options that encourage some communicators to blithely accept[18] design features without thinking through the implications for presenting data accurately. The caveat here is to remember that technology and statistical prowess should never get in the way of the communicator's goals; rather they must be used consciously and deliberately to serve the communicator's intended purpose.[18]

As discussed in Chapters 2 and 3, planning for the presentation of data will occur after the purpose for communication has been determined, attempts have been made to the understand audience(s), contextual factors have been considered, the storyline has been identified, and an assessment has been made as to whether data should be used at all in messages. The ways in which the data are packaged at that point will vary by strategic objective. The "packaging" of messages may be number intensive (such as preparing actuarial tables for decision making by the public or policy makers), or the packaging may be numerically light (such as choosing a few key statistics for giving weight to a persuasive message). In all cases, paying attention to audience' needs is important. Thoughtfully presenting data through the deliberate integration of words, numbers, and symbols will pay dividends by ensuring that communication remains a key aspect of health communication.[37]

Although discussed at length earlier, it is worth reiterating here the importance of ethics when presenting data, as presentation can have a strong effect on audience interpretation and understanding (Figure 4.1). As evidenced by the availability of books titled *How to Lie with Statistics*,[38] *How to Lie with Charts*,[39] and *How to Lie with Maps*,[40] it is easy to mislead audiences. Effective health communicators must adhere to ethical standards when presenting data or risk audience distrust and communication ineffectiveness.[41]

## Knowledge Construction

Research in educational psychology offers a glimpse into the cognitive processes upon which people rely to interpret data presented to them in texts or graphics.[2–4, 42, 43] Eye-tracking studies of students reading science textbooks in laboratory settings have found that most people use a similar process to assemble meaning from similar materials. As people encounter a particular set of data, for example, and look at a line chart presented for the first time, their eyes orient to the center of the picture. They then study the basic elements of the chart, taking stock of the lines, patterns, and shapes making up the figure.[3, 44] At the same time, they begin to interpret the overall meaning of the chart by observing the configuration of basic elements in relationship to each other. Finally, they begin to integrate the meaning of the chart with the written explanations surrounding it in the text.[2]

In many respects, these research findings contradict decades of common wisdom in communication, which has been oriented toward what the communicator tells rather than how and what an audience understands. Instead, research suggests that audience understanding can best be supported by a perspective of "knowledge construction,"[45] much in the same way that the discussion in Chapter 2 illustrated a move away from the one-way model of information delivery to a more interactive model of information processing. Communication is an active process of sense making and knowledge refinement and can be sent off course by unnecessary distractions in the ways in which data are presented.[3, 46–48]

The purpose of designing any presentation, then, is to support audiences as they engage in the automatic process of building knowledge and updating their understanding of the world around them. When formats aid in that process—when they are designed to support knowledge construction in optimal ways—they can enhance understanding and help prevent errors in interpretation. If formats distract from that process, they can increase the time needed to understand the material, muddy comprehension or increase the likelihood for error.[49, 50]

In this chapter, we describe several crucial methods of information design for health communicators' use in creating effective data presentation displays—those that are usable and understood by the audiences who rely on them. First, we detail three basic, semiautomatic perceptual processes that govern the way people understand information.

## Proximity

Proximity refers to the tendency of people to perceive items that are close to each other in a visual field as being related in some way.[51, 52] In charts and graphs, exploiting proximity cues can make data presentation more effective. When the purpose of data presentation is to encourage comparisons, side by side (clustered) bars in a chart can be used to draw the eye to comparison points, which is what the purpose of the task was in Figure 4.1.[3, 53] The bars, placed closely to each other, draw the eye's focus to the comparison data.

In contrast, consider the two charts presented in Figure 4.2. The chart on the left uses the standard comparison of side-by-side columns to illustrate differences between the North and South in a history book detailing economic causes of the U.S. Civil War. In this case, the bar chart did not help tell the story behind the data, which was focused on patterns of change in demographic characteristics of the North and South over time. Experiments demonstrated a clear superiority for presenting the same data as a line chart with a connected line drawing the eye's focus to the trends across years within each region.

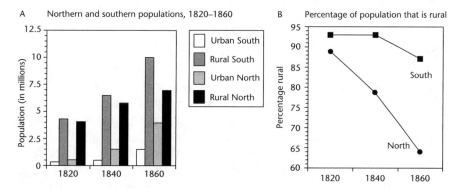

**Figure 4.2** (a) Bar graph used to teach trends leading up to the U.S. Civil War to eighth grade history students reconfigured (b) to make trends more salient. The data showed that the line graph (b) made the growing differences in rurality between the North and South more obvious to students. (Source: Shah P, Mayer RE, Hegarty M. Graphs as aids to knowledge construction: Signaling techniques for guiding the process of graph comprehension. *J Educ Psychol.* 1999;91(4):690–702.)

Experiments such as these reveal that when people try to make sense of a chart or graph, they look first to the center of the image where they evaluate the meaning of individual graphic elements (lines, bars, icons, etc.). Labels placed in proximity to the lines and bars improve comprehension because they give immediate meaning to the trends and patterns being presented. The labels "north" and "south" placed right next to the lines of Figure 4.2(b) make it easy for the reader to construct meaning. Placing a legend in proximity, for example, to the immediate right of a map, does a better job at facilitating understanding than placing a legend at the very bottom of a map away from the main image.[54, 55]

## Continuation

Continuation refers to the eye's tendency to follow lines and directions implied by separate elements within the visual field.[51, 52] Aligning decimal points vertically in a table, for example, helps make it easier for readers to compare numbers. Alternating between shaded and unshaded rows in a table also helps to provide clear continuity cues for readers. The line graph for trends across years in Figure 4.2 took advantage of continuity cues in leading students' eyes to the important patterns to be illustrated by the graphic.

Another implication of continuation has to do with the direction that people from different cultures have been taught to follow when processing information. In Western cultures, readers have been taught to process information from left to right and from top to bottom. Eye-tracking studies suggest that when encountering lines of text or information in tables, people in Western cultures start with the upper left corner, work their way horizontally from left to right, and then proceed to the left side of the next line.[31] On a Web page, this makes information chosen for the upper left corner the most relevant. This space is usually reserved for branding information to tell users what the Web site is and who sponsored it (the first questions most Web users ask of a newly encountered site). Proceeding from left to right on a Web page, the next chunk of information usually answers questions about what the purpose of a particular page might be within the overall Web site, or provides navigational links to frequently performed tasks (menu options). The most effective Web sites take advantage of continuity cues to help users navigate to wanted information quickly and easily.[31, 45, 56, 57]

The same notion applies to written documents. Headlines, headings, and subheadings are most effective when they anticipate readers' needs.[45, 58, 59] Concise headings presented in a hierarchical order allow readers to scan materials quickly and then drill down for details as needed. Familiar headings,

21. In the last five years, have you...

*PLEASE CHECK ONE BOX ON EACH LINE*

| | Yes, I have | No, I have not | |
|---|---|---|---|
| a. ...signed a petition about an environmental issue? | 1 | 2 | |
| b. ...given money to an environmental group? | | 1 | 2 |
| b. ...taken part in a protest or demonstration about an environmental issue? | 1 | 2 | |

**Figure 4.3** A formatting problem on survey instrument for the self-administered International Social Survey Program created a conflict in continuation cues. (Source: Smith TW. *Little Things Matter: A Sampler of How Differences in Questionnaire Design can Affect Survey Responses* (GSS Methodological Report No. 78). Chicago, Ill.: National Opinion Research Center; 1993.)

drawn from commonly shared experience, such as newspapers' section titles, will make it even easier to scan by not slowing down the continuity of a quick overview.[23, 33, 60] Proximity and continuity cues are not just important for data reporting, but are especially critical in instrument design and data collection. Notice in Figure 4.3 how a computer error leads to a misalignment of continuity cues, creating confusion and ultimately invalid responses to a crucial survey item.

## Closure

Closure is the tendency of people to "fill in" information that is not specified in a presentation to make sense of the presentation as a whole. Readers encountering unknown words in written text will use other cues from the text, in conjunction with their own previous experience, to extrapolate meaning from an otherwise confusing sentence. Closure is used frequently to describe visual perception, such as in the common convention in statistical charts of substituting a dashed line for a solid line to help readers distinguish between different categories of data.

One negative effect of people's tendency to use closure to create meaning is that they may fill in the wrong information when they encounter gaps in their understanding. A woman who has tuned in late to a radio broadcast recommending against mammography in a very specific set of circumstances, for example, may make an incorrect set of assumptions about not requiring mammography for early detection of breast cancer in her own circumstance. Several approaches can be used to guard against the tendency of audiences to fill in gaps of information with erroneous assumptions. Acronyms or jargon, no matter how familiar they are among scientists or practitioners within the science (e.g., "NHIS data," "mortality rate," "ACTH," "meds"), should not be used unless they are carefully defined. Elements of a chart or graph should be labeled and the words chosen should be familiar and easy to understand.[23, 58, 61] Include context information for a particular finding, especially if the finding might impact an individual's health behavior, so that members of the audience do not jump to conclusions[45] (see specific examples later in this chapter). If an early finding does not change consensus on medical recommendations, then the communicator should clearly indicate that the findings are premature and do not yet carry with them practical recommendations for change.[62]

## Integrating Words, Numbers, and Symbols

In the remainder of the chapter we discuss recommendations for how to improve the presentation of data through the combined use of words, numbers, and symbols (i.e., graphics). Words are the language (usually in text form) that describe or interpret what the data show, mean, or imply. Numbers are the actual data values themselves (e.g., 150, 2.5, 45%, 1 in 2,500). Symbols, such as bars, lines, icons, colors, and shading, are substitute representations for numbers. Before continuing, it is worth reiterating the point that it is the integration of these three components—woven together to help communicate a compelling storyline—that will make for a good and complete presentation. Studies of educational materials show that a good balance of text, figures, and other illustrations can improve comprehension over text alone.[2, 3] Studies of reference documents and Web sites suggest that a well-crafted balance of text, numbers, and graphic elements will improve usability, satisfaction, comprehension, and decisional quality.[32, 63, 64]

Here, integration implies attention to all the details in a well-orchestrated presentation of information to the public, policy makers, or the press. In health care settings, patient-centered presentations of data that use visual and narrative elements can improve patients' understanding of risk,[65] aid in their understanding of their diagnosis and treatment options,[25, 66] and assist in decision making.[67–69] On the other hand, communicators who present isolated findings with no attempt to synthesize or integrate the information into the broader framework of public health priorities do a disservice to the accuracy of public dialogue.[11]

In Chapter 5, we readdress the topic of integration as a means of ensuring that the public is well served by the science being conducted on its behalf. Although much of the remainder of this chapter emphasizes specific formats for presenting data, studies across several disciplines highlight the importance of integrating the building blocks of effective data presentations (words, numbers, and symbols) to enhance audience perception and comprehension.

## Communicating Findings with Words

Verbal descriptions of findings can be used in two ways: to use words to help communicate a storyline *about* the numbers, or to use words to help communicate a storyline *instead* of numbers. In the first way, verbal explanations can add context and meaning to the "bloodless" presentation of statistics, such as "the amount of alcohol consumed on a college campus in one year is the same as the volume of an Olympic size swimming pool."[70] Labels, explanatory text, verbal qualifiers, metaphors, and narratives can all be used to bolster understanding of the context in which the findings are relevant, and to answer the unspoken question in the audience's mind of "what does this mean for me?"

In the second way, verbal descriptions can be used *instead* of numbers when the presentation of actual data is not advisable. As discussed in Chapters 2 and 3, there are some situations in which presenting numbers, regardless of format, is not advisable. Reasons may include working with audiences who have low quantitative literacy, persons with a narrative orientation who prefer not to be presented with data (Chapter 2), or working in situations where a more authoritarian approach for communicating health information is preferred or warranted (e.g., instruction).

Regardless of clarifying meaning in conjunction with numbers or presenting a finding without using numbers, word choice is important. Most crucial is the necessity to view the communication from the audience's perspective and then craft messages to fit into the audience's frame of reference (there will be more about this under metaphors and narratives discussed later). In the following section, we review a few of the ways in which words can be used to sharpen the presentation of health findings.

## Text Labels

Text labels are as essential as symbols and numbers in helping readers comprehend the implications behind a particular graph, table, or chart. Numbers presented alone are largely meaningless. Numbers couched in the framework of a clear label aid in utility and knowledge construction.[71] Our discussion of proximity suggested that labels are most effective when they are positioned next to the data being displayed in a chart.[3, 4, 42, 45] Labels placed adjacent to trend lines or clustered bars are superior to labels placed in a disconnected legend box. If legends are used, placing them near the data points they are intended to describe, rather than elsewhere on a graph, will help keep the explanatory text near to the object being described.[54, 55]

In no circumstances, though, should labels detract from the reader's task of knowledge construction or decision making.[18, 33] Titles, labels, and headings should be clear and familiar to readers.[7, 23, 33] Using acronyms in a heading, even if explained elsewhere in the text, will increase cognitive demands because the reader is then forced to search for the meaning of the unknown term before coming back to the graph. Labels or legend boxes should not obscure the underlying data they are meant to describe; they should be used frugally, balancing completeness against the distraction of unnecessary clutter.[33]

## Verbal Qualifiers of Data

One way to present data using words is to substitute everyday language to describe the relationship between numbers. Examples include terms such as "much higher," "minimal risk," or "most of the time."[25, 72–75] Verbal qualifiers are less cognitively demanding than numbers, and they fit in with people's tendencies to process data for the overall gist of the argument.[76] In fact, when asked to recall the specifics of a data presentation, most people tend to convert (or interpret) the numeric precision of the data into discrete verbal categories (e.g., remembering that a given number represented a "high" or "low" risk).[26] Content analysis of news coverage suggests that the press tends to make the same sorts of conversions, preferring to use verbal qualifiers to get the point of a story across.[77] Patients often prefer a verbal description of risk, either in addition to a specific numeric estimate or in place of it, when speaking in conversation with their health care providers.[25]

Unfortunately, substituting verbal qualifiers for actual numeric values or visual representations of data can also create problems. As mentioned in Chapter 3, a "low or minimal risk" is often interpreted by lay audiences as "no risk at all."[26] Furthermore, there is much individual variation and ambiguity in the interpretation and meaning of verbal qualifiers among lay and professional audiences.[24, 46, 72, 73, 78–81] There is little agreement, for example, among people as to where to even draw the line between "high" and "low" risk.[74] In one study of genetic risk, lay audiences defined "high risk" as greater than 20%, whereas health professionals defined it as between 12.5% and 25%.[82] In comparison, a study of college students[83] involved in decisions about a prenatal diagnosis of cystic fibrosis suggested that the students interpreted a "moderate chance" of occurring as being around 25% and a "high chance" as around 75%.

The word "frequent" is also subject to much variability in interpretation. A study of lay audiences, for instance, found that when applied to a benefit or risk of a treatment, it was considered to be 70% in numeric terms, on average, but estimates ranged from 30% to 90%.[72] Similar findings have been reported from research on survey questions, with much variability in respondents' numeric interpretations of verbal qualifiers such as "usually," "very often," or "occasionally."[46]

Given the variability of verbal equivalents to numbers, it may be best to err on the side of grounding verbal qualifiers with actual numbers. A physician may offer a specific number to a patient but may then offer a verbal description to help put the number in context.[25] A scientist may offer up a specific odds ratio to the press but may use a verbal qualifier to help couch its impact within the larger framework of scientific evidence. Anchoring statements on actual data may help stave off the tendency to subsequently exaggerate the significance of the finding.[84]

## Metaphors

Scientists are used to a world of abstraction in which real-world phenomena are distilled into numeric measurements for careful analysis and the systematic presentation of conclusions. To the public, policy makers, and the press, however, the recitation of scientific data can be perceived as dull and boring.[85] The following quote from a health reporter sums up many people's reactions when presented with data:

> Public health stories are important, but the problem is that they may be boring...Public health is foremost about people, but officials deal in statistics...The Department of Health and Human Services and state health departments crank out volumes of numbers. So do universities and private research institutes...But phrases like "a two-fold increased risk" and "rate per 100,000" are bloodless...That's why it's so important to find the faces of ordinary people to illustrate the drama buried in the gray numbers of a report.   (Ref. 86, p. 137)

To address this challenge, one approach is to use metaphors and narratives to try to make data "come alive" by using language, phrases, or visual images to provide context and increase audience interest.[87, 88] The word "metaphor" can have different meanings; in this chapter, metaphor is used as a general term for the use of linguistic phrases implying that "A is similar to B." That is, a metaphor makes it possible to understand concept A by bringing in the meaning and feelings associated with concept B.[89] For example, to say that 5 million people die globally each year from smoking cigarettes may or may not drive home the urgency of doing something to curb the statistic. To say that "losing 5 million a year" to smoking is like blowing up atomic bombs in "50 Hiroshimas each and every year" uses a metaphor to evoke strong feelings of avoidable death and loss in the world community.

Metaphors are especially useful in helping public health communicators establish a personalized connection with an audience. They form a type of

**Table 4.1 Examples of metaphors used in public health communication**

"There are 10 times as many gun dealers in California as there are McDonald's restaurants"

"Only 3% of Canadians would prefer a U.S.-type private health insurance model to the single payer model. To put that in perspective, 16% of Canadians believe that Elvis Presley is still alive"

"Think of two twin towers falling from terrorist attacks every day—that's cancer"

*Sources*: Wallack LM. *News for a Change: An Advocate's Guide to Working with the Media.* Thousand Oaks, Calif.: Sage; 1999 (first 2 examples). Rose C. A discussion about cancer in America. *Charlie Rose Show.* April 29, 2004 (third example).

culturally relevant code that lets the audience know the message is relevant to "people like them."[90] Depending on the communication medium, metaphorical language can be complemented by powerful visual images through video, cartoons, or photographs.[89] The images of body bags placed in front of a tobacco company's headquarters during an ad by the American Legacy Foundation's "Truth Campaign" offered a viscerally moving depiction of the mortality statistics underlying cigarette smoking (see Chapter 3, Box 3.1). The images, script, and accompanying voiceover made a deep connection to adolescents who are not accustomed to thinking about their own mortality, and who are seeking to find their own voice in rebelling against the influence of corporate control. If metaphors are used, they are more likely to be effective if the audience has some familiarity with the comparison item, when they have higher levels of novelty, if they are used early in a message, and if they are presented in an audio rather than a written format.[89] In Table 4.1 we offer a few examples of metaphors used to illustrate the concept of numeric magnitude.

## Narratives

A narrative is the use of words, visual images, or both to tell a story[91] that can be fictional or nonfictional. Compared to metaphors, narratives are generally longer, but the length of narratives can vary greatly. Narratives can have many purposes, ranging from entertainment (jokes) to persuasion (personal testimony). Examples of short narratives are anecdotes, quotations, specific examples, vignettes, personal stories/testimonies, and case studies; longer narratives include essays, short stories, books, and scripts for plays, television, movies, and interactive media. Unlike strictly statistical presentations, narratives can increase audience attention to—and level of interest in—new topics because the narratives can "transport" people's minds into different "worlds."[88]

Narratives are widely used by people who work in journalism, business, law, religion, entertainment, and politics.[92] Public health practitioners may balk at the suggestion to consider using narrative formats, as they can easily be used to mislead or manipulate audiences. On the other hand, when used in an ethically responsible manner, they can be quite effective in certain situations. Several studies have found anecdotes without data (narratives) to be more persuasive than statistical evidence alone.[93, 94]

There are several practical reasons for using narratives to help communicate statistical findings. First, as mentioned in Chapter 2, some people have a narrative orientation and simply prefer to receive information in the form of stories. Second, some audiences have great difficulty understanding other types of data presentation formats. Finally, because of the ways in which narratives are processed by the mind (see below), they can increase understanding or persuasiveness in ways not possible through other data presentation formats.

The theoretical reasons for why narratives work so effectively are varied, but most explanations revolve around the notions of schema activation[89] and emotional engagement.[88, 95] Narratives can connect a scientific finding with preexisting schema. Personal schemas are especially powerful constructs; humans as social animals are hardwired to attend to social stimuli and put a lot of stock in narratives about other people. By illustrating a health statistic with the compelling story of an individual, the health communicator will be able to activate attention, evoke emotion, and fill in the gaps for personal meaning. The effect is especially strong if the subject of the narrative is similar to the audience member in some way.[96]

Using narratives also works in such a way that people can more easily organize and make sense of the information that they receive by developing or recalling information through stories they already know.[97] Another explanation for how some narratives work is through their ability to generate emotions in audiences, such as sadness, fear, anger, happiness, humor, love, sympathy, or empathy.[88, 95] As evident in Box 4.1, which contains a description of Guinea worm and its effect on a child in Ghana, this ability of a narrative to describe a health problem using words, and to generate emotions, simply cannot be matched by data presentation.

Regardless of the specific processes by which they work, narratives increase the chance that many lay audiences, especially those with low levels of involvement with health issues, will attend to scientific findings and potentially retain and use that information.[98]

## Communicating Findings Directly with Numbers

Although verbal descriptions of data are good for conveying the gist of a finding, they do not have the precision of numbers. Numbers in a news story convey information concisely, and they serve to quantify assertions. Even in

---

**Box 4.1** Use of a narrative to describe and explain the debilitating effects of Guinea worm

At a Guinea worm containment center in Savelugu, northern Ghana, Assana Mohammed, age 10, cries out in pain. Her eyes are shut and she cannot help but try to remove the health worker's hand from her wound. Little by little, he is extracting a long white Guinea worm from her ankle.

Guinea worm, a parasite, gets into the human body when a person drinks water infested with fleas that have ingested the larvae. The worms grow inside the body, sometimes reaching more than a meter in length and eventually erupting through the skin. The condition causes unbearable pain for weeks and months, preventing the sufferer from engaging in daily activities. Guinea worm therefore has an adverse economic and social impact, in addition to its terrible health effects.

Source: Cozay, "Through their eyes. Poverty in Africa: Stories." Available at http://cozay.com/WORLD-POVERTY-STORIES.php.

---

editorials and feature news, numbers alert the reader to assertions of fact, which can improve the sense of credibility in the argument to come.

From an information design perspective, numbers can be used in a variety of ways. They can have iconic value, as when relating readers to localities on a map; ordinal value, as when leading readers through a list of ranked values; interval value, as when referring to real or implied distances; and ratio value, for describing quantities and multiplicative relationships. The multipurpose nature of numbers along with their relative universality across languages makes their use applicable across a wide range of purposes and contexts. Some of their specific uses are detailed in the following sections.

## Instructing and Informing with Numbers

When the purpose is to instruct or inform in a public health context, the public's safety can be a serious concern. In this context, precision and accuracy are important. The cautionary tale in Chapter 2 about using the word "once" on a prescription pill bottle (as in "take once a day") being misinterpreted as the number 11 in Spanish ("once" means 11 in Spanish) is just one example of how verbal equivalents of numeric quantities can leave room for confusion in a multilingual society.[99] Cognitive testing conducted in a pharmaceutical context suggests that using numbers instead of English equivalents would make prescription instructions clearer.[100] The same finding could easily be applied to other instructional public health contexts in which a prescriptive directive refers to a numeric quantity (such as the amount of bleach to add to drinking water in an emergency situation) or to reading measurements on a gauge or scale (such as determining body temperature above 98.6°F on a thermometer).

When using numbers to instruct or inform, remember that most people have low levels of quantitative and document literacy. Because that is the case, any number used should be simple in nature and given easy-to-understand modifiers to add meaning.[71] To account for this, round most decimals to the closest whole number unless convention requires otherwise (e.g., $3.20 for money, or 98.6°F for body temperature). Create forms that easily allow users to enter numbers (e.g., for monitoring blood glucose levels by persons with diabetes), but test forms with actual users before using them in practice to ensure that instructions are well understood and that data entry is accurate (see Chapter 5). The same also applies when writing instructions for a survey that asks readers to provide numbers. Instructions for collecting numeric data in an interview or questionnaire (e.g., "on a scale of 1 to 10, please rate ...") will influence the quality of data obtained. Cognitive interviewing and pilot testing can improve the reliability and validity of survey questionnaires.[101]

User testing has revealed some surprising discoveries related to the use of numeric content for instructing and informing on the World Wide Web. Recall that most audiences scan online content quickly (see Chapter 3). That tendency is especially pronounced in those with low literacy skills, who are not accustomed to spending much time reading in any setting. Using special equipment to track the eye movements of users looking at Web sites in his laboratory, Nielsen and his colleagues, based on their research, recommend that numbers on the Web always be written as numerals, not as English equivalents. This recommendation contradicts traditional writing style guidelines, Nielsen confesses, but matches more closely what people do. "Numerals often stop the wandering eye," Nielsen writes, because in most people's minds "numbers represent facts."[102] Given users' tendencies, Nielsen makes the following suggestions when using numbers on the Web:

- Write numbers with digits, not letters (e.g., 23, not twenty-three).
- Use numerals even when the number is the first "word" in a sentence or bullet point.
- Use numerals for big numbers up to one billon: "2,000,000" is better than two million, but "two trillion" is better than 2,000,000,000,000 because most people cannot interpret that many zeros. As a compromise, use numerals for the significant digits and write out the magnitude

as a word. For example, write 24 billion (not twenty-four billion or
24,000,000,000).

- Spell out numbers that don't represent specific quantities (e.g., we
  observed "thousands of cases," but we collected data on 2,389
  subjects).[102]


## Using Numbers in Tables

Using tables is an effective way of communicating individual data point values. Tables are mainstays in public health reporting and are especially useful
in presenting snapshots of data across population categories. They can be
used for planning purposes because they facilitate easy navigation to sub-
group sample values through entry points for rows and columns, and they
can be used for individual decision making as in the health care plan selection example presented at the beginning of this chapter. Audiences examine
tables of numbers with basically one of two tasks in mind: (a) to make an
overall comparison of data, often with an eye toward determining relationships, or (b) to search for individual numeric values.[103]

When creating a table, give users the cues and organizational clarity they
need to move through the table as needed.[104] The table should enable selection and drill down, rather than the revelation of overall trends (which can
usually be accomplished more effectively with graphs[105]). Column headings
and row headings need to be clear and understandable. The table should
make strategic use of white space, shading, and border options to channel
the eye easily down columns or across rows (following cues for continuation), and proximity cues should be used to associate clusters of similar
data. Decimal points should be aligned vertically, preferably with the same
number of significant digits presented to the right of the decimal point.
Because of the tendency in Western culture to read from left to right and
from top to bottom, column and row labels that include numeric values
should be presented in sequence (Figure 4.4). Individual cell values that
merit special attention can be bolded (e.g., for statistically significant findings) or presented in a different color, such as showing deficit financial values in red.[103]

Computerization has offered a new level of interactive access to data
tables through public and private use Web sites. Online tables follow
many of the same rules for effective design as print tables—clear headings, strategic use of white space, and careful alignment of decimals.
However, online versions offer additional capacities, such as the use of
hyperlinks to drill down into the data dynamically, "mouse-over" text
to provide on-the-spot definitions of terms, a full color palette, and
on-screen controls.[106]

**The Top 10 Leading Causes of Death in The World, 2004**

| | Percent |
|---|---|
| 1 Ischemic heart disease | 12.2 |
| 2 Cerebrovascular disease | 9.7 |
| 3 Lower respiratory infections | 7.0 |
| 4 Chronic obstructive pulmonary disease | 5.1 |
| 5 Diarrheal diseases | 3.6 |
| 6 HIV/AIDS | 3.5 |
| 7 Tuberculosis | 2.5 |
| 8 Cancer of the lung, trachea, or bronchus | 2.3 |
| 9 Road traffic accidents | 2.2 |
| 10 Prematurity and low birth weight | 2.0 |

Data source: World Health Organization (2008). *World Health Statistics 2008*. Geneva, Switzerland: World Health Organization; 2008.
Table design adapted from Reynolds, R. (2008). *Presentation Zen: Simple Ideas on Presentation Design and Delivery*. Berkeley, Calif.: New Riders; 2008;125.

**Figure 4.4** Example of a table with health data. Note the table has a short title, uses grey shading of alternate rows, and data are ordered from largest to smallest, all of which facilitate easier comprehension.

## Using Numbers to Persuade or Motivate

Recent examples of communicating a few key numbers to lay audiences include statements such as "the economic costs associated with a pandemic flu epidemic are estimated at 800 billion dollars by the World Health Organization,"[107] and "as of April 10, 2006, a total of 515 possible cases of mumps had been reported to the Iowa Department of Health."[108] Using a limited set of numbers is especially common in advocacy, where persuasion is the underlying purpose for communicating with lay audiences; numbers from research studies involving cause-and-effect (e.g., risk factors), evaluation, or prediction are common choices (Chapter 7). Such numbers are often used repeatedly, such as the estimated 400,000 deaths annually from smoking in the United States;[109] and that 1 in 8 women will develop breast cancer in their lifetime;[110] or that 1 in 4 teenage girls in the United States has a sexually transmitted disease.[111] If persuasion is the purpose, research suggests that using more than a few numbers is unlikely to increase message persuasiveness.[93, 94] The persuasive power of numbers is enhanced when the number is perceived as being especially large, because large numbers create a sense of vividness, social pressure, and the magnitude of a problem among audiences.[112]

Numbers are also used in a limited way when trying to increase knowledge among lay audiences, particularly to raise awareness about a health issue[113] that may be new or unfamiliar; such an approach can also be used to contribute to informed decision making. Regularly updating audiences about the number of affected individuals, for example, in an outbreak or some other acute situation, is an example of this (see Chapter 6).

Given the challenges of cognitive burden and limited quantitative literacy discussed in Chapter 3, communicating only a few numbers to lay audiences is highly recommended in many situations. The numbers, however, need to be simple and to be presented in metrics that are familiar to audiences, such as the number of people affected, percentages, or dollars. Using whole numbers (e.g., 16 new cases of tuberculosis) and rounding (e.g., nearly 50%, rather than 48.7%; more than 1 in 4 people, instead of 26.3%; about three times the risk, rather than odds ratios of 2.95; about 14,000 persons were affected, rather than 14,139) will more easily communicate data without adding unnecessary, and possibly confusing, precision.

## Communicating through Visual Symbols

Just as metaphors and narratives can help scientific data come alive, visual presentations and symbols can help bolster understanding, attract attention, and increase information retention more than presentations made through words and numbers alone.[114] For example, news stories that are presented to children in a video format are remembered better than stories presented either in an audio format or in print. News stories that are accompanied by photographs in either a print medium[115, 116] or on the Web[117] can lead to enhanced recall for specific issues over presentations of text alone. Brosius[118] observed that the use of exemplars (visual or narrative illustrations of a fact or trend, e.g., the number of people who die from smoking each year is equivalent to three jumbo jets crashing each day with no survivors) has been shown repeatedly to enhance memory and drive persuasiveness over the presentation of fact alone, and that the effect is robust across media type and recipient characteristics. "Exemplars influence perceptions, opinions, and attitudes," Brosius concluded, "more strongly than statistics, comprehensive overviews, or official information" (see Ref. 118, p. 1).

There are a variety of visual displays available to the scientific presenter, and with the popularity of visually oriented computer programs, the number is increasing all the time. By far, the mainstay for most scientific presentations is the familiar menu of options available through standard analysis programs: pie charts, bar charts, and line graphs. In addition to these, special purpose formats such as icon arrays and scales have emerged as ways

Source of Cancer Information for Adults in the United States, 2005

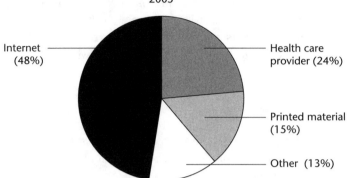

Internet (48%)

Health care provider (24%)

Printed material (15%)

Other (13%)

*Source used for most recent information search among those who had ever sought cancer information. Data source: National Cancer Institute, Health Information National Trends Survey

**Figure 4.5** Pie chart showing source for most recent search for cancer information. Note how the chart uses a short title, contains a limited number of proportions (pie slices), contains legends and lines that point to slices; and has a footnote indicating the source for these data. (Source: Rutten LF, Moser RP, Beckjord EB, Hesse BW, Croyle RT. *Cancer Communication: Health Information National Trends Survey.* Washington, D.C.: National Cancer Institute; 2007. NIH Pub. No. 07-6214.)

of communicating probability and other types of data. The evolution of Geographic Information System (GIS) technologies has made it easier to map health data onto familiar geographic localities. Advances in computer technology have made it possible to experiment with three-dimensional displays. Newer formats, we understand, are on the horizon as health scientists experiment with more compelling ways of presenting data to the public and policy makers. We treat some of these forms individually in the text below.

## Pie Charts

The pie chart, named for its circular geometric shape partitioned into component wedges, is a graphical convention that has a rich history of devotees and detractors. Generally, cognitive studies suggest that the pie chart functions well in supporting estimates of a single proportion or in supporting comparisons between small numbers of proportions[61, 119–121] (Figure 4.5). It does well because the circular shape offers an integrated representation of the whole with individual components set in relationship, something that a bar chart does not immediately convey.[119]

Another significant advantage of the pie chart for illustrating simple relationships is that it is a format familiar to lay audiences. Pie charts are more commonly used in the lay press than they are in scientific or business publications. When it comes to interpreting meaning from charts, familiarity has been shown to play a big role.[42] The pie chart's frequency of use in lay magazines, along with its natural similarity to dials and other readouts,[119] make it an effective tool for conveying part-to-whole relationships when communicating with the public.

## Bar Charts

The bar chart is, by far, the most versatile format for visually displaying numbers.[121] Bar charts comprise narrow rectangles (bars) whose heights or lengths correspond to the intervals of a corresponding scale. Each bar represents grouped data. The heights or lengths of the bars in a chart are measured using a comparative metric, such as counts (frequencies), percentages, dollars, probability estimates (e.g., relative risk data), or some other type of interval-based data.

Bar charts are likely to be the most common format used by public health practitioners and scientists to visually present data to lay audiences. Their greatest value is to demonstrate magnitude in general and comparative magnitude (e.g., relative risk differences) in particular. Bar charts are extremely versatile, as they can be used in many different ways with different types of data, but efforts must be made to ensure that they are displayed simply and clearly in order to enhance audience understanding. There are several reasons why bar charts are an effective visual format for data. First, they allow lay audiences to identify individual numeric values using the vertical ($y$) and horizontal ($x$) axes.[122, 123] Second, they do an excellent job of displaying magnitude (size) of data values. Third, they can be used to make comparisons in magnitude between groups of data (bars), which allows viewers to identify relative differences between the groups or other patterns.[124] This can make them particularly helpful, for example, for comparing data values relative to a baseline, such as national average or recommended maximum levels of exposure.

Bar charts can be oriented either horizontally or vertically (Figure 4.6). One advantage of horizontal placement is that longer text labels can be placed in an easy-to-read position in a space on the chart preceding the data bar. At least in Western cultures, that means viewers can easily scan from left to right and then build meaning by looking at the label for the bar first and then looking for the magnitude by examining the length of the bar.[125] Providing this type of textual information as a cue for interpreting the graphical information in a bar chart has been shown to improve audience understanding.[126] Vertical bar charts are especially common when portraying a comparative rise or fall in counts (frequencies) over levels of one or more variables. Value

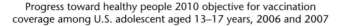

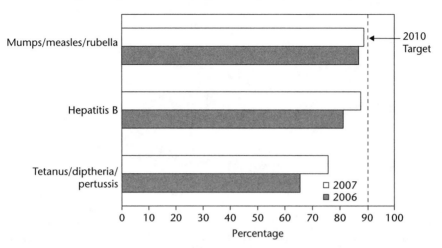

Data source: Centers for Disease Control and Prevention (CDC), National Immunization Survey

**Figure 4.6** Horizontal bar chart with easy-to-read labels, centralized legend placement, and documentation of data source. Note also the inclusion of the dashed line for the Healthy People 2010 goal (further highlighted with an arrow), which helps to provide contextual information for users. (Source: Jain N, Stokley S, Yankey MA. Vaccination coverage among adolescents aged 13–17 years—United States, 2007. *Morb Mort Weekly Rep.* 2008;57:1100–1103.)

labels should be short and to the point so that they can fit within space constraints of a vertically oriented bar chart.[61]

*Dos*

There are several techniques for developing bar charts to enhance lay audience understanding of data. Among these are the following:

- Minimize the total number of bars shown on a given chart to no more than six but preferably fewer.[121]
- Use effective bar colors or shading patterns (optimized for contrast, while minimizing problems for audiences who are color blind).[33]
- Include a bar or a line to indicate a baseline value (to assist with anchoring and comparing).
- Include text, such as short and easily understood titles, labels, or key messages to make the context clear.
- Select beginning and ending values and interval widths for *x*- and *y*-axes that faithfully and ethically represent the patterns in the data without distortion or exaggeration.[39, 121]

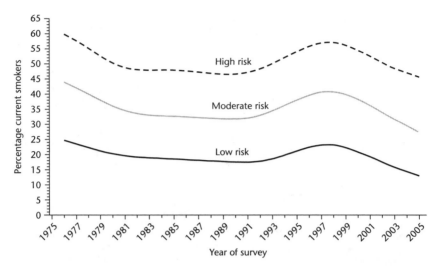

**Figure 4.7** Example of a line graph used to portray long-term trends in smoking among U.S. adolescents. (High, moderate, and low risk refer to adolescents' likelihood of becoming cigarette smokers based on responses to selected survey questions [Reference for "high/moderate/low risk": Nelson DE, Mowery P, Asman K, Pederson LL, O'Malley PM, Malarcher A, Maibach EW, Pechacek TF. Long-term national trends in adolescent and young adults: Meta-patterns and implications. *Am J Public Health.* 2008;98:901–915]). Note the use of labels placed next to trend lines. (Soruce: *Monitoring the Future Survey, 1976–2005.)*

### Don'ts

There are also techniques to avoidx[119–121]:

- Use segmented or stacked bar charts to demonstrate to lay audiences how proportions compare to the whole. Pie charts are better for this.
- Overlay line representations on top of the bars to indicate variance estimates or 95% confidence intervals. There is no evidence that the lines increase lay understanding, and they add unnecessary clutter.

### Line Graphs

Line graphs are a preferred alternative to bar charts when portraying a connected sequence of data, such as trends over time.[61, 121, 122] Line graphs may be composed of straight or curvilinear line segments; typically, lines are drawn between points on a graph to illustrate data patterns.[61] The connected line draws the eye directly to sequential comparisons portrayed across the horizontal axis, thus making the pattern portrayed by the line more salient.[124]

Line graphs are most useful for demonstrating trends and helping to provide audiences with contextual information (Figure 4.7). Showing trends helps audiences answer the question of whether numbers are going up, going down, or remaining the same. In other words, are things getting better, worse, or are they stable? Line graphs are especially helpful for showing before-and-after differences, such as changes in data values that may result from individual- or population-based interventions (e.g., such policy changes). This makes line graphs a good choice for evaluation research because they can demonstrate cause-and-effect relationships to lay audiences by correctly equating correlation with causation (Chapter 3). Studies based on business data have shown that line charts can be equivalent to bar charts in their portrayal of single trends,[123] but are superior to bar charts in portraying multiple trends through juxtaposed lines.[122, 125, 128]

### Dos

There are several practical techniques to use to create effective line graphs:

- Use arrows or text to highlight key events or data, drawing audiences' attention to particularly relevant points.
- Present labels in proximity to the lines they are intended to describe to facilitate better audience comprehension.
- Include baseline data for comparison purposes to help draw the reader's attention to patterns of change.
- Write short and easily understood titles, labels, and key messages to enhance understanding and improve effectiveness.
- Select beginning and ending values and interval widths for y-axis that faithfully and ethically represent the patterns in the data in objective, straightforward ways that do not distort or exaggerate.

### Don'ts

Concerning conventions to avoid, some of the same caveats apply to line charts as they do to bar charts:

- Add unnecessary labels or symbols—this may actually obscure the data.[33]
- Use more than four trend lines.[129]

### Icons and Icon Arrays

Icons, as defined in this book, are individual graphical elements that represent quantitative data. A variety of different types of icons have been used to represent health-related data, with circles, stars, diamonds, and human figure

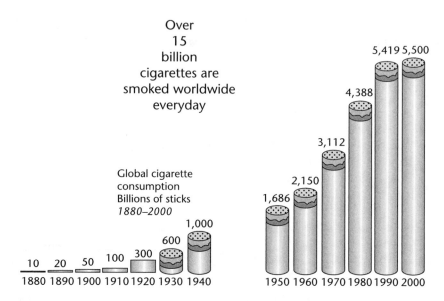

**Figure 4.8** Example of an icon graph with cigarettes used in lieu of bars from the World Health Organization's Tobacco Atlas. (Source: Mackay J, Eriksen M, Shafey E. *The Tobacco Atlas.* 2nd ed. Geneva, Switzerland: World Health Organization, 2006.)

outlines probably the most common choices. More elaborate pictograms of paper or coin currency, national flags, cigarettes, bottles, firearms, and other figures have also been used to represent data in a visually engaging way for lay audiences. The three most common ways in which icons are used to represent health data are as (a) substitutes for vertical or horizontal rectangles in bar charts, (b) rankings or ratings in tabular displays for information seekers, and (c) probability data representing absolute risk in icon arrays.

One of the more creative uses of icons is substituting the icon for the rectangles in vertically or horizontally oriented bar charts. Figure 4.8 provides a good example taken from the World Health Organization's Tobacco Atlas, an educational booklet that uses global data on tobacco consumption and disease to advocate for better tobacco control policies globally. Cigarettes have been used in the figure in place of vertical bars, and the numbers placed next to the cigarettes were used in place of a true *x*- or *y*-axis. In this way, the image has a stylized, eye-catching design. This type of representation tends to be more common in policy making and among the press,[70] as more creative visual images may help to gain the attention or interest of viewers beyond what may be achieved through standard rectangular bars and may be more persuasive.

Because gaining audience attention can be a major challenge in advocacy (Chapter 7), there is merit in considering icons as substitutes for regular bars, as they may help raise or maintain awareness for a public health issue. Give thought to the appropriate picture to be selected. It should be an image that

Annual Estimates of the Resident Population for the
United States: 2004–2008

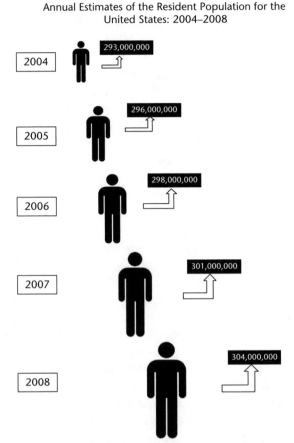

**Figure 4.9.** An example of volume distortion. Notice how the different sizes of human icons and arrows distorts the magnitude of the increase in the United States population from 2004 to 2008.    (Data source:  U.S. Census Bureau, 2008, http://www.census.gov/popest/states/NST-ann-est.html.)

is engaging and emblematic of the topic under discussion. Admittedly, not all topics in public health lend themselves to iconic representation. A substitute icon should not be used if it detracts from the message or if it in any way distorts the findings. One of the biggest concerns in this regard is the issue of volume distortion. Volume distortion occurs when both the horizontal and vertical dimensions are increased to demonstrate larger magnitude, or when data comparisons are made using icons of different shapes (e.g., a cigarette, bottle, and a firearm). The effect, whether intentional or unintentional, is to misrepresent the underlying data upon which the graph is based (see Figure 4.9 as an example).

The second major use of icons is to represent ranking or rating data visually using symbols in some form of tabular display. Probably the most familiar example is the rating system published in the magazine *Consumer Reports*, which uses circles with different colors and levels of shading to rank various characteristics of consumer products and services. Other systems use stars (e.g., with 4 or 5 stars representing higher, and 0 or 1 star representing lower ratings or recommendations), letter grades for evaluation (A through F), dollar signs (for costs), or other icons to indicate magnitude. Icon arrays are primarily used in this way to support decision making by information seekers or to help improve their understanding.

A final use of icons is to display data visually through arrays as a way of helping lay audiences understand probability data presented as absolute risk estimates. These icon arrays are generally used to help with personal health decision making (informed or shared decision making) and are usually presented to lay audiences in clinical settings. However, they could be used in acute public health situations, for example, communicating about outbreaks, environmental exposures, or use of tainted consumer products (see Chapter 6), provided that levels of emotion, such as fear or anger, are not elevated, and careful and adequate explanations about icon arrays are made available.

Icon arrays use individual graphic elements, such as circles or outlines of human figures to portray ratios as discrete counts.[28, 30] Research shows that most people comprehend probability data better when it is presented as discrete counts or natural frequencies (e.g., as 1 in 10 or 1 in 100) rather than as numeric percentages.[130–132] An icon array draws attention to discrete counts by highlighting the implied part of a whole. For example, in the illustrations portrayed in Figure 4.10, icon arrays were used to illustrate how many people with varying preconditions were shown to have developed breast cancer at follow-up. The array used filled-in circles to portray an otherwise complex probability statistical concept in a straightforward way.[133]

Research into the design decisions incorporated into the construction of an effective icon array suggests the following.

*Dos*

- To elicit stronger emotional imagery, which some people prefer, use anthropomorphic figures (e.g., stick figures, portraits, or other representations of humans) rather than abstract symbols like circles or asterisks.[28, 134, 135] (Studies of performance, however, have found the two types of symbols to be equivalent in supporting comprehension and behavior.[28])
- Place icons representing numerator values (e.g., the number "7" out of a denominator value of 200) contiguously, as proximity cues understanding and thus increases overall effectiveness.[136]

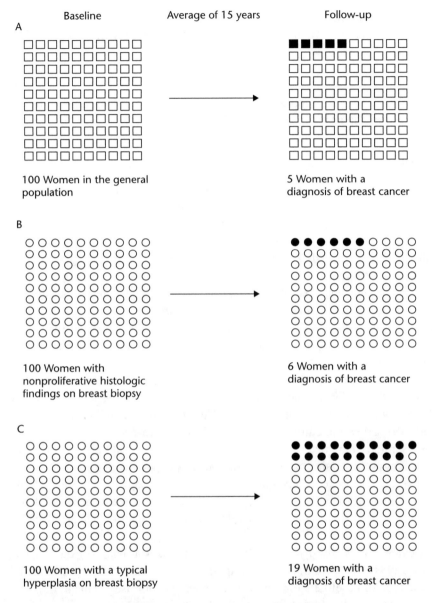

**Figure 4.10** Illustration from Elmore (2005) using natural frequencies to explain differences in risk for being diagnosed with breast cancer for (a) women in the general population compared to (b) women with benign biopsies who exhibit nonproliferative histologic findings, (b) and (c) women with benign biopsies who exhibit atypical findings. (Source: Elmore JG, Armstrong K, Lehman CD, Fletcher SW. Screening for breast cancer. *JAMA*. 2005;293(10):1245–1256.)

- Use a common denominator between two arrays.
- Highlight numerator icons—the number of which will change between the two arrays.

*Don't*

- Randomly place icons representing numerator values unless the sole goal of the array is to demonstrate randomness.[28]


## Visual Scales

Scales are another way to visually present data. They may be used for cardinal data, where numbers are ordered and there are equal distances between intervals (e.g., height), or ordinal data, where data are ordered but the intervals between values may be uneven, such as in a Likert rating scale where values from 1 through 7 represent a varying range from "strongly agree" to "strongly disagree."

As with pie charts, bar charts, and line graphs, some visual scales are simple, giving them the added benefit of being familiar to many lay audiences. Analog thermometers used for measuring air or body temperatures are one such example; vertically aligned scales are sometimes referred to as thermometer representations. Color alone can be used as a type of visual data scale, too. In the United States, red often signifies threat or warning (e.g., "red alert").[121] Visual color scales designed to demonstrate level of threat or danger often use red to signal greater levels of threat, with colors such as yellow or green indicating reduced or minimal threat level.[137]

A semicircular meter with an arrow or line to indicate a range of values from low to high, similar to an automobile speedometer, is yet another way to use a scale to represent data. Note how the design of Figure 4.11 uses a combination of color, a meter, and text to summarize a large number of data measures used to assess current health care quality performance and progress.

Scales can be used to visually represent risk (probability) data.[28] They typically portray a continuum of comparative risk values and they may include some type of baseline comparison risk to help anchor users (Chapter 3). They can be especially helpful for visually demonstrating absolute risk data and provide comparisons to help lay audiences place the health risk (e.g., of an exposure or adverse event) in context. Risk scales can be used in environmental, occupational, or consumer product situations (Chapter 6) (Figure 4.12), such as those involving involuntary exposures to chemical agents[138] and in personal health decision-making situations, such as for disease treatment or prevention decision making.[127]

To create effective scales:

Nevada

Dashboard on Health Care Quality Compared to All States

Overall Health Care Quality

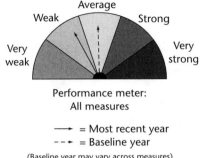

Performance meter:
All measures

⟶ = Most recent year
--➤ = Baseline year
(Baseline year may vary across measures)

**Figure 4.11** Example of a visual scale (a meter or "dashboard") using data available to the U.S. Agency for Healthcare Research and Quality (AHRQ) as of 2007; the summary measure of overall health care quality is based on more than 100 individual data items. On the actual Web site, color gradients are used to highlight the summary score (ranging from dark red for "very weak," to dark green for "very strong"). While somewhat cognitively challenging, at least initially, this visual presentation format synthesizes a great deal of data allowing readers to quickly understand that Nevada's overall health care quality performance is: (a) worse than most states and (b) has gotten worse over time. (Source: Agency for Healthcare Research and Quality, AHRQ, 2008.)

### Dos

- Provide anchoring information, such as lines or arrows, to provide contextual cues to orient people to baseline (comparative) data.
- Include explanatory text, such as short titles and key messages.
- Follow conventional approaches for data presentation, such as using red to indicate higher levels of threat or including the highest levels of risk at the top of a vertical scale.

### Don'ts

- Underestimate the role of emotion and perceived inequity if scales are used in involuntary exposure situations.
- Include too much information, thus increasing cognitive burden.

### Data Maps

Although maps were developed for orientation and navigation, they can also used to represent quantitative findings. Data maps have a long and illustrious history in public health, particularly for outbreak investigations.

| Risk comparisons Risk of death | | | Risk comparisons Risk of death | |
|---|---|---|---|---|
| Level of risk | Activity | | Level of risk (chances out of 1,000) | Activity |
| Higher risk | Smoking 1–2 packs of cigarettes per day | | 35–125 | Smoking 1–2 packs of cigarettes per day |
| | Having 200 chest x-rays per year | | 7–30 | Having 200 chest x-rays per year |
| | Eating 1–10 oz meal per week of mixed Great Lakes Salmonids at 1984 contaminant level | | 5–30 | Eating 1–10 oz meal per week of mixed Great Lakes Salmonids at 1984 contaminant levels |
| | Driving a motor vehicle | | 17 | Driving a motor vehicle |
| Moderate risk | Eating 1–8 oz meal per week of mixed Great Lakes salmonids at 1984 contaminant levels | | 11.12 | Eating 1–8 oz meal per week of mixed Great Lakes salmonids at 1984 contaminant levels |
| | Eating 1–8 oz meal per week of mixed Great Lakes salmonids at 1987 contaminant levels | | 3.6 | Eating 1–8 oz meal per week of mixed Great Lakes salmonids at 1967 contaminant levels |
| | Breathing air in U.S. urban areas at early 1980s contaminant levels | | 0.1–6 | Breathing air in U.S. urban areas at early 1980s contaminant levels |
| | Recreational boating | | 3.5 | Recreational boating |
| Lower risk | Drinking 1–12 oz beer per day | | 1.2 | Drinking 1–12 oz beer per day |
| | Recreational hunting | | 1.5 | Recreational hunting |
| | Complications from insect bite or sting | | 0.014 | Complications from insect bite or sting |

**Figure 4.12** Comparative forms of a risk chart with qualitative descriptions of risk portrayed on the left and quantitative descriptions portrayed on the right. (From Conelly N, Knuth B. Evaluating risk communication: Examining target audience perceptions about four presentation formats for fish Consumption Health Advisory Information. *Risk Anal.* 1998;18:649–659.)

They are used to help illustrate how frequencies (counts) or other types of data are distributed geographically. Most epidemiologists are likely to be highly familiar with map uses in public health, such as describing disease clusters or disease spread by place, raising awareness and increasing understanding about geographic differences, and supporting planning activities.

Studies of how readers process the information contained in a map reveal the same "knowledge construction" process associated with interpreting graphs. First, readers need to orient themselves to the overall map to identify what geographic area is being portrayed; meaningful geographic divisions, such as counties or states; and what the primary symbols (e.g., colors, dots) appear to represent. Next, they attend to legends and labels to help construct a more complete picture of the information the map is designed to

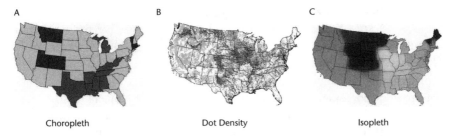

A    B    C

Choropleth    Dot Density    Isopleth

**Figure 4.13** The three types of maps most commonly used in consumer media: (a) the choropleth, (b) the dot density, and (c) the isopleth map. (Note: These maps are not based on the same data). Source: Pickle LW. Usability testing of map designs. In: Braverman A, Hesterberg T, Minnotte M, Symanzik J, eds. *Computing Science and Statistics*. Salt Lake City, Utah: Interface Foundation of North America; 2003.)

communicate. Finally, readers attempt to integrate the information extracted from the map and the surrounding titles, legends, and labels to reach an interpretation or conclusion.[54]

Three mapping forms have promise for communicating data to the public, policy makers, and the press. As depicted in Figure 4.13, they include the choropleth, dot density, and isopleth maps. Choropleth maps use different colors, shades, patterns, or symbols for geographic regions to represent numeric values, for example, by state or county. The ubiquitous "blue state" versus "red state" voting maps used by the press in recent U.S. national elections are familiar examples of choropleth maps; they represent the dominant data mapping format used in public health.

Dot density maps use dots or some other symbol to represent a specified numeric frequency (e.g., one dot = 10 cases of a certain disease); the greater the number of dots clustered in an area, the higher the overall frequency. The famous John Snow map used in the London cholera outbreak is a type of dot density map in which each "x" represented one cholera case. This mapping format is used to present highly localized data (sometimes within one building) and is most common in outbreak or other acute public health situations (see Chapter 6), although it may occasionally be applied for planning purposes.

Isopleth maps, in contrast to choropleth maps, use characteristics of the underlying data set to determine the placement of lines or separation of colors, regardless of geographic boundaries. Weather maps or topographical contour maps are both good examples of isopleth maps. In contrast to choropleth maps, they have the advantage of not forcing data to fit into the somewhat arbitrary confines of geopolitical boundaries.

In addition to the basic geographic orientation function common to all maps, data maps can also be used to support interpretive tasks.[54] One of the most common tasks is simply to demonstrate a data value or range of values for a specific geographic area, often for comparative purposes. For example, state data might be categorized on the basis of quartile ranges (e.g., HIV rates), and different colors or shading might be used in choropleth or isopleths maps to demonstrate numeric values. This is a comparative task that provides contextual information for data, allowing viewers to more easily assess areas where counts or rates are higher or lower than would be possible with numeric tables. This ability of maps to facilitate geographic (place) data comparisons is analogous to the ability of line graphs to facilitate data comparisons over time.

### Dos

Understanding how readers process maps provides clues as to how to support the knowledge construction process:

- Make lines that demarcate discrete entities (such as geographic borders) crisp and clear.
- Use symbols on maps sparingly, but make them memorable and easy to discern.
- Write a clear title for the map.
- Make labels complete but short and to the point.
- Use "call outs" to highlight smaller and potentially unfamiliar geographic regions.
- Use color to make the map more attractive and to illustrate variations in the data.
- Use a multicolor scheme for qualitative data, such as "blue states" and "red states."
- Use a sequential progression of hues from light to dark or dark to light for continuous data.[139, 140]
- Generally, use darker levels of shading to indicate larger levels of magnitude (i.e., bigger numbers) for both choropleth and dot density maps and use lighter shades to demonstrate lower magnitude levels.

### Don'ts

- Include acronyms.
- Juxtapose red and green; the inability to discern these colors from each other is the most common form of color blindness.
- Use more than three or four colors; more will create cognitive burden.
- Assume that color schemes displayed on computer monitors will look the same in print, especially from Web sites. (Recommendations for appropriate color schemes for map printing can be found online at www.colorbrewer.org.)

## Advanced Data Visualization Techniques:
## Approaches and Drawbacks

Although some graphing techniques date back centuries, the mainstream use of graphing techniques to communicate statistical relationships is a fairly recent innovation going back only a century or two.[33, 121, 141] Early displays were more artistic than scientific, with creative license given to the correspondence between the precise nature of the numbers underlying the graph and the spatial characteristics of the geometric shapes used to portray relationships.

As the industrial revolution moved into full force, the need for precision increased. Dials and metering devices were engineered to portray exactingly the spatial characteristics of an underlying quantitative measure on an analog scale. More recently, the evolution of computer technologies not only allowed for an exploration of more advanced data visualization techniques such as charting complex data in three-dimensional space or the advanced use of bioimaging techniques, but led to standardized graphing functions in analytic software packages that allow individual analysts to create technically accurate graphs.

### Presentation Software

One of the most powerful tools for communicating data that is available to most scientists is off-the-shelf presentation software such as Microsoft's PowerPoint® and Apple's Keynote®. Using presentation software has become standard at professional conferences and is a mainstay for top-level policy briefings. Based loosely on a slideshow paradigm, presentation graphics programs now allow a presenter to add highly engaging photographs and graphics to their presentations as well as video, audio, and hyperlinks to the World Wide Web. Professional quality templates and cinematic style transitions can elevate the quality of a presentation to a level of stylized performance previously available only to professional graphic artists.

Used well, presentation software can go a long way in helping professionals communicate complex data to both professional and nonprofessional audiences. Presentation software allows users to create engaging charts and graphs easily and professionally, often by entering data directly into a spreadsheet format. The animation capacity of the programs allows the skilled presenter to build trends dynamically over time or to compare graphs side by side to show similarities and contrasts in numeric trends. Indeed, one of the turning points in the public discussion on the topic of global warming was a documentary created around a PowerPoint file that illustrated numeric trends over time (see Box 4.2).

Used incorrectly, a sloppily assembled PowerPoint presentation might serve to obscure statistical trends rather than reinforce them. For example, a lazy presenter might use the outline function in these programs to create a whole

**Box 4.2 Tips to consider when using presentation software: Lessons learned from "An inconvenient truth"**

Whether you agree or disagree with the viewpoint of former U.S. Vice President Al Gore's "An inconvenient truth" presentation and movie on global warming, there are some key lessons you should take away from a presentation that has become more popular than almost any other presentation in recent memory, even winning an Academy Award.

**Lesson 1: Visuals rule**

One thing you will notice as you watch the presentation is that most slides have no text on them: they are visuals. There is a mix of photographs, diagrams, data graphs and added video clips in the movie. When a slide with text on it is used, it contains very little text compared to the typical number of words on a presentation slide in a business setting. And many of the visuals, especially the graphs, use motion to make the point clear.

**Lesson 2: The number of slides doesn't matter**

After watching the presentation, few people would be able to tell that there were 266 slides in the presentation. They would also say that they didn't feel like Mr. Gore was rushing through slides. So the old lesson of one slide every minute is questionable. Visuals may be used for however long you need in order to make your point.

**Lesson 3: Focus on the audience, not yourself**

As he explains in the movie, Mr. Gore has spent considerable time addressing the objections the audience may have to his message. As he encounters a new objection from an audience, he goes back and works the answer to the objection into subsequent presentations. He has recognized the value of focusing on what an audience needs to hear, instead of simply the messages he wants to communicate.

**Lesson 4: Direct the audience to your point**

When you watch Mr. Gore present in the movie, he has a small screen close by that he uses to point to a part of an image, as a way to focus the audience's attention on a key point of the visual. He also sometimes walks over to the large screen and motions towards a specific part of the visual. In both cases, he is demonstrating that a visual by itself is not sufficient to make a key point: you must direct the attention of audiences to it.

Source: Paradi D. Presentation lessons from "An inconvenient truth." Think Outside the Slide Dave Paradi; 2007.

presentation based solely on an endless recitation of bullet points. When this happens, audiences may no longer recognize or comprehend the most important messages. Likewise, careless presenters might import data tables without paying attention to font size, complexity, or number of data points included, or they might be seduced into thinking that three-dimensional graphics are always better even if they present so much "chart junk"[33] on the screen that they are difficult to interpret (see next section). As illustrated in Box 4.3, an inattention to the overall meta-message of a presentation can lead to disastrous consequences.[18]

---

**Box 4.3** A caveat in the use of presentation software

**PowerPoint: Killer app?**

Did PowerPoint make the space shuttle crash? Could it doom another mission? Preposterous as this may sound, the ubiquitous Microsoft "presentation software" has twice been singled out for special criticism by task forces reviewing the space shuttle disaster.

Perhaps I've sat through too many PowerPoint presentations lately, but I think the trouble with these critics is that they don't go far enough: The software may be as much of a mind-numbing menace to those of us who intend to remain earthbound as it is to astronauts.

PowerPoint's failings have been outlined most vividly by Edward Tufte, a physician and specialist in the visual display of information. In a 2003 *Wired* magazine article headlined "PowerPoint Is Evil" and a less dramatically titled pamphlet, "The Cognitive Style of PowerPoint," Tufte argued that the program encourages "faux-analytical" thinking that favors the slickly produced "sales pitch" over the sober exchange of information.

Exhibit A in Tufte's analysis are PowerPoint slides presented to NASA senior managers in January 2003, while the space shuttle Columbia was in the air and the agency was weighing the risk posed by tile damage on the shuttle wings. Key information was so buried and condensed because of rigid PowerPoint formats (e.g., elaborate bullet outlines, separation of words from data points, poor typography, tables with too much data presented using tiny fonts) as to be useless.

"It is easy to understand how a senior manager might read this PowerPoint slide and not realize that it addresses a life-threatening situation," the Columbia Accident Investigation Board concluded, citing Tufte's work. The board devoted a full page of its 2003 report to the issue, criticizing a space agency culture in which, it said, "the endemic use of PowerPoint" substituted for rigorous technical analysis.

Source: Marcus R. PowerPoint: Killer App? *The Washington Post.* August 30, 2004.

### Three-Dimensional Data Graphics

One of the graphical functions that advanced computer programs offer is the ability to create three-dimensional images from two-dimensional graphics. A pie chart can be set to look like a flattened cylinder with a click of the mouse, bars can be set to look like marble columns, and line charts can be set to look like three-dimensional ribbons. As a general rule of thumb, these three-dimensional techniques for two-dimensional data should be avoided. Figure 4.14 illustrates two charts tested under laboratory conditions: one portraying data using three-dimensional highlights and one presenting data in two dimensions

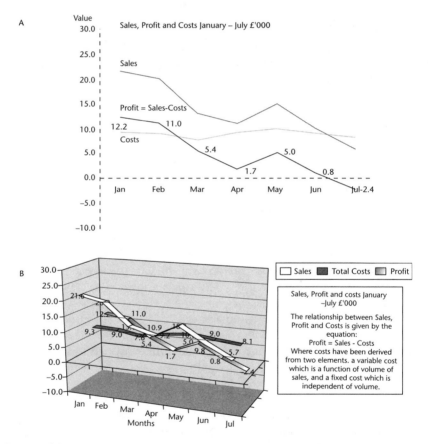

**Figure 4.14** Two versions of line charts: one created with crisp, clean lines in two dimensions, the other created as a "ribbon chart" in three dimensions. Study results showed the three-dimensional graph on the right created a greater information processing burden. (Source: Renshaw JA, Finlay JE, Tyfa D, Ward RD. Understanding visual influence in graph design through temporal and spatial eye movement characteristics. *Interact Comp.* 2004;16(3):557–578.)

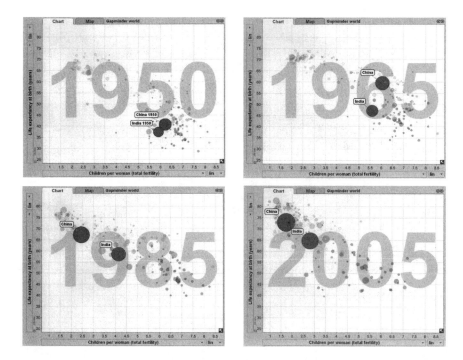

**Figure 4.15** Three-dimensional graphic showing changes in life expectancy by fertility rate for different sized countries. The software program produces a continuously running slide show illustrating changes over time from 1950 to 2005 (notice the public health progress in China and India). (Source: Gapminder Foundation, 2008. Available at http:// www.gapminder.org.)

using crisp, clean lines. Data from the laboratory testing demonstrated better comprehension of the two-dimensional graphic in which the patterns were clear and the extraneous cues (background, dimensionality) were reduced.

A slightly different question to ask is whether two dimensions can be used to present three-dimensional data. Figure 4.15 illustrates a solution introduced by global health expert Hans Rosling in his online Web site at www.gapminder.org. In the chart he set out to explore the relationship between life expectancy and family size (two common indicators of public health) for countries of varying size. The *y*-axis represents life expectancy, whereas the *x*-axis represents family size. He then represented the size of countries with circles instead of single points: the larger the population, the larger the circle. As yet another dimension, enabled by a novel software package created through his not-for-profit foundation, he set the graph in motion across years. Audience members watching the presentation learned first hand how public health interventions globally extended life expectancy while shrinking family size in such populous countries as India and China over a 55-year period. The video-sharing capability of the Web allowed a recorded presentation of the lecture to be downloaded and viewed by over 1 million interested users during a short time following its posting. A similar approach is used by the *New York Times* on its public Web site to present financial information by including selectable parameters for analyzing stock performance. New investments by the National Science Foundation and private sector computer companies, along with expanding capacity on the World Wide Web, promise to produce even more new approaches to visualizing data in the future.[60]

## Data Presentation Considerations

This chapter has covered a wide range of presentation options, ranging from not using data at all to providing extensive amounts of data to audiences

---

**The bottom line**

Contextual cues can go a long way in helping construct meaning from a communication of data. Scientists can help enhance meaning by being sure that sufficient context is provided along with presented charts, figures, tables, and Web pages.

Practical suggestions for dealing with audience limitations include (a) determining whether data should be used, (b) selecting the right data and statistics to present for the audience and purpose, (c) proactively countering misinformation, (d) using data that are familiar, (e) explaining key scientific concepts, (f) striving to reduce the audience's cognitive burden.

Perceptual cues influence the basic ways in which people process information. Three cues that are especially powerful are *proximity*, *continuation*, and *closure*.

Metaphors are most likely to be effective if (a) the audience has some familiarity with the comparison item, (b) the comparison item has a higher level of novelty, (c) they are used early in a message, and (d) if they are presented in an audio format.

Visual presentations can help attract attention, bolster understanding, and facilitate memory. A picture or a well-constructed graph can often be worth a thousand words.

Today's software packages make available a wide range of "extras" in presentation options. These extras should be used thoughtfully and strategically, being careful not to obscure the main message or storyline.

Effective communicators weave words, numbers, and symbols together to create cohesive messages.

---

who have high levels of involvement in order to aid their information seeking. Some formats are more appropriate in public health situations than others.

One final consideration that often confronts those who want to present data to lay audiences occurs when information is to be communicated through longer documents, such as multiple-page pamphlets, reports, or Web-based materials. The communication decision involves whether it is better to present data in such longer materials (a) using only words, (b) using numbers in tables, or (c) using symbols in the form of charts, graphs, or some other visual modality. The answer, as might be expected, depends on the purpose of the presentation.[10]

If data are to be embedded and used as evidentiary matter to support specific arguments for persuasion within an essay, then at least some individual numbers should be included within the text.[8, 61] If the volume of numbers to be included becomes extensive, or if the purpose is either to summarize data findings or to provide audiences with access to specific numbers, then a table is a better choice.[122, 142] Finally, if the intent of the material is primarily to increase knowledge by demonstrating trends, comparing data points, identifying patterns, or showing deviations from expected values, then graphs or charts are preferred choices.[122, 124]

## Conclusion

The selection of data to present, and how they are presented, can have a great influence on lay audiences. Several general guidelines, such as using familiar formats, providing peripheral cues, and adhering to perceptual rules, can greatly enhance data presentation. In this chapter, we reviewed research and provided examples of the presentation formats most commonly used to present data to lay audiences through the elements of words, symbols, and numbers. Effectively integrating two or more of these broad methods is crucial for effective communication. Knowing how to balance these three elements effectively can be elusive at first and may take some trial and error to get right.

With the widespread availability of the World Wide Web to lay audiences, the ready availability of data presentation software to communicators, and the release of increasingly more powerful and advanced tools for data presentation, today's data communicators need knowledge and skills in multiple fields.[10, 16, 143] Nevertheless, effective data presentation will remain strongly dependent upon clearly articulating, in advance, the purpose for communicating, understanding audiences and context, and developing storylines to be communicated, taking into account the need to present data ethically and in a manner easily understood.

## Further Reading

### Texts and Narratives

Brock TC, Strange JJ, Green MC. Power beyond reckoning: An introduction to narrative impact. In: Green MC, Strange JJ, Brock TC, eds. *Narrative Impact: Social and Cognitive Foundations.* Mahwah, NJ: Erlbaum; 2002:1–15.

Dillman DA, Christian L. *The Influence of Words, Symbols, Numbers, and Graphics on Answers to Self-Administered Questionnaires: Results from 18 Experimental Comparisons.* Pullman, Wash.: Washington State University Social and Economic Research Center; 2002.

Koomey J. *Turning Numbers into Knowledge: Mastering the Art of Problem Solving,* 2nd ed. Oakland, Calif.: Analytics Press; 2008.

Reynolds G. *Presentation Zen: Simple Ideas on Presentation Design and Delivery.* Berkeley, Calif.: New Riders; 2008.

Vaiana ME, McGlynn EA. What cognitive science tells us about the design of reports for consumers. *Med Care Res Rev.* 2002;59(1):3–35.

### Presenting Data Graphically

Ancker JS, Senathirajah Y, Kukafka R, Starren JB. Design features of graphs in health risk communication: A systematic review. *J Am Med Inform Assoc.* 2006;13(6):608–618.

Few S. *Show Me the Numbers: Designing Tables and Graphs to Enlighten.* 1st ed. Oakland, Calif.: Analytics Press; 2004.

Robbins NB. *Creating more effective graphs.* Hoboken, N.J.: Wiley-Interscience; 2005.

Tufte ER. *The Visual Display of Quantitative Information,* 2nd ed. Cheshire, Conn.: Graphics Press; 2001.

### Presenting Data on the Web

Albers MJ. *Communication of Complex Information: User Goals and Information Needs for Dynamic Web Information.* Mahwah, N.J.: Erlbaum; 2004.

National Cancer Institute. *Research-Based Web Design and Usability Guidelines.* Bethesda, Md.: U.S. National Institutes of Health; 2003.

Nielsen J. *Designing Web Usability: The Practice of Simplicity.* Indianapolis, Ind.: New Riders; 2000.

### Advanced Techniques

Bederson B, Shneiderman B. *The Craft of Information Visualization: Readings and Reflections.* Boston, Mass.: Morgan Kaufmann; 2003.

Few S. *Information Dashboard Design: The Effective Visual Communication of Data,* Cambridge, Mass.: O'Reilly; 2006.

Marchionini G, Levin M. Digital government information services: The Bureau of Labor Statistics case. *Interactions* 2003;4:18–27.

Murphy T. Research-based methods for using PowerPoint, animation, and video for instruction In: *32nd Annual ACM SIGUCCS (Association for Computing Machinery Special Interest Group on University and College Computing Services) Conference on User Services SIGUCCS '04; 2004.* Baltimore, Md.: ACM Press; 2004:372–374.

## References

1. Einstein A, Calaprice A. *The Expanded Quotable Einstein*. Princeton, NJ: Princeton University Press; 2000.
2. Mayer RE, Bove W, Bryman A, Mars R, Topangco L. When less is more: Meaningful learning from visual and verbal summaries of science textbook lessons. *J Educ Psychol*. 1995;88(1):64–73.
3. Shah P, Mayer RE, Hegarty M. Graphs as aids to knowledge construction: Signaling techniques for guiding the process of graph comprehension. *J Educ Psychol*. 1999;91(4):690–702.
4. Carpenter PA, Shah P. A model of the perceptual and conceptual processes in graph comprehension. *J Exp Psychol Appl*. 1998;4(2):75–100.
5. Fischhoff B. Decision research strategies. *Health Psychol*. 2005;24(4 Suppl): S9–S16.
6. Nelson W, Stefanek M, Peters E, McCaul KD. Basic and applied decision making in cancer control. *Health Psychol*. 2005;24(4 Suppl):S3–S8.
7. Wainer H. *Visual Revelations: Graphical Tales of Fate and Deception from Napoleon Bonaparte to Ross Perot*. New York, NY: Copernicus; 1997.
8. Zwaga HJG, Boersema T, Hoonhout H. By way of introduction: Guidelines and design specifications in information design. In: Zwaga HJG, Boersema T, Hoonhout HCM, eds. *Visual Information for Everyday Use: Design and Research Perspectives*. London, UK: Taylor & Francis; 1998:xvii–xxxiv.
9. Kline K. Popular media and health: Images, effects and institutions. In: Thompson TL, Dorsey AM, Miller KI, Parrott R, eds. *Handbook of Health Communication*. Mahwah, NJ: Lawrence Erlbaum; 2003:557–581.
10. The Royal Institution of Great Britain. *Guidelines on Science and Health Communication*. London, England: The Royal Institution of Great Britain; November 2001.
11. Shenk D. *Data Smog: Surviving the Information Glut*. San Francisco, Ca.: Harper Edge; 1997.
12. Flynn J, Slovic P, Kunreuther H. *Risk, Media, and Stigma: Understanding Public Challenges to Modern Science and Technology*. Sterling, Va.: Earthscan; 2001.
13. Institute of Medicine (US). Committee on Quality of Health Care in America. *Crossing the Quality Chasm: A New Health System for the 21st Century*. Washington, DC: National Academy Press; 2001.
14. Kohn LT, Corrigan J, Donaldson MS. *To Err Is Human: Building a Safer Health System*. Washington, DC: National Academy Press; 2000.
15. Wiklund ME, Wilcox SB. *Designing Usability into Medical Products*. Boca Raton, Fl.: CRC Press; 2005.
16. Gregory J, Miller S. *Science in Public: Communication, Culture, and Credibility*. New York, NY: Plenum Trade; 1998.
17. Alonso W, Starr P, National Committee for Research on the 1980 Census. *The Politics of Numbers*. New York, NY: Russell Sage Foundation; 1987.
18. Tufte ER. *The Cognitive Style of PowerPoint: Pitching out Corrupts Within*. 2nd ed. Cheshire, Conn.: Graphics Press LLC; 2006.
19. Kahneman D, Slovic P, Tversky A. *Judgment under Uncertainty: Heuristics and Biases*. Cambridge, UK: Cambridge University Press; 1982.
20. Hibbard JH, Peters E. Supporting informed consumer health care decisions: data presentation approaches that facilitate the use of information in choice. *Annu Rev Public Health*. 2003;24:413–433.

21. Fiske ST. Schema. In: Kazdin AE, ed. *Encyclopedia of Psychology*. Washington, DC: American Psychological Association, Oxford University Press; 2000:158–160.
22. Morgan MG. *Risk Communication: A Mental Models Approach*. Cambridge, NY: Cambridge University Press; 2002.
23. Albers MJ. *Communication of Complex Information: User Goals and Information Needs for Dynamic Web Information*. Mahwah, NJ: Erlbaum; 2004.
24. Bier VM. On the state of the art: risk communication to decision-makers. *Reliab Eng Syst Saf.* 2001;71:151–157.
25. Epstein RM, Alper BS, Quill TE. Communicating evidence for participatory decision making. *JAMA*. 2004;291(19):2359–2366.
26. Rothman AJ, Kiviniemi MT. Treating people with information: an analysis and review of approaches to communicating health risk information. *J Natl Cancer Inst Monogr.* 1999(25):44–51.
27. Norman DA. *The Psychology of Everyday Things*. New York, NY: Basic Books; 1988.
28. Ancker JS, Senathirajah Y, Kukafka R, Starren JB. Design features of graphs in health risk communication: a systematic review. *J Am Med Inform Assoc.* 2006;13(6):608–618.
29. Woloshin S, Schwartz LM. Reducing the risk that patients get it wrong. *Gastroenterology.* 2005;129(2):748–750.
30. Fagerlin A, Wang C, Ubel PA. Reducing the influence of anecdotal reasoning on people's health care decisions: is a picture worth a thousand statistics? *Med Decis Making.* 2005;25(4):398–405.
31. Dillman DA, Christian L. *The Influence of Words, Symbols, Numbers, and Graphics on Answers to Self-Administered Questionnaires: Results from 18 Experimental Comparisons*. Pullman, Wash.: Washington State University Social and Economic Research Center; 2002.
32. Schnotz W, Kulhavy RW. *Comprehension of Graphics*. Amsterdam: North-Holland; 1994.
33. Tufte ER. *The Visual Display of Quantitative Information*. 2nd ed. Cheshire, Conn.: Graphics Press; 2001.
34. Abrams DB. Applying transdisciplinary research strategies to understanding and eliminating health disparities. *Health Educ Behav.* 2006;33(4):515–531.
35. Lohr S. Dr. Google and Dr. Microsoft. *The New York Times.* August 14, 2007.
36. National Science Foundation. *Cyber-Enabled Discovery and Innovation (CDI)*. Arlington, Va.: National Science Foundation; 2007, November 7.
37. Parrott R. Emphasizing "Communication" in Health Communication. *J Commun.* 2004:751–787.
38. Huff D. *How to Lie with Statistics* (paperback reissue). New York, NY: Norton; 1993.
39. Jones GE. *How to Lie with Charts*. 2nd ed. Santa Monica, Ca.: LaPuerta; 2007.
40. Monmonier MS. *How to Lie with Maps*. 2nd ed. Chicago: University of Chicago Press; 1996.
41. Eng TR, Gustafson DH, United States Department of Health and Human Services. Office of Disease Prevention and Health Promotion. Science Panel on Interactive Communication and Health. *Wired for Health and Well-Being: The Emergence of Interactive Health Communication*. Washington, DC: U.S. Department of Health and Human Services; 1999.
42. Meyer J, Shinar D, Leiser D. Multiple factors that determine performance with tables and graphs. *Hum Factors.* 1997;39(2):268–286.

43. Hastie R, Hammerle O, Kerwin J, Croner CM, Herrmann DJ. Human performance reading statistical maps. *J Exp Psychol Appl.* 1996;2:3–16.

44. Cleveland WS, McGill R. Graphical perception: Theory, experimentation, and application to the development of graphical methods. *J Am Stat Assoc.* 1984;79:531–540.

45. Vaiana ME, McGlynn EA. What cognitive science tells us about the design of reports for consumers. *Med Care Res Rev.* 2002;59(1):3–35.

46. Tourangeau R, Rips LJ, Rasinksi K. *The Psychology of Survey Response.* Cambridge, UK: Cambridge University Press; 2000.

47. Simpkin D, Hastie R. An information processing analysis of graph perception. *J Am Stat Assoc.* 1987;82:454–465.

48. Jacobson RE. *Information Design.* Cambridge, Mass.: MIT Press; 1999.

49. Norman DA. *Things that Make Us Smart: Defending Human Attributes in the Age of the Machine.* Reading, Mass.: Addison-Wesley; 1993.

50. Gigerenzer G. The psychology of good judgment: frequency formats and simple algorithms. *Med Decis Making.* 1996;16(3):273–280.

51. Chang D, Dooley L, Tuovinen JE. Gestalt theory in visual screen design—A new look at an old subject. In: *Seventh World Conference on Computers in Education.* Copenhagen, Denmark; 2002.

52. Wertheimer M. Laws of organization in perceptual forms. In: Ellis W, ed. *A Source Book of Gestalt Psychology.* London, UK: Routledge & Kegan Paul; 1938.

53. Carswell CM, Bates JR, Pregliasco NR, Lonon A, Urban J. Finding graphs useful: Linking preference to performance for one cognitive tool. *Cogn Technol.* 1998;3(1):4–18.

54. Pickle LW. Usability testing of map designs. In: Braverman A, Hesterberg T, Minnotte M, Symanzik J, eds. *Computing Science and Statistics.* Salt Lake City, Utah: Interface Foundation of North America; 2003.

55. Pickle LW, Herrmann D, Wilson B. A legendary study of statistical map reading: The cognitive effectiveness of statistical map legends. In: Pickle LW, Herrmann D, eds. *Cognitive Aspects of Statistical Mapping.* NCHS Working Paper Series. Hyattsville, Md.: National Center for Health Statistics; 1995:233–248.

56. Nielsen J. *Designing Web Usability.* Indianapolis, Ind.: New Riders; 2000.

57. Nielsen J, Tahir M. *Homepage Usability: 50 Websites Deconstructed.* [Indianapolis, Ind.]: New Riders; 2002.

58. Redish J. Reading to learn to do. *IEEE Trans Prof Commun.* 1989;32(4): 289–293.

59. Schriver KA. *Dynamics in Document Design.* New York, NY: Wiley; 1997.

60. Bederson B, Shneiderman B. *The Craft of Information Visualization: Readings and Reflections.* Boston, Mass.: Morgan Kaufmann; 2003.

61. Macdonald-Ross M. How numbers are shown: A review of research on the presentation of quantitative data in texts. *AV Commun Rev.* 1977;25:359–410.

62. Schwartz LM, Woloshin S, Baczek L. Media coverage of scientific meetings: too much, too soon? *JAMA.* 2002;287(21):2859–2863.

63. Houghton HA, Willows DM. *The Psychology of Illustration.* New York, NY: Springer-Verlag; 1987.

64. Mandl H, Levin JR. *Knowledge Acquisition from Text and Pictures.* Amsterdam: Elsevier Science; 1989.

65. Schwartz LM, Woloshin S, Welch HG. Risk communication in clinical practice: putting cancer in context. *J Natl Cancer Inst Monogr.* 1999(25):124–133.

66. O'Connor AM, Fiset V, DeGrasse C, Graham ID, Evans W, Stacey D, et al. Decision aids for patients considering options affecting cancer outcomes: evidence of efficacy and policy implications. *J Natl Cancer Inst Monogr.* 1999(25):67–80.

67. Woloshin S, Schwartz LM, Moncur M, Gabriel S, Tosteson AN. Assessing values for health: numeracy matters. *Med Decis Making.* 2001;21(5):382–390.

68. Zikmund-Fisher BJ, Fagerlin A, Ubel PA. What's time got to do with it? Inattention to duration in interpretation of survival graphs. *Risk Anal.* 2005;25(3):589–595.

69. Fagerlin A, Zikmund-Fisher BJ, Ubel PA. Cure me even if it kills me: preferences for invasive cancer treatment. *Med Decis Making.* 2005;25(6):614–619.

70. Wallack LM. News for a change: an advocate's guide to working with the media. Thousand Oaks, Ca.: Sage; 1999.

71. Viswanathan M, Childers TL. Processing of numerical and verbal product information. *J Consum Psychol.* 1996;5(4):359–385.

72. Edwards A, Elwyn G. Understanding risk and lessons for clinical risk communication about treatment preferences. *Qual Health Care.* 2001;10(Suppl 1):i9-i13.

73. Fischhoff B, Bostrom A, Quadrel MJ. Risk perception and communication. *Annu Rev Public Health.* 1993;14:183–203.

74. Koenig BA, Silverberg HL. Understanding probabilistic risk in predisposition genetic testing for Alzheimer disease. *Genet Test.* 1999;3(1):55–63.

75. Julian-Reynier C, Welkenhuysen M, Hagoel L, Decruyenaere M, Hopwood P. Risk communication strategies: state of the art and effectiveness in the context of cancer genetic services. *Eur J Hum Genet.* 2003;11(10):725–736.

76. Reyna VF, Adam MB. Fuzzy trace theory, risk communication, and product labeling in sexually transmitted diseases. *Risk Anal.* 2003;23(2):325–342.

77. Canales MK, Breslau ES, Nelson DE, Ballard-Barbash RR. Did news reporters get it right? Translation of the 2002 hormone study findings. *Am J Prev Med.* 2008;34(1):61–68.

78. Harding CM. Verbal probability and expected frequency expressions used in relation to immunisation. *Health Educ J.* 1984;42(4):104–108.

79. Mazur DJ, Hickam DH, Mazur MD. How patients' preferences for risk information influence treatment choice in a case of high risk and high therapeutic uncertainty: asymptomatic localized prostate cancer. *Med Decis Making.* 1999;19(4):394–398.

80. Sutherland HJ, Lockwood GA, Tritchler DL, Sem F, Brooks L, Till JE. Communicating probabilistic information to cancer patients: is there "noise" on the line? *Soc Sci Med.* 1991;32(6):725–731.

81. Budescu D, Wallsten T. Dyadic decisions with numerical and verbal probabilities. *Org Behav Hum Decis Process* 1990;46:240–263.

82. Parsons EP, Clarke AJ. Genetic risk: women's understanding of carrier risks in Duchenne muscular dystrophy. *J Med Genet.* 1993;30(7):562–566.

83. Welkenhuysen M, Evers-Kiebooms G, d'Ydewalle G. The language of uncertainty in genetic risk communication: framing and verbal versus numerical information. *Patient Educ Couns.* 2001;43(2):179–187.

84. Schwartz LM, Woloshin S. The media matter: a call for straightforward medical reporting. *Ann Intern Med.* 2004;140(3):226–228.

85. McDonough JE. *Experiencing Politics: A Legislator's Stories of Government and Health Care.* Berkeley, Ca.: University of California Press; 2000.

86. Blum D, Knudson M, eds. *A Field Guide to Science Writing: The Official Guide of the National Association of Science Writers.* New York, NY: Oxford University Press; 1997.

87. Dillard JP, Pfau M, eds. *The Persuasion Handbook: Developments in Theory and Practice*. Thousand Oaks, Ca.: Sage; 2002.

88. Green MC, Strange JJ, Brock TC, eds. *Narrative Impact: Social and Cognitive Foundations*. Mahwah, NJ: Erlbaum; 2002.

89. Sopory P, Dillard JP. Figurative language and persuasion. In: Dillard JP, Pfau M, eds. *The Persuasion Handbook: Developments in Theory and Practice*. Thousand Oaks, Ca.: Sage; 2002:407–426.

90. Siegel M, Doner L. *Marketing Public Health: Strategies to Promote Social Change*. 2nd ed. Sudbury, Mass.: Jones and Bartlett; 2007.

91. Brock TC, Strange JJ, Green MC. Power beyond reckoning: An introduction to narrative impact. In: Green MC, Strange JJ, Brock TC, eds. *Narrative Impact: Social and Cognitive Foundations*. Mahwah, NJ: Erlbaum; 2002:1–15.

92. Pratkanis AR, Aronson E. *Age of Propaganda: The Everyday Use and Abuse of Persuasion*. Rev. ed. New York, NY: W.H. Freeman; 2001.

93. O'Keefe DJ. *Persuasion: Theory and Research*. Thousand Oaks, Ca.: Sage; 2002.

94. Reynolds RA, Reynolds JL. Evidence. In: Dillard JP, Pfau M, eds. *The Persuasion Handbook: Developments in Theory and Practice*. Thousand Oaks, Ca.: Sage; 2002:427–444.

95. Lazarus RS. Progress on a cognitive-motivational-relational theory of emotion. *Am Psychol*. 1991;46(8):819–834.

96. Kreuter MW, Lukwago SN, Bucholtz RD, Clark EM, Sanders-Thompson V. Achieving cultural appropriateness in health promotion programs: targeted and tailored approaches. *Health Educ Behav*. 2003;30(2):133–146.

97. Bennett P, Calman, K. *Risk Communication and Public Health*. New York, NY: Oxford; 1999.

98. Petty RE, Cacioppo JT. Communication and persuasion: central and peripheral routes to attitude change. New York, NY: Springer-Verlag; 1986.

99. Nielsen-Bohlman L. *Health Literacy: A Prescription to End Confusion*. Washington, DC: National Academy Press; 2004.

100. Wolf MS, Davis TC, Shrank W, Rapp DN, Bass PF, Connor UM, et al. To err is human: patient misinterpretations of prescription drug label instructions. *Patient Educ Couns*. 2007;67(3):293–300.

101. Willis GB. *Cognitive Interviewing: A Tool for Improving Questionnaire Design*. Thousand Oaks, Ca.: Sage; 2005.

102. Nielsen J. *Show Numbers as Numerals when Writing for Online Readers* [Online]. Available at: http://www.useit.com/alertbox/writing-numbers.html. Accessed November 5, 2007.

103. Warren TL. Prolegomena for a theory of table design. In: Zwaga HJG, Boersema T, Hoonhout HCM, eds. *Visual Information for Everyday Use: Design and Research Perspectives*. London, UK: Taylor & Francis; 1999:203–208.

104. Zwaga HJG, Boersema T, Hoonhout HCM. *Visual Information for Everyday Use: Design and Research Perspectives*. London: Taylor & Francis; 1999.

105. Davis AJ. Presenting visual information responsibly. *SIGGRAPH (Special Interest Group on Graphics and Interactive Techniques) Computer Graphics Newsletter*. August 1999.

106. Koyani S, Bailey RW, Nall JR. *Research-Based Web Design and Usability Guidelines*. NIH Publication No. 03–5424. Bethesda, Md.: National Institutes of Health; 2003.

107. World Health Organization. *WHO Strategic Action Plan for Pandemic Influenza 2006–2007*. Geneva, Switzerland: World Health Organization.

108. Quinlisk P, Redd S, Dayan G, et al. Exposure to mumps during air travel—United States. *MMWR* 2006;55:401–402.

109. Adhikari B, Kahende J, Malarcher A, Pechacek T, Tong V. Annual smoking-attributable mortality, years of potential life lost, and productivity losses—United States, 2000–2004. *MMWR* 2008;7:1226–1228.

110. Ries L, Harkins D, Krapcho M. *SEER Cancer Statistics Review, 1975–2003.* Bethesda, Md.: National Cancer Institute; 2006.

111. Forhan S. Prevalence of sexually transmitted infections and bacterial vaginosis among female adolescents in the United States: Data from the National Health and Nutritional Examination Survey (NHANES) 2003–2004. In: *2008 National STD Prevention Conference.* Chicago, Ill.; March 11, 2008.

112. Gilovich T, Griffin DW, Kahneman D. *Heuristics and Biases: The Psychology of Intuitive Judgement.* Cambridge, UK, New York, NY: Cambridge University Press; 2002.

113. Stone DA. *Policy Paradox: The Art of Political Decision Making.* Rev. ed. New York, NY: Norton; 2002.

114. Zillmann D. Exemplification effects in the promotion of safety and health. *J Commun.* 2006;56(Suppl 1):S221–S237.

115. Zillmann D, Knobloch S, Yu H-S. Effects of photographs on the selective reading of news reports. *Media Psychol.* 2001;3(4):301–324.

116. Zillmann D, Gibson R, Sargent SL. Effects of photographs in news-magazine reports on issue perception. *Media Psychol.* 1999;1(3):207–228.

117. Knobloch S, Hastall M, Zillmann D, Callison C. Imagery effects on the selective reading of Internet newsmagazines. *Commun Res.* 2003;30(1):3–29.

118. Brosius H-B. Toward an exemplification theory of news effects. *Doc Des.* 2000;2(1):19–27.

119. Spence I. No humble pie: The origins and usage of a statistical chart. *J Educ Behav Stat.* 2005;30(4):353–368.

120. Spence I, Lewandowsky S. Displaying proportions and percentages. *Appl Cogn Psychol.* 1991;5:61–77.

121. Lipkus IM, Nelson DE. Visual communication. In: Nelson DE, Brownson RC, Remington PL, Parvanta C, eds. *Communicating Public Health Information Effectively: A Guide for Practitioners.* Washington, DC: American Public Health Association; 2002:155–172.

122. Jarvenpaa SL, Dickson GW. Graphics and managerial decision making: Research-based guidelines. *Commun ACM.* 1988;31(6):764–774.

123. Culbertson HM, Powers RD. A study of graph comprehension capabilities. *A.V. Commun Rev.* 1959;7(2):97–100.

124. Zacks J, Tversky B. Bars and lines: A study of graphic communication. *Mem Cogn.* 1999;27(6):1073–1079.

125. Muscatello DJ, Searles A, MacDonald R, Jorm L. Communicating population health statistics through graphs: A randomised controlled trial of graph design interventions. *BMC Med.* 2006;4:33.

126. Zacks J, Levy E, Tversky B, Schiano DJ. Reading bar graphs: Effects of extraneous depth cues and graphical context. *J Exp Psychol Appl.* 1998;4(2):119–138.

127. Lipkus IM, Hollands JG. The visual communication of risk. *J Natl Cancer Inst Monogr.* 1999(25):149–163.

128. Schutz HG. An evaluation of methods for presentation of graphic multiple trends. *Hum Factors.* 1961;3(2):108–119.

129. Nelson DE. Translating public health data. In: Nelson DE, Brownson RC, Remington PL, Parvanta C, eds. *Communicating Public Health Information Effectively: A Guide for Practitioners.* Washington, DC: American Public Health Association; 2002:33–45.
130. Gigerenzer G, Edwards A. Simple tools for understanding risks: From innumeracy to insight. *BMJ.* 2003;327(7417):741–744.
131. Edwards A, Elwyn G, Covey J, Matthews E, Pill R. Presenting risk information—A review of the effects of "framing" and other manipulations on patient outcomes. *J Health Commun.* 2001;6(1):61–82.
132. Edwards A, Elwyn G, Mulley A. Explaining risks: Turning numerical data into meaningful pictures. *BMJ.* 2002;324(7341):827–830.
133. Elmore JG, Armstrong K, Lehman CD, Fletcher SW. Screening for breast cancer. *JAMA.* 2005;293(10):1245–1256.
134. Slovic P, Peters E, Finucane ML, Macgregor DG. Affect, risk, and decision making. *Health Psychol.* 2005;24(4 Suppl):S35–S40.
135. Schapira MM, Nattinger AB, McHorney CA. Frequency or probability? A qualitative study of risk communication formats used in health care. *Med Decis Making.* 2001;21(6):459–467.
136. Royak-Schaler R, Blocker DE, Yali AM, Bynoe M, Briant KJ, Smith S. Breast and colorectal cancer risk communication approaches with low-income African-American and Hispanic women: Implications for healthcare providers. *J Natl Med Assoc.* 2004;96(5):598–608.
137. Markel M. *Technical Communication.* 8th ed. New York, NY: Bedford/St. Martin's.
138. Johnson B, Slovic P. Presenting uncertainty in health risk assessment: Initial studies of its effects on risk perception and trust. *Risk Anal.* 1995;15:485–494.
139. Lewandowsky S, Behrens JT, Pickle LW, Herrmann DJ, White AA. *Perception of Clusters in Mortality Maps: Representing Magnitude and Statistical Reliability.* NCHS Working Paper Series Report No. 18. Hyattsville, Md.: National Center for Health Statistics; 1995.
140. Lewandowsky S, Herrmann DJ, Behrens JT, Li SC, Pickle LW, Jobe JB. Perception of clusters in statistical maps. *Appl Cogn Psychol.* 1993;7:533–551.
141. Spence I, Wainer H. Who was Playfair? *Chance* 1997;10:35–37.
142. Marchionini G, Hert C, Liddy L, Schneiderman B. Extending understanding of federal statistics in tables. In: *2000 Conference on Universal Usability.* Arlington, VA; November 16–17, 2000.
143. Miller JD, Kimmel LG. *Biomedical Communications: Purposes, Methods, and Strategies.* San Diego, CA: Academic Press; 2001.

# 5

## Putting it All Together: Communicating Data for Public Health Impact

> In science the credit goes to the man who convinces the world, not to the man to whom the idea first occurs.
>
> Sir Francis Darwin (son of Sir Charles Darwin)[1]

### Introduction

The previous chapters provided a broad overview of the many aspects of and influences on communication, in general, and on communicating data, in particular. The focus of this chapter, however, is decidedly different: it emphasizes practical application of how to communicate data to a lay audience in situations that public health scientists and practitioners are most likely to face.

There are myriad situations for communicating health data, and no two are exactly the same. The opportunity may come about unexpectedly from a journalistic inquiry, it may be part of a planned campaign to raise public awareness about an issue, or it may involve "hidden" communication that comes about when someone finds health information on a Web site or inadvertently learns of a story from a friend or a news report. Communication may be a one-time occurrence; it may occur over a period of weeks, months, or years (e.g., in acute public health situations, such as outbreaks or for serious personal health issues, such as diabetes or HIV), or it may even be part of routine daily interactions, as when physicians interpret medical evidence for their patients.[2, 3]

Whatever the situation, there are a set of basic principles that, if followed, can help improve the meaningfulness of research and public health surveillance findings.[4, 5] Following these principles is important, we believe, to achieve real population-wide health gains. Using the principles can help structure the communication of data-based findings in ways that are planned and organized, and they can help make it easier for intermediaries (such as journalists) to extrapolate the most important elements to share with others. Being mindful of these basic principles offers a starting place for considering how solid communication practices can be used to support an audience's comprehension of complex issues.[6]

In this chapter, we offer a set of practical steps to guide the communication of data to most audiences and throughout most circumstances. The steps can be scaled back when demand for quick turnaround is high or the budget is limited, or they can receive more systematic attention when timelines are more generous and organizational resources are readily available. To put these steps into context, we offer a description of some of the overarching issues confronting scientists and practitioners as they engage in the work of communicating their findings to lay audiences. We then offer some real-world applications of these steps in practice.

### Overview of the OPT-In Framework

A central point to remember throughout this book is that presenting health data to any lay audience is, in essence, a communication task. Effective communication requires careful attention to the sources, audiences, purposes, channels, storylines, and messages that comprise the context for the undertaking (Chapter 2). This simple but powerful notion can often get lost when looking at only a small piece of information, such as a data table or figure. In striving to ensure accuracy and completeness in data analyses and reports, it is often easy to lose sight of whether data are needed, how they may be perceived, or how they may best be used.

The field of communication in general and health communication in particular is replete with books and other materials designed to help health professionals communicate more effectively to public audiences. Needless to say, a thorough review of this literature is beyond the scope of this book (see Further Reading at the end of this chapter for a helpful list of relevant sources). However, to help guide users in thinking about whether and how to present health data to lay audiences in the broader backdrop of communication writ large, we have developed a simple framework that uses the mnemonic OPT-In. OPT-In stands for

- **O**rganize
- **P**lan
- **T**est
- **I**ntegrate.

This mnemonic serves not only as a memory device to help recall the facets of communication to bear in mind when presenting data, but also conveys a sense of proactively participating in the scientific/public discussions that surround public health issues.

The OPT-In framework, as discussed over the next several pages, represents a best-case scenario. Many communication activities with lay audiences about data or other types of health information are informal. Resource and time constraints are very real in public health, medical care, and other situations, and may prevent implementing all aspects of the framework, or at least not at the level desired by communicators. Nevertheless, it provides a practical way to approach communicating about data with lay audiences and ensuring that the most important factors involved are considered.

### Organize

Regardless of the situation, the crucial first step involves organizing. Organizing has several aspects. It is essential to have a clear understanding of scientific knowledge, and the level of consensus among scientists, about a particular health topic. This may involve a formal review of the literature if the state of the science is not known, but in many cases—such as in describing known risk factors for a particular disease—there will already be a strong consensus among public health scientists. In most cases, this means that review and synthesis may require little time commitment; however, in situations where new information is available that may warrant communicating with lay audiences, it needs to be seen in the context of prior scientific knowledge: that is, is the information completely new because no prior knowledge exists (as in some acute situations [Chapter 6]), does it confirm prior knowledge, or is it contradictory to what is believed?

After reviewing and synthesizing, the next aspect of organizing is to identify the storyline. The concept of storyline was introduced in Chapter 2. A storyline can best be described as the major conclusion, based on the review and synthesis of the science, that communicators would like audiences to understand.

The easiest storylines are based on "settled science," that is, there is a clear scientific consensus based on many studies over time. Examples include the effectiveness of hand washing in reducing the transmission of certain infectious diseases (especially in health care settings), that condom use reduces the risk of contracting sexually transmitted diseases, and that fluoridating public water supplies reduces the risk of dental caries. But many storylines in public health are not this simple, as science is dynamic in nature. Research may result in discovery of new explanations or refute prior explanations.

There may be limited or no scientific knowledge, let alone consensus among scientists, on a topic.

It is at this point that the communicator needs to determine whether data would be helpful in developing messages that convey the storyline to lay audiences. If they determine that communicating data is warranted, then they need to become familiar with the findings to be discussed, especially with an eye toward identifying what can be said, and what cannot be said, with the data. Recall that audiences will generally process health information for the gist or overall meaning.[7] Too much nuance, equivocation, or extraneous detail—although important in the scientific community—may interfere with the audience's ability to remember the take-away points from the communication. Too much tentativeness on the periphery of the finding may interfere with the contribution of what is known. Identifying what the potential contribution of the data is ahead of time will help guide responses to questions and will help steer evaluation efforts later on.

During the organization phase it is also worthwhile to become familiar with the reasons why certain data elements were collected in the first place, what methods were used, and what assumptions went into their reporting. Knowing the limits of the data will give the communicator confidence in those trends that are supported statistically and will also prevent the communicator from giving an answer to a question that may overreach the scientific bounds of confidence.[8–10] Being prepared to defend the validity of a number or describe the statistical methods used to create an estimate, if asked, will help strengthen the argument when communicating to policy makers, for example.[11]

Clearly, tying data back to the broader foundation of an existing scientific knowledge base is easiest when considering data that are noncontroversial or supportive of settled science. Compelling health promotion material can easily be organized to support public campaigns around established guidelines for smoking cessation, diet, or exercise. What is more problematic is what happens when communicators attempt to persuade audiences when situations are not so clear-cut. They may have a tendency to use data in the interest of gaining the attention of audiences, using language such as "revolutionary" or "surprising" or that "change everything we know" about a particular health issue. In actual practice, most new scientific findings are evolutionary in nature, not revolutionary and may at best offer a slight modification to what is already known about a particular health behavior.

Organizing for communication also means identifying the scope and depth of resources needed to support the effort. Most large institutions will have a press office that can assist in developing an accurate but engaging press release to communicate a new finding. Press offices can also help identify related materials and links that can be placed on Web sites to support follow-up interactions. As we described in Chapters 1 and 2, communication in the twenty-first century is becoming more interactive over time. Communication efforts are less frequently a matter of simple "push," but are a matter of "push/pull" as the public struggles to understand the implications of a health finding for the decisions they make in their own lives.[12] Newspapers, news magazines, and professional organizations are all moving toward an interactive model in which consumers are invited to visit their Web sites for links to community resources, supporting documentation, transcripts, and more.[13, 14]

## Plan

After organizing, the next step is planning. The main role of communication planning is to ensure that storylines are accurately and strategically presented to audiences. The plan may be brief, as when preparing for an interview with a journalist to discuss findings from a particular study[15] or the plan may be very involved, as when preparing for a major public health campaign on a particular topic.[5] The five components of planning are

1. determine the purpose for communication;
2. analyze the audience(s);
3. considering the context in which communication will occur;
4. develop a preliminary message (which may or may not include data); and
5. plan a strategy to reach audiences.

Details about most of these components were discussed previously and will only briefly be reviewed here.

The first aspect of planning, which follows directly upon storyline development, is defining the purpose for communicating with the lay audience. Purpose represents the "why" of communication, which can include increasing knowledge (or awareness), instructing (helping people "learn how to do"[16]), facilitating informed decision making, or persuading (see Chapters 1 and 2 for details about communication purpose). A clear definition of the objective will be influential in decisions about whether, what, when, and how to communicate data or other types of health information to lay audiences. Values and ethics also come into play when deciding the purpose of a communication. Clearly identifying the purpose during the planning process should help reduce the chances of miscuing lay audiences about why the communication is happening.

The second aspect of planning is audience analysis. As introduced in Chapter 2, lay audiences differ in many ways, which makes audience analysis crucial to effective communication.[5, 17, 18] Although demographic differences such as age, gender, race/ethnicity, and education level seem most obvious, many other audience factors can greatly influence the entire communication process when it comes to health. Among these are general interest level in health, involvement with a specific issue, lay health beliefs, worldviews, past experience, personal health behavior, social networks, culture, structural factors such as health insurance, and occupational and institutional factors.

For example, learning that an audience has limited or no knowledge about a public health topic would guide communicators to develop initial communication messages and materials that are designed to raise awareness.[19] If audience analysis revealed that a lay audience had an existing but mistaken health belief, communicators might decide to develop messages that acknowledge the belief prior to presenting counterarguments (see Box 3.4 in Chapter 3 for an example).[20] When it comes to deciding whether to use data or not in messages, the audiences' quantitative literacy, document literacy, and general comfort with scientific thinking are important additional considerations.

Audience analysis is also needed in less formal situations and extends to audience preferences. For example, when practitioners or scientists are asked to make an oral presentation to policy makers or members of the public, asking the organizers for information about audience characteristics constitutes a type of informal audience analysis.[21] Understanding the audience with which they are communicating allows public health practitioners to understand the sources and channels through which those audiences prefer to receive information (Chapter 2), taking into account credibility, availability, and audience preferences (e.g., considering access to and the extent to which an audience uses Internet Web sites). Several of the references included in the Further Reading section at the end of this chapter provide extensive guidance on audience analysis for communication planning.

The next aspect of planning involves a consideration of the context in which communication will occur, and involves consideration of the situation, venue, and timing factors associated with the opportunity to communicate. Keep in mind that many issues of concern to public health scientists and practitioners are not at the forefront of the minds of many lay audiences, as they have competing, short-term priorities (Chapter 2). For example, in the absence of a focusing event,[22] such as finding a suspicious mole, there are only rare situations that prompt lay audiences to consider preventing skin cancer, motor vehicle injuries, or other public health issues. Communication efforts for these types of issues often involve trying to raise or maintain awareness over the din of competing priorities.

Context can include emotions (Chapter 3).[23, 24] Emotion levels, such as fear, confusion, or anger, can be especially pronounced in personal health care situations that involve decision making about serious illnesses (e.g., cancer) in clinical settings,[25] or in acute public health situations, such as suspected illness clusters or outbreaks (Chapter 6). Public health and clinical professionals must be aware of these emotions and take them into account when planning for communication.

The venues in which communication occurs are another contextual factor. Venues differ in their support for one-way versus interactive communication and the types of exhibits that can be used to illustrate a numerical trend. Face-to-face meetings can be the most interactive. Depending on the formality or protocol of the situation, a speaker may be able to take advantage of presentation software to add a sense of dynamism and life to a presentation. In a one-on-one interview, a health care provider might be able to use risk charts or other exhibits in a "teachable moment" for patients.[26, 27] Telephone calls are most limited in using exhibits to illustrate trends, but can be supported by materials sent to the caller ahead of time.[15] Likewise, small meetings with policy makers may provide an opportunity to supply them with short written summaries of key points ahead of time (e.g., one pagers).[11] On the other hand, broader population-based efforts involve attempting to communicate with audiences through more diffuse venues, such as Web sites, mass media, iPods, or information kiosks.[28, 29]

Deciding whether, how, and in what formats to communicate information also depends upon timing. Pragmatically, the venues and channels chosen for a particular communication event may depend entirely on timing. If there is an emergency there may simply not be enough time to consider compelling graphics. The public health communicator will probably need to rely heavily on narrative skills to translate the meaning of data into a message the audience can understand and use. Events that are planned well in advance, such as the release of a lengthy, data-heavy report, can afford the communicator more time to think creatively about how the data will be released. Packets of information materials created in advance can be used to complement the speaker's oral messages when speaking directly to journalists in a press conference or when doing personal interviews.

The fourth aspect of planning is to develop a preliminary message or messages. Note that although many public health messages are short and straightforward, especially those that are for persuasion, this need not be the case. There may be multiple potential messages developed for communication, depending on the audience and their level of interest, understanding, and needs. This is particularly true for materials developed for the purpose of increasing knowledge with no intention to influence (e.g., explanations about disease causation or the scientific discovery process) or to support individual-level decision making (e.g., Web sites with "look up" tables; written or visual materials on risks and benefits for health care treatments, screening, or services).

A critical aspect to remember is that most health messages will be considered by lay audiences in terms of their functionality, particularly for themselves or their loved ones[30] (Chapters 2 and 3). Offering a one-time press release of a new health finding may be of little use to the public if there is no indication of what to do next.[31] Simply portraying data that are stark and frightening (e.g., that 1 in 4 African American women are at risk for HPV infection) may grab headlines but will not go far in supporting health behavior change. An action message is useful in helping the affected persons understand what they can do to deal with the risk, which in this case might consist of preventing HPV through safer sexual practices or recommending speaking with a health care provider about the appropriateness of a HPV vaccination. A useful starting point in message development is to recognize some of the questions that lay audiences are likely to have in mind when processing the communication: what do these numbers describe, what does it mean for me, and what can be done about it (e.g., personal actions by members of the public, funding decisions for programs, policy decisions).[6]

The final aspect of planning is strategy (Chapter 2). Strategy consists of the approach(es) used by communicators to reach audiences with messages[5] and can be considered active, passive, or some combination of the two.[32] A passive strategy relies on the repository or "library" model and consists of placing information in one or more places (e.g., on Web sites, in printed reports) and relying on information seekers to find it on their own. An active communication strategy requires making an effort to gain the attention of audiences (e.g., through mass or small media or by attempting to activate interpersonal social networks), and requires more resources in terms of time or money.

For larger communication efforts some combination of active and passive strategies (i.e., "push–pull") is typically used, for example, providing a link to a Web site for journalists or gatekeepers who work for policy makers to obtain more information in conjunction with a single press-oriented event, such as a press conference or press release. More details about strategy are included in Chapter 2.

## Test

The third part of the OPT-In mnemonic refers to testing. Unfortunately, in spite of the best planning efforts, nothing goes perfectly all the time. Obviously, whether testing is feasible at all, as well as the extent to which communicators conduct testing, is highly variable depending on the scope of the communication efforts, time, and resources. Testing of decision aids for the public, for instance, can be especially useful in helping to align the materials to the demands of the task; for example, risk charts can be evaluated in terms of their ability to support personal decision making for treatment options. Unfortunately, far too many communication activities fail because of skipping the testing phase.

Formative and usability testing represent the major ways in which communication materials are tested. The techniques can be as informal (and quick and inexpensive) as asking members of the target audience to review a statement and offer input, or they can be as formal as implementing usability engineering techniques into the design of online, consumer-based tools.[5] Testing gives communication message developers early and frequent opportunities to incorporate feedback from audiences' perspectives into development and adjust communication plans accordingly.[33–35]

Formative testing (or formative evaluation) refers to obtaining input and feedback from people who can be considered typical target audience members before beginning communication activities, that is, during the development of messages, communication materials, or during final decision making about communication channels.[36] Popular techniques for formatively testing printed materials include (a) conducting interviews, (b) holding focus groups, (c) administering surveys, and (d) collecting feedback cards. Such techniques are usually used to gather information about audience preferences and basic understanding of messages, and one or more are commonly used whenever materials are being developed for wider scale use with public audiences.

Usability testing borrows from a suite of techniques developed from the field of human factors research to evaluate a product's ability to support a user's task, such as supporting decision making, knowledge management, or similar tasks. What usability methodologies have in common is using observational techniques in structured ways to catch errors and to improve communication functionality.[33–35, 37] Usability testing or related types of performance testing should be used to ensure that the decision aid, Web site, or software application does not generate unanticipated errors in usage.[38, 39]

The distinction between usability testing and preference-based methodologies (e.g., focus groups or interviews commonly used in formative testing) is extremely important: studies of data presentations for risk communication have shown that audiences' preferred presentation formats do not always result in improved outcomes, such as understanding.[40]

It is strongly recommended that communicators conduct testing whenever possible (even informally) in an attempt to determine whether messages and presentation formats are likely to be effective with intended audiences, and to avoid costly mistakes and optimize reach.[5] Testing, especially early, reduces cost, guards against errors, and improves efficiency by calibrating the communication process (i.e., messages, channels, and products) to audiences' understanding, goals, and capabilities.

## Integrate

The last major component of the OPT-In mnemonic is integration. Integration refers to two distinct concepts: integration of communication efforts, and integration of messages within a broader context of what those messages mean based on current scientific understanding.

Synchronization is the process of coordinating efforts within and across communication channels for a defined communication effort. Integration in this sense builds upon synchronization and means moving away from focusing on a single communication within a single channel to emphasize the total range of communication messages people experience, *over time*, across channels. Within a clinical practice setting, for example, it is not just the 15-min clinical encounter that is important to a patient but every conversation the person has with receptionists, nurses, and technicians about a particular topic or recommended course of action over time.[41]

The format and type of information presented to lay audiences should, when possible, include additional resources that may be of use to audience members desiring more information. For example, if the communication purpose is to support or facilitate decision making and the audience is the general public, then a one-page summary of key information could include a Web site address or telephone number for readers to use if they had further questions.[42] If the audience consists of policy makers and the purpose is to persuade, integration may consist of providing them with a complete scientific report supplemented with an easy-to-understand executive summary.[11]

The other aspect of integration is that communicators have a responsibility not only to portray scientific findings and conclusions accurately, but also to convey them in such a way as to be clear and useful to lay audiences. Whatever the purpose and whoever the audience, findings will have more of an impact if integrated into a frame of reference that is easy to understand. As one technical communication specialist put it: "The ability to create effective verbal and visual information for people to use according to their own needs is the heart of the communicator's role."[43]

In the era of "data smog"[44] and information overload,[38, 45–47] using clear and concise terminology and selecting a presentation format that does not create a large cognitive processing burden on the audience (Chapters 3 and 4) is an absolute requirement. Web site designers should be acquainted with the principle of "universal design"[48, 49]; that is, creating content that can be universally accessed and used by as many people as possible (Chapter 3). Common techniques are available to make visual content on Web sites easily accessible to users with sight limitations in accordance with Section 508 of the Americans with Disabilities Act. Adhering to principles of "plain language" will improve the readability of materials across a multitude of audiences.[50] Developing culturally relevant formats may be appropriate to improve accessibility in some situations and for some audiences.[45]

Lay audiences need help to understand how a particular finding fits within the larger scheme of health and science. Is a finding consistent with ongoing guidelines or does it represent a shift in thinking? If it is contrary to scientific consensus or health care practice, how strong is the evidence for suggesting personal change; for example, is it the first anomalous finding that defies conventional wisdom (with more research needed for confirmation) or does it highlight an accumulation of a well-known solid stream of evidence? In addition, lay audiences need to know what to do next with the information. Is a change in a behavior or policy warranted? Is there somewhere else to go to learn more about what to do next?

After all phases of the OPT-In model are completed, final decisions can then be made about sources and channels, messages, strategies, and products to use to communicate with audiences. As well as being a practical and useful approach, the OPT-In model is a useful reminder that decisions about presenting data, let alone what data to present and how to present them, represent merely one part of a much larger communication chain of events.

## Overarching Issues

The rationale and reasons for communicating data to lay audiences were described in Chapters 1 and 2. To briefly recap, scientific data are used as a form of evidence to support a conclusion.[51–53] In Western societies, data are often viewed as "cultural icons of objectivity" and audiences usually expect data to be used to support science-based conclusions.[54, 55]

In many situations, data can enhance source credibility and increase the believability of messages (Chapter 2); moreover, they can positively influence personal and population health.[4] Data can influence what the public and policy makers discuss (agenda setting),[11, 45, 56–59] what they understand about science-based health findings,[60, 61] and how they make decisions.[12] Well-communicated data can also support decision making and minimize excess risk-related activities.[62–65]

There are positives and negatives to the ways that data can be used in the clinical setting. Data-based decision making is becoming an integral part of medical practice.[66–71] On the other hand, profit-oriented direct-to-consumer advertising, such as by pharmaceutical companies, continues to "push" data to the public, which may foster naïve overestimations of drug efficacy.[72–74]

Research has shown, for example, that the manner in which data are communicated can directly influence patients' emotional responses, understanding of possible next steps, adherence to treatment recommendations, and sense of personal efficacy.[2, 24]

Recall from Chapter 2 that quantitative data messages are more likely to be understood by lay audiences with

1. higher levels of involvement;
2. lower levels of emotion (especially fear or anger);
3. higher levels of education;
4. higher levels of mathematical, science, and document literacy;
5. a rational orientation; and
6. agreement with the position advocated, which data support (in persuasive situations).

Data messages are also more likely to be effective for topics or situations that are complex or that are unfamiliar to audiences. Despite the many challenges faced by lay audiences when exposed to mathematics and science, most people are capable of increasing their understanding of science and data if their involvement levels are high and also if science and data are well communicated using clear definitions and explanations of scientific and mathematical principles, appropriate analogies, and readily understandable visual formats.

However, given the multidimensionality of communication, this does not mean that attempting to communicate data to lay audiences is always effective or worthwhile (Chapters 2 and 3). For example, if an audience is unlikely to understand data, prefers not to receive information in the form of data, or when an acute public health situation exists that requires urgent action (Chapter 6), then data should not be used in messages. Thus, a critical first consideration is deciding whether data should even be used in messages. More specifically, are data needed to support the storyline that communicators want audiences to understand?

## Roles for Data in Health Messages

If communicators believe that including data will strengthen their storylines, then selecting data to present to lay audiences depends on what role(s) data may play. Data as part of public health messages usually serve one or more of seven defined roles, although there is some overlap, especially for explanatory data (Table 5.1). (More details and recommendations about using data in acute situations are presented in Chapter 6, and program or policy advocacy situations are discussed in Chapter 7.)

**Table 5.1** Roles for data in messages when communicating with lay
audiences

Raise awareness
Reduce level of concern
Explanation (cause and effect)
Provide contextual information
Predict
Evaluate
Maintain awareness

*Source*: Spasoff RA. *Epidemiologic Methods for Health Policy.* New York, N.Y.: Oxford University Press; 1999. Blum D, Knudson M, Henig RM, eds. *A Field Guide for Science Writers: The Official Guide of the National Association of Science Writers.* 2nd ed. New York, N.Y.: Oxford University Press; 2006. Rossi PH, Lipsey MW, Freeman HE. *Evaluation: A Systematic Approach.* 7th ed. Thousand Oaks, Calif.: Sage; 2004. Abelson RP. *Statistics as Principled Argument.* Hillsdale, N.J.: Lawrence Erlbaum; 1995. Albers MJ. *Communication of Complex Information: User Goals and Information Needs for Dynamic Web Information.* Mahwah, N.J.: Lawrence Erlbaum; 2004. Petticrew M, Whitehead M, Macintyre SJ, Graham H, Egan M. Evidence for public health policy on inequalities: 1: The reality according to policymakers. *J Epidemiol Community Health.* 2004;58(10):811–816. Slovic P. *The Perception of Risk.* London; Sterling, VA: Earthscan; 2000.

Perhaps the most common role of public health data in messages to lay audiences is to raise awareness. Some health issues are not on the "radar screen" for lay audiences; data can be used to gain attention and help to demonstrate that a problem exists, to explain why it exists, or to describe option(s) available for addressing it. Many public health communication programs involve efforts, often long term, to raise awareness among the public, policy makers, or journalists that a public health problem warrants attention because it affects a lot of people; has serious effects; is costly; or that some type of action is needed to address it.

Data useful for raising awareness are often simple descriptive findings from public health surveillance systems. The data usually selected demonstrate the large magnitude or seriousness of a problem, or the predicted effectiveness of an intervention or other action. Examples include frequencies showing the number of persons affected ($X$ number of people were diagnosed last year with disease $Y$), percentages, dollars, or attributable deaths. Trend data demonstrating that the extent of the problem is worsening may also be helpful to raise awareness.

Associative or causal data from etiologic research or evaluation studies (i.e., cause and effect), often in the form of relative risk estimates, can also be used in efforts to raise awareness. Such data can help communicate effective solutions for prevention or treatment and the magnitude of their expected effect. Not surprisingly, larger numbers are more likely to be effective at raising awareness than smaller numbers.[52, 55, 75] Data selected for raising awareness, particularly for program or policy advocacy, are usually part of a gloom theme, stressing negative aspects, including decline, inequity, or disparity.[55]

Another way of raising awareness is to communicate data-containing messages that encourage lay audiences to consider credible scientific evidence when making decisions (support informed decision making), particularly in clinical situations.[75] Given the many factors discussed in Chapter 3, and the amount of inaccurate or misleading information to which lay audiences may be exposed, data can be provided in various ways (e.g., using tables, figures, or icon arrays) to raise awareness about the comparative effectiveness of screening or treatment options.

Reducing levels of concern is another important role for data[55, 75–77] and this role contrasts sharply with the raising awareness role. Given the 24-hr news cycle and the omnipresence of fear-related stories about many topics, including health, lay audiences (the public, in particular) may lose perspective about what constitutes a substantial level of health risk. Much of the debate about whether to communicate probability data in terms of relative or absolute risk stems from whether the question of data should be used to raise awareness or reduce concern.

Communicating data messages in clinical settings in such a way as to provide people with a realistic perspective about their levels of risk or the potential risks and benefits of prevention or treatment can involve attempting to reduce levels of concern. Similarly, data may be used to try to reduce levels of concern among lay audiences in community or broader population settings, such as when certain environmental or consumer product exposures occur.[76, 77] In contrast to the role of data in raising awareness, data that show absolute differences, such as absolute risk, percentage point differences, or numbers needed to treat, can be used in efforts to reduce levels of concern.

A third, and especially common, role for providing data messages to lay audiences is to provide explanations. Explanation is a classic role for scientific research: data can demonstrate or refute associative or cause-and-effect relationships and their magnitude (e.g., disease etiology, preventive behaviors) and provide the basis as to why scientists reached certain conclusions or make certain recommendations. Causal data can be communicated to support storylines of hope or success: there is something that can be done to address or control a problem. Action may range from recommending that policy makers support a new program or policy to encourage the public to receive a screening test, treatment, or change a behavior.[55, 78, 79]

Data that support causal explanations are commonly part of persuasion messages to the public, as they help provide the rationale for recommended actions.[55, 78–81] The data measures most likely to be effective are relative difference measures, such as relative risk or relative percentage change. Scientific research designed for explanation, however, can also be used to support decision making or to increase knowledge for its own sake.

Providing contextual information is yet another role for data. As discussed in Chapter 3, people seek contextual cues to improve their understanding, and they are also subject to anchoring and adjustment bias. Thus, data can provide contextual information to increase lay audiences' understanding of a public health issue; this is typically done by providing some type of comparison.

Time trends are probably the most common way of using data to provide contextual information (Chapter 4). They provide comparisons over time, demonstrating whether a measure of a particular health issue is getting worse, better, or staying the same. Geographic data can also provide contextual information. For example, mentioning the national prevalence estimate for diabetes can help lay audiences understand and interpret the diabetes prevalence estimate in their own state. Data that represent baseline information, or standards, based on limits set by independent organizations (e.g., published exposure limits in occupational settings from the National Institute for Occupational Safety and Health) can provide context for understanding exposure data (Chapters 3 and 4).

Patient-oriented reports or decision aids can serve a similar use by providing a range of acceptable (normal) limits for a medical laboratory test that will help people interpret their own laboratory data. In selected instances, comparisons can sometimes be made between health risks as a way to provide contextual information, being careful to avoid comparing voluntary with involuntary health risks. The use of comparative risk data in acute public health situations is discussed in more detail in Chapter 6.

Related to explanation, data can serve the roles of prediction or evaluation in messages. As used in this book, prediction and evaluation refer to programs and policies influencing populations. Prediction refers to the projected or expected effects of a policy or program, or conversely, of changing or ending a program or policy.[82] Evaluation is the flip side of prediction, referring to the observed effects of programs or policies or of changes to them, such as discontinuation.[36] Many debates about programs or policies involve projecting or evaluating the effect(s) of a proposed policy or program.[36, 55, 83] Data can provide the scientific underpinnings to conclude that "if we do $X$, we believe this will be the effect on $Y$,"[84] or that "we did $A$, and these data show the effect on $B$."[36]

Different data measures may be used for prediction or evaluation, depending on the issue, program, or policy. They may range from simple to complex, such as frequencies (e.g., number of people projected to receive screening tests because of a new program), relative or absolute differences (e.g., relative risk difference or absolute percentage change in persons vaccinated after a new program was implemented), or statistical modeling (e.g., the projected costs and benefits over many years after ending a policy).[55, 82, 83, 85] More details about communicating prediction and evaluation data to lay audiences are included in Chapter 7.

The last role for data in messages to lay audiences is to maintain awareness. There are many issues, risk factors, interventions, and programs with which lay audiences may be familiar (e.g., hand washing to reduce the risk of infectious disease transmission, the benefits of physical activity, screening for breast cancer, requiring mandatory school immunizations). A major challenge for communicators is to try to keep an issue, risk factor, or intervention in the minds of lay audiences.[80, 81]

This role is similar to the raising awareness role for data, and the types of data that are most useful are similar. For example, a data-oriented awareness maintenance message encouraging people to use motor vehicle safety belts might stress the increase in use over time ("safety belt use more than doubled in our state since 1985"), but remind people to keep using them regularly ("Regular safety belt use reduces the risk of a serious motor vehicle injury by about 40%. It remains the most effective way of reducing your risk of a motor vehicle injury") (Chapter 3).

Although the roles for data were described separately, data serving different roles can be combined in messages.[55] For example, when developing a message to encourage people to take a specific action, it could include (a) data to help raise awareness about a preventable public health problem (a gloom theme) and (b) explanatory data to demonstrate the effectiveness of an intervention (a hope theme).[55, 86]

## Other Considerations

In addition to considering the roles that data-related messages may play, there are a few other major factors to remember for data selection and presentation, most of which were discussed in detail in Chapters 3 and 4 and will only be briefly reviewed here.

First, given the limited science, mathematical, and document literacy of lay audiences, if data are used, they should be used sparingly to minimize cognitive burden (Chapter 3) and presented in formats likely to be familiar, such as pie charts or certain types of icon arrays (Chapter 4). Given the technological advances that make it easy and inexpensive to rapidly present data to audiences through multiple communication channels, there is a serious possibility that too much information will be presented at too fast a pace for many individuals to process.

Second, the way in which data-oriented messages are framed as gains (benefits) or losses (negative effects) is highly influential, particularly if the purpose of the communication is to persuade or to support informed decision making. As noted in Chapter 3, data used for primary prevention purposes, such as attempting to persuade lay audiences to adopt safer sexual behaviors or to reduce their risk of skin cancer, should be selected and presented in such a manner as to emphasize the positive effects of the recommended action or behavior. Conversely, for secondary prevention, such as recommending screening to identify diabetes or treatable types of cancer, data should stress the potential negative effects of the health condition or the effect of failing to be screened.

Third, the order or sequence in which data are presented will have an influence on how information is remembered. Numbers presented first (primacy) and last (recency) are much more likely to be remembered than numbers presented in the middle of a list.[87] Furthermore, numbers presented first as part of efforts to assist audiences in estimation will heavily influence (anchor and adjust) subsequent estimates (Chapter 3). The implication of these tendencies is that communicators need to pay particular attention to the numbers being presented first (and last, if more than two numbers are presented) because they are more likely to be remembered by audiences and influence subsequent judgments.

Fourth, it is important to identify and make numbers "stand out" by showing what is unique or novel about them. This will help gain audiences' attention[88] and may indicate what is potentially most newsworthy for journalists.[89] For example, effectively communicating science sometimes requires communicators to challenge traditionally held beliefs.[90, 91] Reporting a counterintuitive data finding may be helpful not only to gain an audience's attention, but also to promote deeper levels of cognitive processing (i.e., central processing of messages as in the Elaboration Likelihood Model)[92] to understand an anomaly.[93]

Finally, the importance of integrating words, numbers, and symbols cannot be overstated (Chapter 4). This usually requires using text or symbols, in conjunction with numbers, to summarize the key messages that communicators are attempting to demonstrate. This is often done by using data-oriented metaphors or providing peripheral cues in visual presentations.

This chapter contains a great deal of information about selecting a presenting data to lay audiences. Using the OPT-In framework and overarching issues just reviewed, Table 5.2 provides a brief and practical checklist summary of major steps to consider.

## Applying OPT-In: Case Studies of Communicating Health Data to Lay Audiences

There are many public health issues and specific situations, ranging from one-on-one interpersonal interactions to large-scale public health campaigns, in

**Table 5.2 Summary Checklist of Factors to Consider when Selecting and Presenting Data to Lay Audiences**

**OPT-In Framework**

• **Organize**

✓ Review/synthesize state of scientific knowledge and consensus
✓ Identify storyline
✓ Determine if messages need to contain data to help convey storyline
✓ Become familiar with data (why they were collected, possible limitations)
✓ Tie data back to broader context of existing scientific knowledge
✓ Assess scope and resources needed to support communication effort

• **Plan**

✓ Determine purpose for communication: increase knowledge/awareness, instruct, facilitate informed decision making, or persuade
✓ Analyze audience(s)
✓ Consider communication context for audiences, such as competing issues for their attention, emotion level, venue, timing
✓ Develop preliminary message(s), taking into consideration functionality
✓ Select strategy (active, passive, or both) to reach audiences

• **Test**

✓ Conduct informal or formal testing of communication messages, materials, and channels
✓ Conduct usability testing or related performance testing of communication materials and presentation formats

• **Integrate**

✓ Integrate the total range of communication messages and channels over time
✓ Provide additional resources for information seekers
✓ Convey messages clearly and make them useful to audiences
✓ Help audiences understand what scientific findings mean within larger scheme of health and science, and recommend action(s) to take

**Overarching Issues**

✓ Recognize data can enhance source credibility and increase message believability, but may not be necessary or helpful
✓ Determine what role(s) data can play in messages (raise awareness, reduce levels of concern, explanation, provide contextual information, predict, evaluate, or maintain awareness)
✓ Use data sparingly to minimize cognitive burden, and present them in formats likely to be preferred and familiar to audiences
✓ Consider framing effects (gains [benefits] or losses) when selecting data to present
✓ Consider the order in which data are presented (primacy and recency effects)
✓ Make key data stand out by emphasizing what is unique or important about them
✓ Integrate numbers with words and symbols

which translating data is part of the communication process. In this section, we present six case studies that use the OPT-In framework and demonstrate the process through which communicators consider selecting and presenting health data to lay audiences. Although these case studies all use the four phases of the OPT-In framework (organize, plan, test, integrate), they do not include all of the aspects within each level. In particular, they generally include less information about testing.

These examples were chosen because we believe they represent fairly typical situations that public health practitioners and researchers face when considering whether, and how, to communicate data to lay audiences in situations involving some type of individual-level change (e.g., in knowledge, beliefs, attitudes, intentions, or behaviors) among members of the general public. As such, the lay audiences for these communications are generally the public or the press, rather than policy makers.

## Mass Media Public Health Campaigns: Telephone Quitlines for Smoking Cessation

A common public health activity is health promotion—encouraging people to adopt healthier behaviors or discontinue unhealthy behaviors (persuasion)—with prevention or delaying an adverse outcome as the goal.[94] Public health mass media campaigns are commonly used for large-scale health promotion in attempts to improve health behavior among the public and have been successful at gaining attention and influencing behavior change for many public health issues.[56] Mass media campaigns generally occur when there is strong scientific consensus about what is effective, as is the case for using safety belts, being immunized, using condoms, screening for colorectal cancer, hand washing and related behaviors to reduce the risk of infectious disease transmission in clinical settings, increasing physical activity, and screening for cholesterol.

Many mass media smoking cessation campaigns have been conducted to encourage smokers to quit (especially at the state level) and have been shown to be effective at reducing tobacco use when used as part of multicomponent (comprehensive) tobacco prevention and control efforts.[95] They often use television, radio advertisements, or public service announcements to encourage smokers to call a telephone quitline (e.g., a toll-free telephone number) to get help from a professional with quitting. Persons in most states have access to a toll-free quitline.[96]

### Organize

The organize phase of the OPT-In framework (reviewing and synthesizing scientific information and developing a storyline) in this case is straightforward. There is little need to extensively review or synthesize the science, given the research on the benefits of quitting smoking,[97] the availability of effective approaches for quitting,[97, 98] and the evidence that cessation campaigns increase the number of calls to telephone quitlines.[95] The science-based storyline is that quitting smoking can reduce health risks. A key aspect of the message to smokers, however, is providing them a telephone number to call to get help to quit (Figure 5.1). Note the importance of including this action step (Chapter 3)—providing people with something to do—as a way to help them address the problem raised by the storyline.

*Plan*

The plan phase involves considering the purpose for communication, context, strategy, conducting audience analysis, and developing preliminary messages. Two of these components of planning are straightforward for a mass media quitline campaign and do not require much elaboration. The purpose for a quitline campaign is persuasion; that is, trying to get smokers to quit smoking. An active strategy would be used, as by definition, a mass

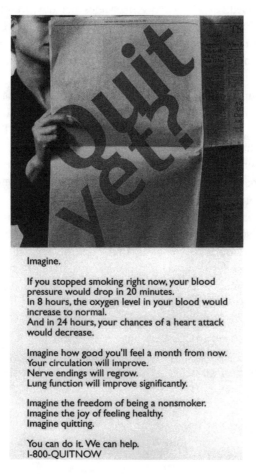

**Figure 5.1** Source: Adapted from a smoking cessation campaign poster used in New York City.

media public health campaign involves active efforts to reach intended audiences with messages.

Audience analysis is an important component of planning. Cigarette smokers are clearly the intended audience.* However, smokers' attitudes and beliefs about smoking can vary by demographics; furthermore, not all smokers are interested in, or intend, to quit.[99] For example, some smokers have fatalistic attitudes and believe that they have already done themselves irreparable damage or not care much about the adverse health effects from smoking.[100] Another audience consideration making it difficult to reach smokers with messages about cessation is that they are aware that their behavior is unhealthy and not socially condoned, and they often try to avoid being exposed to antismoking messages.[101]

Context is a major concern for all public campaigns, given that people are exposed to hundreds of advertising messages per day, making it difficult to "break through" and gain audience attention (Chapter 2). Another challenge is that there are many "pro-tobacco" messages, as tobacco companies spend billions on advertising and marketing to help encourage smokers to continue using their products.[102]

The next component of planning is to develop preliminary messages. As discussed throughout this book, many factors are involved in decisions about what messages to use and how to present them to audiences. Data, or messages based on data that do not use actual numbers, may not be needed for messages used in public health campaigns designed to increase use of quitlines. Obviously, letting audiences know that a quitline exists to help them and what the telephone number actually is are essential to include in messages.

But in a campaign to increase the use of quitlines, data in messages could play a role in raising awareness, maintaining awareness, or explanation (cause and effect). Data could be included that mention how many smokers have successfully quit or let audiences know about the health benefits of quitting with which they may not be familiar. Here are a few data-containing, or data-based, messages that could be used:

- More than half of all smokers have successfully quit.
- Regardless of your age, quitting smoking can improve your health.
- Within 1 year of quitting, a smoker's chance of having a heart attack is reduced by about 50%.

These messages do not use data to stress the health risks of continuing to smoke, many of which are known to smokers. The second message contains

---

* Although family members and friends of smokers sometimes call quitlines, they are not the primary audience.

no actual numbers but is based on a synthesis of research studies (similar to the approach used in Figure 5.1). Note how messages are framed in a positive manner (Chapter 3) and stress the benefits of quitting. Coupled with a message about the quitline number itself, the overall role of these messages is to help give smokers hope: it's not too late to quit and there's somewhere to turn to get help.

### Test

Public health mass media campaigns are expensive, and using ineffective messages must be avoided at all costs. Thus, formative and usability testing, the two components of the test phase of OPT-In, are especially critical. If communication channels besides mass media, such as Web sites, are part of a campaign to increase quitline use, then usability testing would be important. However, the test phase would mainly involve formative testing of preliminary messages, using one or more techniques, such as focus groups with intended audience members.

After completing the testing phase, messages, whether they contain data or not, would be finalized before beginning a quitline mass media campaign.

### Integrate

Integration for a quitline campaign would involve ensuring that communication efforts are coordinated and that messages are consonant with current scientific understanding. The latter is not an issue here, as smoking cessation is a well-studied and established component of tobacco control and prevention efforts. Integrating a quitline mass media communication campaign is also well understood. It might include ensuring that written or other types of materials with consistent messages are widely available through multiple communication channels, and working with health care providers and their organizations to ensure that they are aware, and supportive, of the quitline campaign.

## Community Health Promotion: Colorectal Cancer Screening among African Americans

Health promotion in community settings is another common public health activity, and it is conducted by health, community, professional, and other organizations for a variety of public health issues.[94] Communication for health promotion may involve using a wide variety of approaches, such as using earned or paid media; distributing materials widely (e.g., brochures, posters, products, coupons); or sponsoring community events.[94] Data messages can play a role in each of these approaches.

Colorectal Cancer is a leading cause of cancer death in the United States.[103] Screening (e.g., fecal occult blood tests, colonoscopy) can substantially reduce the risk of developing advanced colorectal cancer,[104] but these tests are underused.[103] In a recent experimental study, Nicholson and his colleagues[105] examined the effects of having African American adults read differently framed messages about colorectal cancer in newspaper stories. They found that message framing colorectal cancer (impact, disparity, or progress over time), which included the use of data-oriented messages, was highly influential and demonstrated the importance of message testing.

The findings and implications of this important research are discussed in this case study. We apply the OPT-In model, but because this example is based on an experimental research study of messages, the plan and test phases are discussed together. Also, as this was not an actual public health communication activity or intervention, some aspects of OPT-In are not applicable (e.g., context and strategy components of the planning phase, usability testing for the testing phase, and the integration phase).

### Organize

A review and synthesis of research and surveillance findings demonstrate that colorectal cancer is an important health problem and that effective screening tests exist to identify and treat it at early stages of the disease. African Americans currently underuse colorectal cancer screening tests and they are more likely than other racial/ethnic populations to be diagnosed with this type of cancer at later stages of disease.[103] The basic storyline used in this study was, "Colorectal cancer is a serious health problem that can be prevented." As with the smoking cessation example, it was also important to incorporate some type of action step in messaging, such as "resources are available in this community to help you get screened for this health problem."

### Plan and Test

As in the quitline case study, understanding several components of the OPT-In framework's plan phase for colorectal cancer community health promotion are straightforward. Although Nicholson's study had an element of attempting to increase knowledge about colorectal cancer and how to prevent it, the primary purpose for communication was persuasion: African American adults aged 40 years or older would be encouraged to get screened for colorectal cancer in a community setting. Because this was an experimental study, there are no contextual factors to consider, nor is there a communication strategy. However, if it were an actual community health promotion effort, clearly an active strategy would be employed.

Understanding the middle-aged and older African American audience is especially important for health promotion. Past history and level of distrust are critical determinants used by audiences when assessing the source and content of messages (Chapter 2). Many African Americans have low levels of trust for the health care "establishment" and its representatives.[106] Furthermore, there are abundant news media messages about the relative disadvantages that African Americans experience in areas other than health, such as education or finance,[107] which could be perceived as negative or discouraging.

The major emphasis of the study itself was on preliminary message development (plan phase) and formative testing of messages (test phase) and are discussed together here. The researchers set out to determine African Americans' responses to differently framed messages about colorectal cancer. The responses included the effects of messages on emotions, as well as whether messages influenced intent to obtain colorectal cancer screening. Messages effects were assessed through questionnaires completed by study participants.

Different message frames (Chapter 3) were used in mock newspaper articles that were written in a format similar to those found in *USA Today* (Figure 5.2). Each article contained a headline, subheadline, data on colorectal cancer mortality (including a visual modality, such as a bar chart or line graph), and interpretive text about the findings. The role of data in these stories was to help raise awareness. News stories were further contextualized for audiences by including a quote from a fictitious community member; at the end of each story, a list of available local community resources was included that could help an audience member who wanted to be screened.

Study participants were randomly assigned to read an article about colorectal cancer among African Americans that contained one of three message frames: (a) *impact* on African Americans, (b) *disparity* among

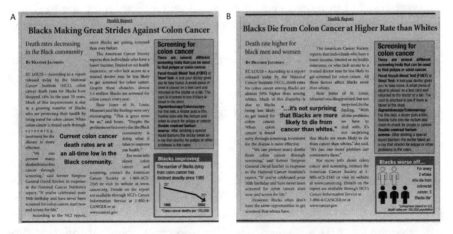

**Figure 5.2** Two ways of framing the health disparities issue. The (b) "progress" framed story led to a significantly greater degree of positive emotion and intentions to be screened than the (a) "disparities" framed story. (Source: Courtesy of the Saint Louis Center of Excellence in Cancer Communication Research, 2008.)

African Americans compared to whites (based either on current differences or differences over time), or (c) *progress* over time, emphasizing the declining rate of African American deaths from colorectal cancer during the past two decades. Data were selected and presented for each article in such a way as to support the underlying message's frame. These examples demonstrate the use of data in the mock news stories:

- *Impact*   African Americans have a high rate of colon cancer, with thousands dying each year. This disease kills more African American men and women annually than all other cancers except lung cancer. An estimated 7,000 African Americans will die this year from colon cancer.
- *Disparity*   African Americans are more likely to die from colon cancer than whites, with much of the disparity a result of African Americans being less likely to be tested for this disease.
- *Progress*   African Americans are making great strides, as death rates from colon cancer are decreasing in the African American community. Rates of colon cancer deaths for African Americans have decreased by 14% over the past 20 years. Much of the improvement is a result of the growing number of African Americans being tested. Despite obstacles, more than 5 million African Americans are screened each year for colon cancer.

The researchers found that the news story with the progress-framed message resulted in more positive emotions and a greater intention to obtain colorectal cancer screening, whereas the story with a disparity-framed message resulted in more negative emotions and a lesser intention to obtain colorectal cancer screening; findings for impact-framed messages were intermediate. The implications for communication would be that messages using a progress frame would likely be more effective for encouraging colorectal cancer screening than other types of frames for African Americans, and that data should be selected and presented to support the progress-framed message, such as showing trends using a line graph.

### Comments

Because this was an experimental study, no final messages were ultimately developed or communicated to lay audiences. It is important to realize that this was only one study, so readers should be cautious about concluding that colorectal cancer messages emphasizing disparity or impact are less effective among African Americans. The important points of this study for messages in general, and for the selection and presentation of data-oriented messages, are the importance of conducting audience analysis and message testing before developing communication materials. It also demonstrates the close relationships between storyline, purpose, audience, and framing when it comes to selecting and presenting data to lay audiences (Figure 5.2).

## Shared Decision Making in Clinical Settings: Angina Treatment

Communicating with lay audiences about data can occur in clinical settings. Although there are those who prefer that their health care providers use a paternal approach and make decisions for them, most people desire a two-way communication process for health care decisions that takes into account their values and preferences (shared decision making).[108, 109] Shared decision making is especially helpful when people need to make decisions about serious health problems, such as treatment for cancer. A broad array of patient decision aids have been developed and tested,[25, 110] many of which involve selecting and presenting data as part of shared decision making.[25, 109]

Coronary heart disease is a serious health problem that has long been the leading cause of death in the United States.[111] Angina, a symptom of this disease, is characterized by sharp or severe chest pain that may radiate to other parts of the body, such as the arms, jaw, or abdomen, and is caused by narrowed coronary arteries.[112] Several options are available for treating angina, including medication, coronary artery bypass surgery, or angioplasty (a procedure that involves threading a balloon-like device to "open up" coronary arteries and placing stents to help keep arteries open).[113]

There are individuals for whom medication alone is not very successful in treating angina, which can limit their choice to bypass surgery or angioplasty. Although bypass surgery is the most effective treatment, it causes substantially greater short-term disability (e.g., postoperative pain, more hospitalization days, longer time away from work) than angioplasty.[114–117] Which treatment is "best" for individuals involves many considerations, including the severity of underlying disease, presence of other medical conditions, risk of serious side effects, and expected length of disability. This case study applies the OPT-In framework for selecting and presenting data to support patient decision making in a clinical setting when the angina treatment choice is between bypass surgery and angioplasty.[†]

### Organize

Reviews and syntheses have been conducted based on the substantial research literature on angina treatment.[113] They indicate that although there is generally consensus among scientists that bypass surgery is the most

---

[†] Although discussed here as a dichotomous choice, another option for persons with angina is to make bypass surgery a last resort, that is, use it only if angioplasty is unsuccessful.

effective treatment, angioplasty is also effective. As mentioned above, bypass surgery creates greater short-term disability; it also has a slightly higher risk of serious side effects than angioplasty.[113, 116]

Storyline development is the next component of the organize phase. The storyline for angina treatment in this situation is, "Given your specific set of circumstances, there are two treatment options for treating your angina: bypass or angioplasty. Considering your specific situation, weigh the scientific evidence before making your decision about treatment."

### Plan

The communication purpose is informed decision making, that is, having individuals with angina make treatment decisions based on scientific evidence–based messages and in consultation with their health care providers. However, there is at least some element of persuasion, given that health care providers are trying to persuade people to consider scientific evidence before deciding about treatment.

The audience consists of individuals in clinical settings with angina. The decision-making processes of people can vary greatly. For instance, individuals may have widely different attitudes toward surgery, with some strongly opposed to it while others hold more favorable attitudes. The role of scientific data in decision making by lay audiences in clinical or other settings can also vary greatly. Although most lay audiences have difficulty understanding numbers, especially probability (risk) estimates, many people can, with some instruction, learn "statistical reasoning." On the other hand, there are people who strongly prefer not to view or consider data as part of their decision-making process (Chapters 2 and 3).

Regarding contextual factors, treatment decisions about life-threatening forms of disease can generate intense emotions, especially fear (Chapter 3).[108] Health care providers need to be prepared to address fear or confusion among individuals facing a potentially life-threatening decision. Timing is another relevant contextual factor for people facing important health decisions and experiencing high levels of emotion. They may need additional time (e.g., another office visit) to think about their options. Financial considerations can be another major concern: not only is bypass surgery more expensive than angioplasty, but the length of disability is also longer and may result in greater loss of employment income.

The next component of planning, and the major emphasis of this case study, is preliminary message development. The storyline ("Weigh the scientific evidence before making a treatment decision") and the preliminary message are essentially the same; the key decision communicators must make about the message is how to present the scientific evidence to patients about treatment options. This involves making decisions about (a) whether to include data, (b) what data to include, and (c) how to present data most effectively to support patient decision making.

For most people, data about the effectiveness of different angina treatment options should be included in messages, as research has shown that health data can play an important role in decision making by members of the general public in clinical settings.[118] The roles that data might play in messages will vary, depending on individuals and their preexisting attitudes or beliefs. Data clearly are used, first and foremost, for predicting the anticipated outcome of treatment, but may also serve other roles, such as raising awareness or reducing levels of concern.

There is growing research suggesting that presenting absolute risk (probability) data in the form of natural frequencies (e.g., 1 out of 60 people) is more effective than using percentages or other types of data in clinical settings (Chapter 3). Furthermore, for treatment decisions, data messages framed positively (i.e., in terms of the likelihood of success) are likely to be more effective with lay audiences than negatively framed messages. This means that data messages for persons considering angina treatment options should be framed and presented to predict the likelihood of reducing or eliminating their angina symptoms.

Much research has been conducted on presenting data in clinical settings using different formats, especially visual presentations of data.[40] Visual data displays that demonstrate natural frequencies such as "part-to-whole" relationships for predicted outcomes are likely to be more effective than other presentation format. Icon arrays (Chapter 4), such as the one shown in Figure 5.3,[119] would be a particularly appropriate format for presenting data on scientific research about the angina treatment options of bypass surgery and angioplasty. As shown in this icon array, bypass surgery has a higher success rate.

Several design features of this icon array contribute to the effectiveness of this visual presentation. First, the text associated with the graphic is framed in terms of the likelihood (probability) of success. Second, all the darkened icons are adjacent to each other, as opposed to being randomly scattered, which allows viewers to rapidly assess proportion size with minimal cognitive burden. Third, the two arrays are placed one above the other, providing the opportunity for patients to easily make comparisons.

Strategy is the final component of planning. In clinical settings, communication strategies can be active or passive, but usually involve both. For individuals with symptoms or certain conditions who have sought health care, the communication strategy can, on one level, be considered passive, as people seek the advice of health care providers about their specific problem. But health care providers also actively provide additional information about the same health care problem, as well as potentially discuss other health care issues unrelated to the major reason patients sought care. For example, a health

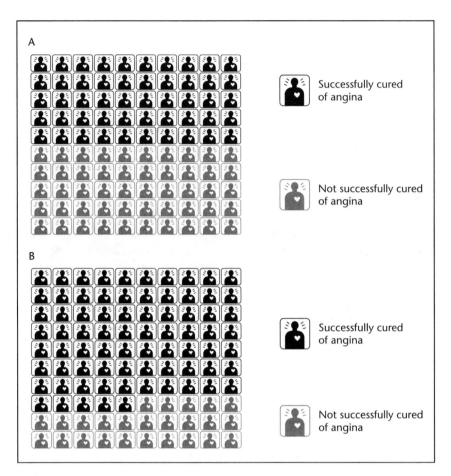

**Figure 5.3** Pictographs used to illustrate comparisons in cure rate between (a) balloon angioplasty and (b) bypass surgery. (Source: Fagerlin A, Wang C, Ubel PA. Reducing the influence of anecdotal reasoning on people's health care decisions: Is a picture worth a thousand statistics? *Med Decis Making.* 2005;25(4):398–405.)

care provider may educate a patient about previously undiagnosed hypertension. Both active and passive strategies are likely to be used regarding angina treatment options for angina. Persons with angina may arrive unexpectedly in health care settings because medication alone failed to relieve their symptoms and seek advice from health care provider. Conversely, through active questioning, health care providers may discover that their patients with angina experience symptoms unrelieved by medication alone.

### Test

Testing and finalizing data-containing messages is highly informal in clinical settings. Whether individuals prefer not to receive data-oriented messages about angina treatment options can be learned by simply asking them if they are opposed to such messages. If so, verbal descriptors (e.g., higher chance, lower chance) can be used to describe the likelihood of successful outcomes from angioplasty versus bypass surgery. Usability testing is unlikely to be relevant in most clinical settings.

### Integrate

Integration refers to both the synchronization of communication efforts and meaning within the broader context of scientific understanding. In clinical contexts, such as communicating with patients about angina treatment options, they are essentially one and the same. As part of the process of explaining treatment options and success rates, patients can be provided with additional materials or told of other science-based information outlets such as written materials, DVDs, podcasts, or Web sites.

## Releasing a Major Data Report: National Estimates of Tobacco, Alcohol, and Other Drug Use among Adolescents

One common type of situation in which government health agencies, and some nongovernmental organizations (NGOs), attempt to communicate data to lay audiences is when a major data report is released. The annual report to the nation on cancer,[120] and survey findings on selected topics by the Pew Foundation[121] and the Kaiser Family Foundation,[122] are examples of reports that contain substantial amounts of data of interest to some lay audiences. Cross-cutting or topic-specific public health reports may also be published at the state, regional, and local level by public health agencies and NGOs. Sponsoring organizations often seek news media coverage about their findings in the hope that their messages will reach, and potentially influence, the public and policy makers.

One example of the release of a report that contains extensive amounts of public health data occurs every December when the national data on prevalence and trends for tobacco, alcohol, and other drug use among adolescents are released at a press conference. These data come from the University of Michigan's Monitoring the Future (MTF) surveys, which have been conducted annually since 1975[123] with funding from the National Institute on Drug Abuse.

### Organize

Reviewing and synthesizing in this example is somewhat different than in previous case studies, as it does not usually entail reviewing the scientific literature. (Research has clearly shown the health hazards of tobacco, alcohol, and other drug use with the exception of newly developed drugs, for which the health risks may not be familiar to lay audiences.) Instead, organizing consists of (a) examining current prevalence and trend data in the form of tables, line graphs, or bar charts, (b) determining if the prevalence for each substance and adolescent population group has increased, decreased, or is unchanged, and (c) explaining prevalence estimates or trends. This last point is especially important to remember, as lay audiences look to experts to explain why something is happening (Chapters 2 and 3).

Because MTF surveys collect data about multiple substances, there are several potential storylines that could be used as the basis for developing messages (e.g., separate storylines about cigarettes, alcohol, marijuana, cocaine, or other drugs) depending on prevalence or trends.

### Plan

The next phase of the OPT-In framework is planning. The purpose for communicating the findings or conclusions from a public health data–oriented report to lay audiences is usually to increase knowledge or to persuade, depending on the organization and its goals. For government agencies, research institutions, and some NGOs, the communication purpose is more likely to be to increase knowledge. Advocacy groups are most interested in communicating findings to lay audiences for the purpose of persuasion, for example, to try to influence decisions by policy makers about policies, programs, or resource allocation (Chapter 7).

But data reports may have both an increased knowledge and persuasion purpose; for example, reporting the numbers themselves may serve to increase knowledge, while the interpretation or explanation of the findings may have a more persuasive purpose. Data themselves may play any, and sometimes all, of the roles listed in Table 5.1, that is, raising awareness, explaining, providing context, predicting, evaluating, or maintaining awareness, depending on the issues and audiences.

The major audience for the annual release of the MTF report is the press, as a conduit to reach the public and policy makers. Audience analysis involves first understanding journalists and the type of messages most likely to gain their interest and to encourage them to create news stories that will disseminate the new information (Chapter 2). Those responsible for planning the release of the annual MTF report are well aware of the characteristics and needs of reporters, and the type of information most likely to garner their attention. They provide, or make them aware, of written materials, such as press releases and visual presentations, that highlight key data points. Press releases often also include statements from the leading scientists involved with the surveys. Such information subsidies help to address the tendency of reporters to satisfice (Chapters 2 and 3). Finally, the press conference includes high-level federal agency officials, such as the Secretary for the

U.S. Department of Health and Human Services, which helps to gain the interest of reporters.

The major contextual factor for releasing a report designed to get the attention of reporters is timing. Competing news stories about other topics can gain reporter interest; conversely, a major breaking story about adolescents and drug use may increase interest in data. The release of MTF data and press conference usually occurs in mid-December just before the Christmas and New Year holidays,[124, 125] which historically is a slower time of the year for certain types of news events and stories. This increases the likelihood that the press conference and press release with the latest MTF findings on adolescent use of tobacco, alcohol, and other drugs will be of interest to reporters.

The final components of planning are developing the preliminary message and the strategy. In a data report such as the annual MTF survey data release, unlike most other situations involving communicating public health information to lay audiences, data themselves, and their interpretation (explanation), constitute the messages. As in the angina treatment case study, preliminary messages are essentially equivalent to storylines. For MTF data, given that data are collected about adolescent use of many types of substances, many different messages are possible. Selecting data to present to lay audiences depends on prevalence estimates, trends, and other factors that may influence the findings.

For a press-oriented event based on the release of a data report, an active strategy is necessary to gain the attention of reporters. For the MTF annual data release, and typical of the approach used for the release of other major reports, the investigators themselves, as well as public affairs personnel, press officers, or other communication liaisons, create written materials for journalists (e.g., press releases, tables and figures), as well as information about a Web site where more information is available. Communication liaisons attempt to reach reporters by email or telephone to notify them about the report and provide details about the press conference and press releases.

For the MTF report, two press releases are created by the research team at the University of Michigan: one for tobacco and another for alcohol and illicit drugs. In addition, a parallel press release is prepared by the sponsoring federal agency. The texts of these releases are five to six pages in length and contain major data highlights and interpretation; quotes are also included from the scientists who produce the report. Press release text is supplemented with data tables and figures, which ranged in 2005 and 2006 from 15 to 51 pages in length.[124, 125]

*Test*

When the primary audience is journalists, as it is with the release of MTF reports, it is rare to conduct formal or informal testing before preliminary messages are finalized. It is usually impractical to conduct formative research or usability testing with journalists for a specific report release: their work load is heavy, and there is the possibility that information may inadvertently be "leaked" before the planned release date.

Thus, it is essential that communication liaisons be knowledgeable about the interests and needs of journalists, for example, what journalists are likely to consider newsworthy and the type of information in a data report most likely to be considered compelling.[126] Communication liaisons at the University of Michigan and the National Institute on Drug Abuse have substantial experience working with journalists and a good understanding of messages likely to resonate with reporters.

### Integrate

Integration is essential when rolling out a report for which organizations would like to gain widespread interest among journalists. For a press conference or press release, synchronization is crucial; materials need to be provided or made available (e.g., on Web sites) to reporters in a timely manner so that they have what they need to help them write news stories or videotape interviews. For the MTF report, written materials, tables, and figures are made available on a Web site on the date and time of the press conference and press releases.

Messages contained in the MTF materials are carefully considered in the context of what they will mean for those involved in the fields of drug, alcohol, or tobacco use among adolescents, given earlier scientific research, surveillance findings from other data sets, and activities in areas such as public health, clinical medicine, and education.

Below are slightly modified examples of final messages included in the 2005 MTF press release about tobacco,[124] and the 2006 MTF press release about alcohol and illicit drug use.[125, 127] It is worth noting several characteristics of these messages that are likely to make them effective, such as the use of natural frequencies, description of trends, interpretation, and prediction.

- At present, about 1 in 11 eighth graders (9%) indicate smoking in the prior 30 days, as well as 1 in every 7 tenth graders (15%), and nearly 1 in 4 twelfth graders (23%).
- Teen smoking had been in steady decline from the recent peak levels of use reached in the mid-1990s through 2004...but the rate of decline in their use of cigarettes has been decelerating over the past several years; in 2005 the decline halted among eighth grade students.
- Furthermore, the rise in the proportion of students seeing smoking as dangerous leveled this year in both eighth and tenth grades...None

of these changes bodes well for future progress in reducing smoking among youth.

- This year's survey reveals that a fifth (21%) of today's eighth grade students, over a third (36%) of tenth graders, and about a half (48%) of all twelfth graders have ever taken any illicit drug during their lifetime.
- Marijuana, by far the most widely used of the various illicit drugs, showed the fifth consecutive year of decrease among tenth- and twelfth-grade students, but it appears the recent declines in marijuana use have stopped among eighth graders.
- "Perceived risk is often a leading indicator of changes in actual use" [Lloyd] Johnston (principal investigator of the MTF surveys) said, "So, when we see a change like this, we take it as an early warning of trouble ahead.
- Not all drugs have shown appreciable declines from their recent peaks. In particular, the use of prescription-type drugs like narcotics, tranquilizers, and sedatives remains at relatively high levels.

### Publication of Research Study in a Scientific Journal: Alcohol Use Disorders (AUD) among Adults

Although scientific studies are of most interest to researchers and practitioners, there are times when a study in a scientific journal contains findings that warrant communication to lay audiences. A published research study showing low levels of adult immunization, for example, could include recommending approaches for increasing immunizations and ultimately become a springboard for messages to lay audiences. A few examples of research studies that could lead to communication efforts about personal (individual-level) health with lay audiences include nutrition (e.g., diet, obesity), cancer, reproductive health, child and adolescent health, immunization, or substance use (alcohol, tobacco, or other drugs). (Communication about issues potentially relevant to lay audiences for acute public health situations and policy debates are discussed in Chapters 6 and 7.)

A study on national estimates of alcohol abuse and alcohol dependence (AUD) among adults published in the July 2007 issue of the *Archives of General Psychiatry* provides a good example of communicating data findings from a scientific article to lay audiences.[128] The article contained seven detailed data tables and one figure on a range of estimates, including prevalence of AUD, contributing factors, comorbid conditions such as other drug use or psychiatric disorders, average age of onset and duration of episodes, disability, and treatment. Active efforts by the scientific journal, the National Institute on Alcohol Abuse and Alcoholism, study authors, and communication liaisons were successful in achieving extensive news media coverage about the study's findings.

### Organize

The review and synthesis of the science occurs mainly within the scientific journal article itself (through reviews of the literature and the context and implications of the research findings included in the Introduction and Discussion sections). This was true for this study on alcohol. The authors reviewed health and other impacts of AUD and findings from prior surveys, compared their findings with prior research, provided possible explanations, discussed potential implications, and included a call to action for better education of the public and policy makers about AUD, and also encouraged persons with AUD to seek help.

Several storylines were evident based on prior research and the findings from this study: (a) a large proportion of adults experience AUD during their lives, (b) some population groups are at greater risk than others (e.g., younger adults, American Indians), (c) there are often long delays between the onset of AUD and treatment, and that (d) most people with AUD fail to receive any treatment.

### Plan

As with the prior case study on the release of data reports, the news media is the primary lay audience in the hope that news stories will reach the public or policy makers. The three components of the planning phase of the OPT-In framework—audience analysis, context, and strategy—are essentially the same as in the previous case study about releasing a major data report and will not be reviewed again here in depth. Thus, understanding journalists well, the context in which they work, and the types of information they need is essential. An active strategy is needed to reach them. For the alcohol study, press releases were developed and distributed to reporters by staff members of both the *Archives of General Psychiatry* and the National Institutes of Health (NIH).[129, 130]

The purpose for communicating research findings from a scientific journal article to lay audiences is usually to increase knowledge or to persuade. For the alcohol study, the primary purpose for communication was to increase knowledge about AUD.[128–130] However, there appears also to have been a persuasion purpose, shown by statements such as a call to action to change public and professional attitudes about alcohol use, the need to destigmatize (alcohol use) disorders, and encouraging earlier identification and treatment of persons with alcohol problems, all of which were included in the article and the NIH press release.[128, 130]

The preliminary message development component of planning is when decisions must be made whether data are needed to support the storyline. For a quantitative research study, such as this scientific article on AUD in which data are prominent parts of storylines, data provide valuable support for storylines (in fact, storylines and preliminary messages may be equivalent). Further decisions must then be made about which data to select and how to present them.

Depending on the study, data may play one or more of the roles discussed earlier in the chapter (raising awareness, explaining, providing context, predicting, evaluating, or maintaining awareness) when communicating with lay audiences. For the alcohol study, the major role that data could play in messages was to raise awareness, and to a lesser extent, maintain awareness. The major challenge was deciding which data to select (and by extension, which to exclude). Given the desired roles for data to play in messages, selecting and presenting a few large numbers was likely to be more effective (e.g., the AUD lifetime prevalence of 30%). Larger numbers have the benefit of helping to gain audience attention (Chapters 2, 3, and 7).

### Test and Integrate

Because journalists are the primary lay audience, the test and integrate phases for communicating findings from a scientific journal article are similar to the data report case study and will not be discussed again in detail. As mentioned previously, testing of messages (e.g., formative research or usability testing) is rarely practical to conduct with journalists before preliminary messages are finalized. Communication liaisons at the *Archives of General Psychiatry* and NIH were knowledgeable about journalists and their work environments. They were experienced in developing press releases and other written materials, and created messages that both gained the attention of journalists and were useful for journalists in crafting their news stories.

For the alcohol study, the scientific journal and NIH staff were experienced in synchronizing the release of relevant materials in conjunction with press releases. Separate press releases about this study were issued on the same day (July 2, 2007); before issuing the releases, potentially interested parties were notified in a timely manner. Messages were developed that were consistent with the review and synthesis of the scientific literature, and were well integrated within the broader sense of current scientific understanding about AUD. One indication of this type of integration was that the study was published in a peer-reviewed journal that is highly respected among scientists.

The final messages communicated to reporters were contained in the press releases. Only a selected set of actual data points were included, with the largest numbers featured most prominently; no visual formats were used.

There were many similarities in data included in the press releases issued by the *Archives of General Psychiatry* and NIH (integration).[129, 130] Early in the text, both releases included the estimate for lifetime prevalence of AUD (30%). The *Archives* release referred to it in the headline, "Almost one-third of adults report having some form of alcohol use problem during their lifetime," and again in the first sentence of the first paragraph, "About 30 percent of Americans…" The first sentence of the NIH press release began with "At some time during their lives, more than 30 percent of U.S. adults surveyed in 2001–2002 had met current diagnostic criteria for an alcohol use disorder."

Both press releases noted that only 24% of those with AUD received any treatment, the average age of onset for AUD (22.5 years), and the presence of a lengthy gap in time (8–10 years) between the age of developing AUD and age of first treatment (this long gap between onset and treatment was included in the headline of the NIH press release). Both releases went on to mention which demographic groups had higher estimates without including actual percentage estimates for most of them; a similar approach was used when mentioning associations between AUD and disability and between AUD and co-occurring mental health disorders.

There was extensive news media coverage about the study,[131–133] and stories prominently featured the larger data estimates. For example, headlines in the Associated Press[131] and Reuters[132] wire service stories both stressed lifetime prevalence ("Study: Over 30 percent report alcohol use" [Associated Press]; "One-third of Americans abuse alcohol: Survey" [Reuters]), and both mentioned early in their articles that only 24% of persons were ever treated. Both wire service articles mentioned current prevalence of AUD, although these data were placed in later paragraphs. The Associated Press story also mentioned in the first paragraph the average of an 8-year gap between the age at which AUD first occurred and the age of first treatment.

## Helping the Public Find Credible Information Sources on the Internet: The Consumer Reports Best Buy Web Site and Antidepressant Medications

The Internet has vastly expanded the ability of the public to access information and has influenced the nature of the relationship between patients and health care providers.[134] Information seeking (Chapters 2–3) is common among persons with high levels of involvement. Web sites have become an important source of health information for many people.[12, 134, 135] A growing role for those working in health fields is to help members of the public make more informed decisions by locating Web site information sources that (a) come from credible organizations, (b) contain content useful for meeting audience needs, and (c) are designed in such a way that people can rapidly find the information they desire.

One area that can be a challenge for lay audiences is evaluating prescription drug information for their personal health decisions. Several factors are involved for people weighing their choices about prescription drugs, such as cost and side effects.[136] Information about prescription drugs on the Consumer Reports Best Buy Drugs© (CRBBD) Web site is one example of an organization's attempt to assist the public.[137]

This prescription drug information project is sponsored by the independent and nonprofit Consumers Union (publisher of the magazine *Consumer Reports*).[138] Information on antidepressants is available on this Web site to the public at no cost. The OPT-In framework is used in this case study to examine the effectiveness of the CRBBD Web site in communicating antidepressant data to lay audiences for personal health decision making.[‡]

### Organize

Unlike previous case studies, the organize phase is more complicated when applied to Web sites. Audiences have a wide variety of expectations and needs; furthermore, there is no one definitive storyline, such as "quitting smoking reduces health risks." For a practitioner, scientist, or lay person evaluating the quality of health information on a Web site, review and synthesis involves assessing credibility. This assessment applies to evaluating the sponsoring organization for potential biases resulting from financial conflicts of interest or ideology; the quality of the scientific information included on the site (the process used to identify research and the sources cited); and currency of the information (when it was posted or last updated). In the case of the CRBBD Web site, Consumers Union strives to maintain its reputation for independence and trustworthiness by attempting to avoid actual or perceived conflicts of interest.[137, 138] For example, this organization does not accept paid advertising.

Scientific information included on the CRBBD Web site is based on a review and synthesis of research about antidepressants for their effectiveness, safety, and adverse effects conducted by the Oregon Health Sciences University's Center for Evidence-Based Policy (CEBP).[137] Data on average monthly costs for antidepressants were obtained from Wolters Kluwer

---

[‡] This case study uses the OPT-In framework to assess this Web site from the perspective of persons working health fields. Applying the OPT-In framework would be different if it were being used prospectively to aid the development of a health-oriented Web site.

Health, which is a company that tracks prescription drug costs data nationally. The site went live in 2005 and was updated in 2006.[137]

As mentioned above, there is no one definitive storyline. On the other hand, simply providing lay audiences with a lot of data and hoping that they can effectively interpret the information and apply it to their own situation is problematic because of low quantitative literacy and high cognitive burden (Chapter 3).

To help address these challenges, CRBBD staff took into account various factors to identify and highlight those antidepressants considered to be "best buys" for consumers and used them in their messages,[137] including helping provide guidelines for antidepressant users or potential users.[§] Criteria used for determining best buy antidepressants were that the drug had to

- be in the top tier of effectiveness
- have a safety record similar to, or better than, other antidepressants
- have an average price for a 30-day supply that was significantly lower than the most costly antidepressant meeting the first two criteria.

*Plan*

Assessing an existing health information Web site for planning primarily consists of considering the original purpose and audience analysis.

The communication purpose for most personal health–oriented Web sites is informed decision making, although any or all of the other three purposes for communication (increasing knowledge, instructing, or persuading) may be present. For the CRBBD project, informed decision making is the primary purpose: it is designed to allow people to make their own comparisons based on effectiveness, safety and tolerability (side effects), convenience (frequency of use), and average monthly cost. But there is also an element of persuasion: three medications were considered to be "best buys" (generic fluoxetine, generic citalopram, and generic bupropion) and were featured prominently in all materials.

The members of the general public who are taking, or considering taking, antidepressant medications are the intended audience for the CRBBD Web site. But it is evident that when deciding what information to include, the site developers recognized that other factors besides research on antidepressant drug effectiveness and safety are important to audiences.

Consistent with research about issues that people consider when selecting medications,[136] these factors include (a) whether they need to be used at all (are there effective alternatives?), (b) effectiveness (comparisons between

---

[§] Realizing, of course, that there can be much variability among people as to how much weight they give the importance of these CRBBD criteria due to the potential influence of personal experiences or the recommendations of health care providers in their decision making.

types of drugs or between brand name and generic versions of the same drug), (c) cost, (d) safety (potential side effects), and (e) ease of use (e.g., dosing schedules). These factors were used to develop the approach for organizing the information (taxonomy) included on the Web site.

Considering the preliminary message development, context, and strategy components of planning can only be done retrospectively for an existing Web site. Besides creating the taxonomy for presenting information just mentioned, we are not aware of the specific processes or steps used by the CRBBD staff for most of these components. We can speculate, however, that they were based on Consumers Union's 60 years of experience providing consumer-oriented technical information to lay audiences.[138]

Because there is not one specific message or messages, the key consideration is selecting what information to include and emphasize, and deciding how best to present it so that audiences can readily locate and understand key points. This involves Web site content and design, and depends on communication purpose(s) and audience analysis, guided by research-based Web development practices.[139] Obviously, for a Web site designed to share data as a major part of the communication activity, data were included. The major role data play for consumer-oriented personal health Web sites is to raise awareness. For a site with substantial amounts of data that involve searching (look-up function), well-designed tables that include peripheral cues and contextual information to assist with interpretation are the best format for presentation (Chapter 4).

Context and strategy are clear cut. The most relevant aspects of context are access and preferences for information sources (Chapter 2), as the Internet is not universally available and many people prefer not to use Web sites to find information. The strategy is mainly passive, relying on information seekers to find the site, although an active strategy was also used to reach readers of *Consumer Reports* magazine through announcements of the availability of the CRBBD Web site.

### Test and Integrate

As with the preliminary message development and strategy components of planning, assessing the testing phase of the OPT-In framework for an existing Web site is also a retrospective exercise—we do not know about formative or usability testing conducted by this organization. Suffice to say that both types of testing with intended audiences are important before finalizing Web site content and design, and are especially important when selecting and presenting data, given difficulties that many audiences have in understanding numbers (Chapter 3).

Assessing the integration phase involves considering the integration of the communication activities themselves and integrating meaning within a broader sense of understanding. For the former, integration of the CRBBD Web site material for antidepressants was achieved by using consistent messages across communication products (45-s and 10-min videos; 2-, 9-, and 22-page summaries and reports). For example, a summary of recommendations with bulleted text listing dosages and costs for the three recommended antidepressant medications is included on the first page of all three written reports.

The decision to rely upon a detailed report about antidepressants produced by independent scientific researchers at an academic institution meant that the information and recommendations provided on the Web site are consistent with current scientific thinking. Substantial amounts of background information are included to help users place these data in the broader context of treatment for depression. Examples include short explanations and descriptions of the symptoms of depression, treatment options besides medication, types and levels of depression, side effects, and drug–drug interactions. Furthermore, suggestions were included for communicating with health care providers.

Each of the written products contained tables that followed the principles discussed in Chapter 4. Figure 5.4 contains a table from the nine-page report. Note the use of a concise title and short column headings, which are clearly delineated from the body of the table through the use of shading. Within the body of the table, row shading is used to distinguish medications. Small rectangular boxes labeled "CR Best Buy" next to the far left column and bolding of text for the generic name and dose indicate recommended choices.

## Conclusion

Communicating data to lay audiences occurs within the broader aspects of communication in general. It involves carefully considering several factors and taking interim steps before deciding whether data should be used in messages at all, let alone what data to select and how to present them more effectively. The OPT-In framework, which stands for organize, plan, test, and integrate, provides a useful way to remember the major communication factors and steps for communicating with lay audiences in general, and about data in particular. The mnemonic also can assist communicators in realizing the importance of quantitative health findings needing to enter into public discourse.

As shown in these case examples, the selection and presentation of data messages can play several important roles, such as raising awareness or demonstrating cause-and-effect relationships for lay audiences in many types of communication situations. In the next two chapters, further discussion and examples are provided about selecting and presenting data to lay audiences in acute public health situations (Chapter 6) and for advocacy (Chapter 7).

| | Antidepressant Cost Comparison | | | | |
|---|---|---|---|---|---|
| Generic Name and Dose | Brand Name[1] | Drug is a Generic | Frequency of Use per Day | Average Monthly Cost[2] | |
| Bupropion 75mg tablet | Wellbutrin | No | Three | $148 | |
| **Bupropion 75mg tablet** | Generic | Yes | Three | $60 | BEST BUY |
| Bupropion 100mg sustained release tablet | Wellbutrin SR | No | Two | $154 | |
| Bupropion 100mg sustained release tablet | Budeprion SR | No | Two | $105 | |
| Bupropion 100mg sustained release tablet | Generic | Yes | Two | $86 | |
| Bupropion 100mg tablet | Wellbutrin | No | Three | $194 | |
| **Bupropion 100mg tablet** | Generic | Yes | Three | $71 | BEST BUY |
| Bupropion 150mg sustained release tablet | Wellbutrin XL | No | Two | $223 | |
| Bupropion 150mg sustained release tablet | Wellbutrin SR | No | Two | $157 | |
| Bupropion 150mg sustained release tablet | Budeprion SR | No | Two | $114 | |
| Bupropion 150mg sustained release tablet | Generic | Yes | Two | $96 | |
| Bupropion 300mg sustained release tablet | Wellbutrin XL | No | One | $144 | |
| Citalopram 20mg tablet | Celexa | No | One | $94 | |
| **Citalopram 20mg tablet** | Generic | Yes | One | $50 | BEST BUY |

**Figure 5.4** Excerpt from *Consumer Reports Best Buy Drugs* table allowing for easy comparisons between types of antidepressant products.

**The Bottom Line**

Presenting health data to any lay audience is, in essence, a communication task: most people are capable of increasing their understanding of science and numbers if their involvement levels are high, and if information is communicating using clear definitions and explanations, appropriate analogies, and readily understandable visual formats.

The OPT-In framework (**O**rganize, **P**lan, **T**est, **In**tegrate) helps to plan for communicating data, and also conveys a sense of scientists and practitioners proactively participating in discussions with lay audiences about health issues.

Formative testing of information materials before presenting them to audiences is a crucial, yet often overlooked, step in communication planning.

Roles for data in messages include: (a) raising awareness, (b) reducing levels of concern, (c) explaining (cause and effect), (d) providing contextual information, (e) predicting, (f) evaluating, and (g) maintaining awareness.

The OPT-In framework can readily be used to communicate data and other health information across a variety of different situations.

## Further Reading

### Planning Communication Activities

Lundgren RE, McMakin AH. *Risk Communication: A Handbook for Communicating Environmental, Safety, and Health Risks.* 3rd ed. Columbus: Battelle; 2004.

National Cancer Institute. *Making Health Communication Programs Work.* Washington, D.C.: U.S. Department of Health and Human Services, National Institutes of Health, National Cancer Institute; 2002. NIH Pub. No. 02–5145.

Nelson DE, Brownson RC, Remington PL, Parvanta C. eds. *Communicating Public Health Information Effectively: A Guide for Practitioners.* Washington, D.C.: American Public Health Association; 2002.

Witte K, Meyer G, Martell DP. *Effective Health Risk Messages: A Step-by-Step Guide.* Thousand Oaks, Calif.: Sage; 2001.

### Integrating Consumer Feedback

CDC. *CDCynergy*, Basic edition 3.0. Atlanta, Ga.: Centers for Disease Control and Prevention; 2004.

Koyani SJ, Bailey RW, Nall JR. *Research-Based Web Design and Usability Guidelines*, Washington, D.C.: U.S. Department of Health and Human Services; 2003.

Nielsen J. *Designing Web Usability.* Indianapolis, Ind.: New Riders; 2000.

Rossi PH, Lipsey MW, Freeman HE. *Evaluation: A Systematic Approach*. 7th ed. Thousand Oaks, Calif.: Sage; 2004.

## References

1. Darwin F. First Galton lecture before the Eugenics Society. *Eugen Rev.* 1914;6:1.
2. Kreps GL, Thornton BC. *Health Communication: Theory and Practice*. 2nd ed. Prospect Heights, Ill.: Waveland Press; 1992.
3. Wright KB, Sparks L, O'Hair D. *Health Communication in the 21st Century*. Malden, Mass.: Blackwell; 2008.
4. The Royal Institution of Great Britain. *Guidelines on Science and Health Communication*. London, England: The Royal Institution of Great Britain; 2001.
5. National Cancer Institute. *Making Health Communication Programs Work*. Washington, D.C.: U.S. Department of Health and Human Services, National Institutes of Health, National Cancer Institute; 2002. NIH Pub. No. 02–5145.
6. Nelson DE, Brownson RC, Remington PL, Parvanta C, eds. *Communicating Public Health Information Effectively: A Guide for Practitioners*. Washington, D.C.: American Public Health Association; 2002.
7. Reyna VF, Adam MB. Fuzzy-trace theory, risk communication, and product labeling in sexually transmitted diseases. *Risk Anal.* 2003;23(2):325–342.
8. Baum M. What is newsworthy? Frenzy to feed the media can be bad for patients. *BMJ.* 2002;325(7367):774.
9. Woloshin S, Schwartz LM. What's the rush? The dissemination and adoption of preliminary research results. *J Natl Cancer Inst.* 2006;98(6):372–373.
10. Zuckerman D. Hype in health reporting: "Checkbook science" buys distortion of medical news. *Int J Health Serv.* 2003;33(2):383–389.
11. Brownson RC, Malone BR. Communicating public health information to policy makers. In: Nelson DE, Brownson RC, Remington PL, Parvanta C, eds. *Communicating Public Health Information*. Washington, D.C.: American Public Health Association; 2002:97–114.
12. Fox S, Rainie L. *Vital Decisions: How Internet Users Decide What Information to Trust When They or Their Loved Ones Are Sick*. Washington, D.C.: Pew Research Center; 2002.
13. Brown J. NBC Universal undergoes restructuring that will cut 700 at the network. In: Lehrer J, ed. *Lehrer News Hour: Public Broadcasting System*; 2006. Available online at http://www.pbs.org/newshour/bb/media/july-dec06/nbc_10–19.html, Accessed February 20, 2008.
14. Conn J. Health 2.0: The next generation of Web enterprises. In: *Modern Health Care Online*. Chicago, Ill.; 2007. Available online at http://modernhealthcare.com/apps/pbcs.dll/article?AID=/20071211/FREE/312110003, Accessed February 20, 2008.
15. Greenwell M. Communicating public health information to the news media. In: Nelson DE, Brownson RC, Remington PL, Parvanta C, eds. *Communicating Public Health Information Effectively*. Washington, D.C.: American Public Health Association; 2002:73–96.
16. Redish J. Reading to learn to do. *IEEE Trans Prof Commun.* 1989;32(4):289–293.
17. Maibach E, Parrot RL. eds. *Designing Health Messages: Approaches from Communication Theory and Public Health Practice*. Thousand Oaks, Calif.: Sage; 1995.

18. Rice RE, Atkin CK. eds. *Public Communication Campaigns*, 3rd ed. Thousand Oaks, Calif.: Sage; 2001.
19. Prochaska JO, Velicer WF. The transtheoretical model of health behavior change. *Am J Health Promot.* 1997;12(1):38–48.
20. McGuire WJ. *Persuasion and Social Control* [sound recording]. Washington, D.C.: American Psychological Association; 1976.
21. Payne JG. Oral presentations. In: Nelson DE, Brownson RC, Remington PL, Parvanta C, eds. *Communicating Public Health Information Effectively: A Guide for Practitioners.* Washington, D.C.: American Public Health Association; 2002:141–154.
22. Birkland TA. Focusing events, mobilization, and agenda setting. *J Public Policy.* 1998;18:53–74.
23. Leventhal H, Brissette I, Leventhal EA. The common-sense model of self-regulation of health and illness. In: Cameron LD, Leventhal H, eds. *The Self-Regulation of Health and Illness Behaviour.* New York, N.Y.: Routledge; 2003:42–65.
24. Croyle RT. *Psychosocial Effects of Screening for Disease Prevention and Detection.* New York, N.Y.: Oxford University Press; 1995.
25. Epstein RM, Alper BS, Quill TE. Communicating evidence for participatory decision making. *JAMA.* 2004;291(19):2359–2366.
26. McBride CM, Emmons KM, Lipkus IM. Understanding the potential of teachable moments: The case of smoking cessation. *Health Educ Res.* 2003;18(2):156–170.
27. McBride CM, Puleo E, Pollak KI, et al. Understanding the role of cancer worry in creating a "teachable moment" for multiple risk factor reduction. *Soc Sci Med.* 2008;66(3):790–800.
28. Maibach EW, Abroms LC, Marosits M. Communication and marketing as tools to cultivate the public's health: A proposed "people and places" framework. *BMC Public Health.* 2007;7:88.
29. Maibach EW, Weber D, Massett H, Hancock GR, Price S. Understanding consumers' health information preferences: Development and validation of a brief screening instrument. *J Health Commun.* 2006;11(8):717–736.
30. Nielsen-Bohlman L. *Health Literacy: A Prescription to End Confusion.* Washington, D.C.: National Academy Press; 2004.
31. Cameron LD, Leventhal H. *The Self-Regulation of Health and Illness Behaviour.* New York, N.Y.: Routledge; 2003.
32. Johnson JD. *Cancer-Related Information Seeking.* Cresskill, N.J.: Hampton Press; 1997.
33. Dumas JS, Redish J. *A Practical Guide to Usability Testing.* Rev. ed. Exeter, England; Portland, Or.: Intellect Books; 1999.
34. Nielsen J. *Designing Web Usability.* Indianapolis, Ind.: New Riders; 2000.
35. Nielsen J. *Usability Engineering.* Boston, Mass.: Academic Press; 1993.
36. Rossi PH, Lipsey MW, Freeman HE. *Evaluation: A Systematic Approach.* 7th ed. Thousand Oaks, Calif.: Sage; 2004.
37. Norman DA. *The Design of Everyday Things.* 1st Basic paperback ed. New York: Basic Books; 2002.
38. Institute of Medicine. *Crossing the Quality Chasm: A New Health System for the 21st Century.* Washington, D.C.: National Academies of Science; 2001.
39. Institute of Medicine. *To Err Is Human: Building a Safer Health System.* Washington, D.C.: National Academies of Science; 2000.
40. Ancker JS, Senathirajah Y, Kukafka R, Starren JB. Design features of graphs in health risk communication: A systematic review. *J Am Med Inform Assoc.* 2006;13(6):608–618.

41. Zuboff S, Maxmin J. *The Support Economy: Why Corporations Are Failing Individuals and the Next Episode of Capitalism.* New York, N.Y.: Viking; 2002.
42. Kemper DW, Mettler M. *Information Therapy: Prescribed Information as a Reimbursable Medical Service.* 1st ed. Boise, Idaho: Healthwise; 2002.
43. Smudde P. Downsizing technical staff: The risk to corporate success. *Tech Commun.* 1993;40(1):35–41.
44. Shenk D. *Data Smog: Surviving the Information Glut.* New York, N.Y.: Bantam; 1997.
45. Institute of Medicine. *Speaking of Health: Assessing Health Communication Strategies for Diverse Populations.* Washington, D.C.: National Academy Press; 2002.
46. Cohn M. Politics, pragmatism and the information overload. *Aust Fam Physician.* 1996;25(5):660–661.
47. Light L. Cancer and diet: Helping the consumer cut through the information overload. *Promot Health.* 1987;8(1):4–5, 10.
48. Iezzoni LI. Toward universal design in assessing health care experiences. *Med Care* 2002;40(9):725–728.
49. Hesse BW, Shneiderman B. eHealth research from the user's perspective. *Am J Prev Med.* 2007; 32(5 Suppl):S97-S103.
50. Hemming HE, Langille L. Building knowledge in literacy and health. *Can J Public Health.* 2006;97(Suppl 2):S31–S36.
51. Parrott R, Silk K, Dorgan K, Condit C, Harris T. Risk communication and judgments of statistical evidentiary appeals. When a picture is not worth a thousand words. *Human Commun Res.* 2005;32:423–452.
52. Ramage JD, Bean JC, Johnson J. *Writing Arguments: A Rhetoric with Readings.* 6th ed. New York, N.Y.: Pearson/Longman; 2003.
53. Weston A. *A Rulebook for Arguments.* 3rd ed. Indianapolis, Ind.: Hackett; 2000.
54. Reinard JC. The persuasive effects of testimonial assertion evidence. In: Allen M, Preiss RW, eds. *Persuasion: Advances through Meta-Analysis.* Cresskill, N.J.: Hampton Press; 1998:69–85.
55. Stone DA. *Policy Paradox: The Art of Political Decision Making.* Rev. ed. New York, N.Y.: Norton; 2002.
56. Hornik RC. ed. *Public Health Communication: Evidence for Behavior Change.* Mahwah, N.J.: Lawrence Erlbaum; 2002.
57. Kline K. Popular media and health: Images, effects and institutions. In: Thompson TL, Dorsey AM, Miller KI, Parrott R, eds. *Handbook of Health Communication.* Mahwah, N.J.: Lawrence Erlbaum; 2003:557–581.
58. Schwartz LM, Woloshin S. News media coverage of screening mammography for women in their 40s and tamoxifen for primary prevention of breast cancer. *JAMA.* 2002;287(23):3136–3142.
59. McCombs M, Ghanem S. The convergence of agenda setting and framing. In: Reese SD, Gandy OH, Grant AE, eds. *Framing Public Life: Perspectives on Media and Our Understanding of the Social World.* Mahwah N.J.: Lawrence Erlbaum; 2001:67–82.
60. Demers D, Viswanath K, eds. *Mass Media, Social Control and Social Change: A Macrosocial Perspective.* Ames, Iowa: Iowa State University Press; 1999.
61. Woloshin S, Schwartz LM. Press releases: Translating research into news. *JAMA.* 2002;287(21):2856–2858.
62. Kittler AF, Hobbs J, Volk LA, Kreps GL, Bates DW. The Internet as a vehicle to communicate health information during a public health emergency: A survey analysis involving the anthrax scare of 2001. *J Med Internet Res.* 2004;6(1):e8.

63. Lundgren RE, McMakin AH. *Risk Communication: A Handbook for Communicating Environmental, Safety, and Health Risks.* 3rd ed. Columbus, Ohio: Battelle; 2004.

64. Morgan MG. *Risk Communication: A Mental Models Approach.* Cambridge; New York, N.Y.: Cambridge University Press; 2002.

65. Tinker T, Vaughn E. Risk communication. In: Nelson DE, Brownson RC, Remington P, Parvanta C, eds. *Communicating Public Health Information Effectively.* Washington, D.C.: American Public Health Association; 2002: 185–203.

66. Nelson W, Stefanek M, Peters E, McCaul KD. Basic and applied decision making in cancer control. *Health Psychol.* 2005;24(4 Suppl):S3–S8.

67. Brailer D. Action through collaboration: A conversation with David Brailer. The national coordinator of HIT believes that facilitation, not mandates, are the way to move the agenda forward. Interview by Robert Cunningham. *Health Aff (Millwood).* 2005;24(5):1150–1157.

68. Zerhouni E. Extracting knowledge from science: A conversation with Elias Zerhouni. Interview by Barbara J. Culliton. *Health Aff (Millwood).* 2006;25(3):w94–w103.

69. Hesse BW. Harnessing the power of an intelligent health environment in cancer control. *Stud Health Technol Inform.* 2005;118:159–176.

70. Nelson R, Ball MJ. *Consumer Informatics: Applications and Strategies in Cyber Health Care.* New York, N.Y.: Springer; 2004.

71. Shortliffe EH, Cimino JJ. *Biomedical Informatics: Computer Applications in Health Care and Biomedicine.* 3rd ed. New York, N.Y.: Springer; 2006.

72. Kaphingst KA, Rudd RE, Dejong W, Daltroy LH. Comprehension of information in three direct-to-consumer television prescription drug advertisements among adults with limited literacy. *J Health Commun.* 2005;10(7):609–619.

73. Weissman JS, Blumenthal D, Silk AJ, et al. Physicians report on patient encounters involving direct-to-consumer advertising. *Health Aff (Millwood).* 2004;(Suppl Web exclusives):W4-219-33.

74. Weissman JS, Blumenthal D, Silk AJ, Zapert K, Newman M, Leitman R. Consumers' reports on the health effects of direct-to-consumer drug advertising. *Health Aff (Millwood).* 2003;(Suppl Web exclusives):W3-82-95.

75. Gigerenzer G. *Calculated Risks: How to Know When Numbers Deceive You.* New York, N.Y.: Simon & Schuster; 2002.

76. Sandman P. Crisis communication best practices: Some quibbles and additions. *J Appl Commun Res.* 2006;34:257–262.

77. Slovic P. ed. *The Perception of Risk.* London; Sterling, Va.: Earthscan; 2000.

78. Blum D, Knudson M, Henig RM. eds. *A Field Guide for Science Writers.* 2nd ed. New York, N.Y.: Oxford University Press; 2006.

79. Cohn V, Cope L. *News and Numbers: A Guide to Reporting Statistical Claims and Controversies in Health and Other Fields.* 2nd ed. Ames, Iowa: Iowa State Press; 2001.

80. Advocacy Institute. *By the Numbers: A Guide to the Tactical Use of Statistics for Positive Policy Change.* Washington, D.C.: Advocacy Institute; no date.

81. Wallack L, Dorfman L, Jernigan D, Themba M. *Media Advocacy for Public Health.* Newbury Park, Calif.: Sage; 1993.

82. Spasoff RA. *Epidemiologic Methods for Health Policy.* New York, N.Y.: Oxford University Press; 1999.

83. Longest B. *Health Policymaking in the United States.* Ann Arbor, Mich.: Health Administration Press; 2005.

84. Petticrew M, Whitehead M, Macintyre SJ, Graham H, Egan M. Evidence for public health policy on inequalities: 1: The reality according to policymakers. *J Epidemiol Community Health.* 2004;58(10):811–816.

85. Birkland TA. *An Introduction to the Policy Process: Theories, Concepts, and Models of Public Policy Making.* Armonk, N.Y.: M.E. Sharpe; 2001.

86. Nisbet MC, Mooney C. Framing science. *Science.* 2007;316(5821):56.

87. Hastie R, Dawes RM. *Rational Choice in an Uncertain World: The Psychology of Judgment and Decision Making.* Thousand Oaks, Calif.: Sage; 2001.

88. Chinn CA, Brewer WF. The role of anomalous data in knowledge acquisition: A theoretical framework and implications for science instruction. *Rev Educ Res.* 1993;63:1–49.

89. Stryker JE. Reporting medical information: Effects of press releases and news-worthiness on medical journal articles' visibility in the news media. *Prev Med.* 2002;35(5):519–530.

90. Albers MJ. *Communication of Complex Information: User Goals and Information Needs for Dynamic Web Information.* Mahwah, N.J.: Erlbaum; 2004.

91. Rowan KE. When simple language fails: Presenting difficult science to the public. *J Tech Writ Commun.* 1991;21:369–382.

92. Petty RE, Cacioppo JT. *Communication and Persuasion: Central and Peripheral Routes to Attitude Change.* New York, N.Y.: Springer-Verlag; 1986.

93. McCrosky JC. The effects of evidence as an inhibitor of counter-persuasion. *Speech Monogr.* 1970;37:188–194.

94. Kreuter MW. *Community Health Promotion Ideas that Work.* 2nd ed. Sudbury, Mass.: Jones and Bartlett; 2003.

95. Zaza S, Briss P, Harris K. *The Guide to Community Preventive Services: What Works to Promote Health?* New York, N.Y.: Oxford University Press; 2005.

96. North American Quitline Consortium. *Quitlines of North America and Europe.* Phoenix, Ariz.: North American Quitline Consortium; 2007.

97. Fiore M, Bailey W, Cohen S. *Clinical Practice Guidelines: Treating Tobacco Use and Dependence.* Rockville, Md.: Public Health Service, U.S. Department of Health and Human Services; 2000.

98. Wu P, Wilson K, Dimoulas P, Mills EJ. Effectiveness of smoking cessation thera-pies: A systematic review and meta-analysis. *BMC Public Health.* 2006;6:300.

99. Pearlman M, Thorndike F, Haaga D. Stages of change in smoking cessation: A com-parison of expectancies among precontemplators and contemplators. *J Ration Emotive Cognit Behav Ther.* 2004;22:131–147.

100. Schnoll RA, Malstrom M, James C, et al. Correlates of tobacco use among smokers and recent quitters diagnosed with cancer. *Patient Educ Couns.* 2002;46(2):137–145.

101. Witte K, Allen M. A meta-analysis of fear appeals: Implications for effective pub-lic health campaigns. *Health Educ Behav.* 2000;27(5):591–615.

102. Federal Trade Commission. *Cigarette Report for 2004 and 2005.* Washington, D.C.: Federal Trade Commission; 2007.

103. American Cancer Society. *Cancer Facts and Figures for African Americans 2007–2008.* Atlanta, Ga.: American Cancer Society; 2007.

104. U.S. Preventive Services Task Force. *Screening for Colorectal Cancer: Recommendations and Rationale.* AHRQ Pub No. 03–510A. Rockville, Md.: Agency for Healthcare Research Quality; 2002.

105. Nicholson R, Kreuter MW, Lapka C, Wellborn R, Clark E, Sanders-Thompson V. Unintended effects of emphasizing disparities in cancer communication to African Americans. *Cancer Epidemiol Biomarkers Prev.* 2008;17:2946–2953.

106. Williams DR, Rucker TD. Understanding and addressing racial disparities in health care. *Health Care Financ Rev.* 2000;21(4):75–90.

107. Gandy O. Framing comparative risk: A preliminary analysis. *Howard J Commun.* 2005;16:71–86.

108. Roter D, Hall J. *Doctors Talking with Patients/Patients Talking with Doctors: Improving Health Communication in Medical Visits.* 2nd ed. Westport, Conn.: Praeger; 2006.

109. Willis C, Holmes-Rovner M. Patient comprehension of information for shared treatment decision making: State of the art and future directions. *Patient Educ Couns.* 2003;50:285–290.

110. O'Connor A, Stacey D, Entwistle V, Llewellyn-Thomas H, Rowner D, Homes-Rovner M. Decision aids for people facing health treatment or screening decisions. *Cochrane Database Syst Rev.* 2003(2):CD001431.

111. National Center for Health Statistics. *Health, United States 2007 with Chartbook on Trends in the Health of Americans.* Hyattsville, Md.: Centers for Disease Control and Prevention, National Center for Health Statistics; 2007.

112. National Heart, Lung, and Blood Institute. *What Is Angina?* Bethesda, Md.: National Institutes of Health; National Heart, Lung, and Blood Institute Disease and Conditions Index. Available at: http://www.nhlbi.nih.gov/health/dci/Diseases/Angina/Angina_WhatIs.html. Accessed December 9, 2008.

113. Stanger O, Unger F. Surgical treatment of coronary multivessel disease. *Expert Rev Cardiovasc Ther.* 2006;4(4):569–581.

114. Boudrez H, De Backer G. Recent findings on return to work after an acute myocardial infarction or coronary artery bypass grafting. *Acta Cardiol.* 2000;55(6):341–349.

115. Bradshaw PJ, Jamrozik K, Gilfillan IS, Thompson PL. Return to work after coronary artery bypass surgery in a population of long-term survivors. *Heart Lung Circ.* 2005;14(3):191–196.

116. Kuukasjarvi P, Malmivaara A, Halinen M, et al. Overview of systematic reviews on invasive treatment of stable coronary artery disease. *Int J Technol Assess Health Care.* 2006;22(2):219–234.

117. Stroupe KT, Morrison DA, Hlatky MA, et al. Cost-effectiveness of coronary artery bypass grafts versus percutaneous coronary intervention for revascularization of high-risk patients. *Circulation.* 2006;114(12):1251–1257.

118. Trevena LJ, Davey HM, Barratt A, Butow P, Caldwell P. A systematic review on communicating with patients about evidence. *J Eval Clin Pract.* 2006;12(1):13–23.

119. Fagerlin A, Wang C, Ubel PA. Reducing the influence of anecdotal reasoning on people's health care decisions: Is a picture worth a thousand statistics? *Med Decis Making.* 2005;25(4):398–405.

120. Espey DK, Wu XC, Swan J, et al. Annual report to the nation on the status of cancer, 1975–2004, featuring cancer in American Indians and Alaska Natives. *Cancer.* 2007;110(10):2119–2152.

121. Pew Research Center. *Are We Happy Yet?* Washington, D.C.: Pew Research Center; 2006.

122. The Kaiser Commission on Medicaid and Underinsured. *Racial and Ethnic Disparities in Access to Health Insurance and Health Care.* Menlo Park, Calif.: Kaiser Family Foundation; 2000.

123. Johnston L, O'Malley P, Bachman J, Schulenberg J. *Monitoring the Future National Survey Results on Drug Use, 1975–2006. Vol. I: Secondary School Students.* Report No. NIH Publication No. 07-6205. Bethesda, Md.: National Institute on Drug Abuse; 2007.

124. University of Michigan News Service. *Decline in Teen Smoking Appears to Be Nearing an End* (press release, December 19, 2005). Ann Arbor, Mich.: University of Michigan; 2005.

125. University of Michigan News Service. *Teen Drug Use Continues Down in 2006, Particularly Among Older Teens, But Use of Prescription-Type Drugs Remains High* (press release, December 21, 2006). Ann Arbor, Mich.: University of Michigan; 2006.

126. Heath R, ed. *Handbook of Public Relations*. Thousand Oaks, Calif.: Sage; 2001.

127. Johnston LD, O'Malley PM, Bachman JG, Schulenberg JE. *Monitoring the Future. National Results on Adolescent Drug Use: Overview of Key Findings, 2005.* Bethesda, Md.: National Institute on Drug Abuse; 2006.

128. Hasin DS, Stinson FS, Ogburn E, Grant BF. Prevalence, correlates, disability, and comorbidity of DSM-IV alcohol abuse and dependence in the United States: Results from the National Epidemiologic Survey on Alcohol and Related Conditions. *Arch Gen Psychiatry.* 2007;64(7):830–842.

129. JAMA & Archives. *Almost One-Third of Adults Report Having Some Form of Alcohol Use Problem in Their Lifetime* (press release, July 2, 2007). Chicago, Ill.: JAMA; 2007.

130. National Institutes of Health News. *Alcohol Survey Reveals "Lost Decade" between Ages of Disorder Onset and Treatment.* Authors Call for National Campaign to Change Public and Professional Attitudes (press release, July 2, 2007). Bethesda, Md.: National Institutes of Health; 2007.

131. Associated Press. *Study: One Third of Americans Report Alcohol Abuse* (press release, July 2, 2007). New York, N.Y.: Associated Press; 2007.

132. Reuters. *One Third of Americans Abuse Alcohol* (press release, July 2, 2007). London, UK: Reuters; 2007.

133. Yahoo! News. *Study: Over 30 Percent Report Alcohol Abuse.* Sunnyvale, Calif.: Yahoo.com; 2007.

134. Hesse BW, Nelson DE, Kreps GL, et al. Trust and sources of health information: The impact of the Internet and its implications for health care providers: Findings from the first Health Information National Trends Survey. *Arch Intern Med.* 2005;165(22):2618–2624.

135. Beckjord EB, Finney Rutten LJ, Squiers L, et al. Use of the Internet to communicate with health care providers in the United States: Estimates from the 2003 and 2005 Health Information National Trends Surveys (HINTS). *J Med Internet Res.* 2007;9(3):e20.

136. Shikiar R, Rentz AM. Satisfaction with medication: An overview of conceptual, methodologic, and regulatory issues. *Value Health.* 2004;7(2):204–215.

137. Consumer Reports. *Consumer Reports Best Buy Drugs.* Yonkers, N.Y.: Consumer Union; 2007.

138. Consumers Union. *About Consumers Union.* Yonkers, N.Y.: Consumers Union; 2007.

139. Wathen C, Burkell J. Believe it or not: Factors influencing credibility on the Web. *J Am Soc Inform Sci Technol.* 2002;53:134–144.

# 6

## Communicating Data in Acute Public Health Situations

> Two problems with the public [concerning health risks] are their
> desire for zero risk and their thirst for certitude.
> Keeney and von Winterfeldt, "Improving risk
> communication," *Risk Analysis*[1]

## Introduction

Acute public health situations represent a special communication situation. Acute situations can occur not only because of infectious disease etiologies, but also for many other reasons, such as with many environmental or other actual or perceived exposures (e.g., disease clusters), or when strongly held beliefs or previous scientific consensus recommendations are challenged or changed (scientific bombshells) (Table 6.1).[2–7] They can occur anywhere from the local level, such as mass psychogenic illness in one school,[8] to the international level, such as the multinational severe acute respiratory syndrome (SARS) epidemic in 2003.[9]

The major concern of most lay audiences in acute situations, especially initially, is on potentially serious acute, long-term, or chronic health effects; this is in contrast to most other public health situations, where many other concerns or factors besides health are involved (Chapter 2; salience of the issue, worldviews, economic interests). In addition, compared to communications for other types of public health situations, these can quickly gain the attention of lay audiences because they may generate fear (even terror), anger, anxiety, or other strong emotions (Chapter 3).[10–13] Acute situations can result in potentially serious consequences beyond those directly related to

**Table 6.1 Types and examples of acute public health situations**

| Type | Examples |
|------|----------|
| Infectious disease outbreaks | • Listeria<br>• Influenza<br>• West Nile Virus<br>• Diphtheria |
| Natural disasters | • Blizzards<br>• Floods<br>• Hurricanes |
| Explosions or fires | • Chemical plant explosions<br>• Hotel fires |
| Possible adverse effects of pharmaceutical products or medical devices | • Prescription or nonprescription drug recalls<br>• Defective implantable heart defibrillators |
| Possible disease clusters | • Cancer<br>• Birth defects |
| Intentional adverse health events | • Health care worker mercy killings<br>• Chemical, biological, or radiological terrorist events |
| Actual or perceived adverse effects of immunizations | • Intussusception associated with rotavirus vaccine<br>• Perceived link of childhood vaccines to autism |
| Psychological events | • Mass psychogenic illness |
| Unexpected scientific findings or influential reports (bombshells) | • 1964 Surgeon General's Report on Smoking<br>• 2002 study on adverse effects of hormone therapy for postmenopausal women |

health. They can cause environmental contamination, severe financial losses, or changes in employment or physical location.[14–16] More intangible consequences may also occur, such as reduced levels of trust or declines in the reputations of organizations or individuals.[17]

Effective communication with lay audiences is a critical activity during such situations,[3, 4, 7, 9, 11, 12, 16–23] as among other impacts, poor communication practices can adversely affect the beliefs and emotions of lay audiences (e.g., by inappropriately increasing levels of concern). Poorly handled situations can result in the public and policy makers taking inappropriate actions and diversion of limited public health resources.[3, 14, 16, 21, 24–26] There is an extensive literature on risk perception, risk communication, and crisis communication (see Further Reading at the end of this chapter); readers desiring more specifics should review this literature or consult with experts experienced in these fields.

Communicating data is only one part (and often only a small part) of communication with lay audiences in acute situations. As with other types of situations, effective communication of data requires that the entire communication process be effective. Furthermore, in many instances no data need to be communicated (e.g., instructing people not to consume certain types of foods, providing recommendations on preparing for natural disasters).

This chapter briefly describes the major aspects of acute situations and communication issues, and then provides recommendations on selecting and presenting data to lay audiences. Because the responsibility for addressing these types of situations usually resides with public health or other government agencies, communication is considered from the perspective of government agency employees (or their representatives).

## Background

### Characteristics and Definitions

Acute public health situations have certain distinguishing characteristics.[7, 16, 21, 24, 27–30] First, they involve a discrete event or discovery that is unexpected, unplanned, or out of the ordinary. Second, there is an actual or perceived serious or widespread health problem, or a new understanding or recommendation about a health issue from scientists that is likely to affect, or be of interest to, a substantial number of people within the general public. Third, the acute situation has the potential to generate intense emotions, especially fear and anger. Fourth, it is likely to receive news media attention. Fifth, the public, policy makers, and the press expect public health professionals to identify the health problem rapidly and take appropriate action to resolve it.

Many terms have been used to describe communication in acute public health situations, such as disaster, crisis, emergency, or risk communication. For this book, we use the broader terms crisis and risk communication, as they include principles inherent in similar types of situations. Crisis communication, which involves providing messages to stakeholders and the public when there is an unexpected threat, has some distinctive characteristics.[14, 16, 17, 19, 21] It can be required when a threat occurs to an organization that may be beyond its control and potentially threatens its reputation or survival; the situation may involve moral or legal culpability (e.g., a financial or other type of scandal involving high level officials). Another type of crisis communication situation involves factual communication about a specific issue or topic with some sense of urgency, without reference to an organization's reputation or culpability from a moral or legal perspective[7, 21, 30, 31]; it is this type of situation that is covered in this chapter.

Risk communication refers to the interactive exchange of information about the expected type and magnitude of an outcome associated with an exposure or behavior.[4, 7, 19, 26, 28, 32–37] It is typically applied in one of three situations: (a) disease prevention related to individuals' risk behaviors, (b) exposure to potentially toxic occupational or environmental agents, or (c) product safety and consumer protection.[35] Relevant issues involving communicating about disease prevention and individual risk behaviors were covered in Chapter 5; select aspects of risk communication in the last two types of situations are covered in this chapter.

There is overlap between risk and crisis communication.[7, 21, 30, 31, 37] The Centers for Disease Control and Prevention (CDC) has developed a hybrid term, crisis and emergency risk communication, which is applicable to most acute situations.[7, 30] This is defined as communication efforts by health experts to provide information to individuals, stakeholders, and communities to make the best possible decisions for situations in which there are narrow time constraints and a perceived urgent health risk, recognizing that the available information may be incomplete, outcomes may be uncertain, and decisions may be irreversible.

## Contributing Factors to the Development of Acute Situations

Several major factors are known to increase the likelihood that an acute public health situation will develop and can strongly influence communication (Table 6.2).[19, 26, 33, 34, 38–42] Three factors in particular—involuntary risk, trust, and uncertainty—can be especially influential on communication and are discussed here in more depth.

*Involuntary risk* means that exposed or potentially exposed people did not willingly choose to be in harm's way (e.g., discovering that one's family

**Table 6.2 Factors increasing the chance that an event will become an acute public health situation**

Dread disease, condition, or catastrophic potential
Irreversibility of effects
Identifiable victims
Large magnitude (number of people affected)
Children involved or at risk
Uncontrollability
Local relevance
Involuntary risk
Trust/distrust
Uncertainty
Questionable or unclear benefits (inequity)
Values and worldviews
News media coverage

*Source*: Covello VT, Peters RG, Wojtecki JG, Hyde RC. Risk communication, the West Nile virus epidemic, and bioterrorism: Responding to communication challenges posed by the intentional or unintentional release of a pathogen in an urban setting. *J Urban Health* 2001;78:382–391. Koenig BA, Silverberg HL. Understanding probabilistic risk in predisposition genetic testing for Alzheimer disease. *Genet Test* 1999;3(1):55–63. National Research Council. *Improving Risk Communication*. Washington, D.C.: National Academy Press; 1989. Renn O. Perceptions of risks. *Toxicol Lett*. 2004(149):405–413.

members have been drinking water contaminated by a potential carcinogen). This is in sharp contrast to voluntary risk, such as hang gliding or using recreational drugs.[26, 43] But even when individuals are voluntarily exposed, such as to consumer products, acute situations can still occur when an unexpected or higher than expected health risk is identified, such as the association between heart disease and the prescription drug Robecoxib® (Vioxx®).[44] Involuntary risk exposure can result in intense anger or rage because of a strong sense of inequity and unfairness.

*Trust (or distrust)* of the individuals, organizations, or institutions potentially responsible for the situation itself, or in those trying to remedy the situation, has a powerful impact on communication (Chapter 2).[16, 21, 24, 31, 38, 39, 41, 42, 45–47] Distrust may stem from inequitable or questionable risks and benefits (e.g., when a corporation financially benefits from the presence of the potentially harmful exposure, while employees or community residents, who may be members of disadvantaged populations, are at risk for the adverse health effects).

Audiences' trust of messages will be strongly influenced by past experiences with, or reports about, individuals, organizations, and institutions.[24, 29, 37, 42] Organizations with a history of successfully addressing acute or other types of public health situations in the past, especially if they have communicated in an open and honest manner and empathized with lay audiences, are more likely to be trusted and have their messages believed (Box 6.1). In contrast, some private and public organizations have histories of being perceived as

---

**Box 6.1** Positive effects of trust on communication: The Johnson & Johnson Company and their response to cyanide-contaminated Tylenol® capsules

Johnson & Johnson is a well-established personal products company with a long history of strong and open relationships with their employees and with news media representatives. In the fall of 1982, seven deaths in the Chicago area were tied to cyanide-contaminated Tylenol® capsules produced by this company. Once organizational leaders learned of the deaths, they met to discuss what to do. Although Johnson & Johnson did not have a formal crisis communications plan, they quickly created a team of individuals to deal with communication issues and decided that their first priority was to warn the public.

The communication team defined four audiences that they wanted to reach: (a) the public (consumers); (b) health professionals; (c) employees; and (d) the U.S. Food and Drug Administration. The company

*(continued)*

made extensive efforts to notify each audience that they had recalled all Tylenol® capsules from stores in the Chicago area and elsewhere. They kept each audience aware of other decisions they had made to address the situation. For example, to reach the public, they worked closely to address the needs of news media representatives by sending out electronic information packages; employees were shown a video describing what was happening during the crisis and told that their jobs were secure.

There was intensive news media coverage about the cyanide-related deaths, although the first major newspaper articles reporting on them made little mention of Johnson & Johnson. As the crisis continued, the company placed a full-page ad in major Chicago newspapers offering to exchange Tylenol® capsules for tablets (tablets were not implicated in any of the deaths). As can occur in crisis communication situations, although the company effectively handled hundreds of thousands of telephone calls from the public, news media members, and others, there were challenges. The company's corporate vice president initially had said there was no cyanide present in manufacturing plants. As soon as he learned that tiny amounts of cyanide were used in quality testing, he immediately called an Associated Press news wire service representative and admitted his mistake. He informed reporters that the cyanide used for testing purposes was stored and used in a completely separate facility than the Tylenol® production line and that it could not be the source of the poisoning. When newspapers ran the story, they reported it as described by the corporate vice president without accusations.

Not surprisingly, sales of all nonaspirin painkillers by Johnson & Johnson and other companies plummeted in the wake of the murders and widespread publicity (law enforcement officials were not able to determine the individual or individuals implicated in causing the cyanide-related deaths). Eventually Johnson & Johnson reintroduced their extra strength Tylenol® product in tablet form, widely publicizing the presence of new and much more secure packaging. Because of the company's past reputation, rapid response to the situation, openness about decision making, and emphasis on ensuring consumers' safety, they were seen by most audiences as honest and trustworthy. Johnson & Johnson suffered no long-term adverse effects, as Tylenol® sales eventually returned to previous levels.

Source: Fearn-Banks K. *Crisis Communications: A Casebook Approach*. Mahwah, N.J.: Lawrence Erlbaum; 2002.

distrustful or not understanding or addressing lay concerns. Box 6.2 provides an example of the role that distrust and other factors can have on communication in an acute situation.

Certain communication approaches can result in reducing trust dramatically. The decide, announce, and defend (DAD) communication

---

**Box 6.2** The negative effects of distrust on communication: The Valdez tanker oil spill crisis in Prince William Sound, Alaska

When the Exxon Valdez oil tanker hit the rocky reef that tore an enormous hole in its hull in March 1989, spilling crude oil into Alaska's Prince William Sound, the company was completely unprepared for the communications crisis it faced. Local media reports of the 11-million gallon spill that killed wildlife and washed up on the shores of the sound quickly spread to all three major television networks. Within 36 hr, Exxon was inundated with three audiences desiring information—concerned environmentalists, angry local citizens, and media representatives from around the world—all wanting answers about how the accident could have happened.

Exxon's first communication responses were to blame the tanker's captain and stress that their immediate priority was action to control the oil spill, not provide explanations as to how the spill occurred. When further asked about what they were specifically doing, an Exxon spokesperson said that he could not verify the extent of the damage or what the company was doing about it. Exxon's chief executive officer (CEO) actively avoided making any comment to the press. (At that time, the company had no history of a relationship with the news media; it was not until after Exxon's CEO resigned in 1993 that the company reorganized and created a public relations department.) Articles in the *Anchorage Daily News* newspaper accused Exxon of reacting slowly and conducting an inadequate clean-up.

People's trust in the company waned—clients began canceling their Exxon credit cards, and even some employees were disillusioned. Some people blamed the accident on Exxon's corporate culture and its total focus on "moving the oil." With no history of cooperation with the media, and no public relations department at the time, Exxon enjoyed no prior public trust. Environmentalists questioned the effectiveness of the company's clean-up efforts, and the federal government levied a $5 billion fine. Exxon never publicly took responsibility for the spill.

Source: Ref. (71).

---

model[38] is especially likely to reduce trust. Furthermore, organization leaders may provide a façade of active listening to concerns of individuals, giving an appearance of shared decision making when, in reality, no sharing actually occurs. Unfortunately, trust is easy to lose and hard to regain.[24, 26] When low levels of trust are present, improving communication will require spending much time and effort to try to increase trust.

*Uncertainty* (Chapter 3) plays a major role in determining whether an acute situation occurs and how long it lasts.[28, 32–34, 36–39, 41, 43, 45, 48, 49] Uncertainty, in this sense, refers to scientific uncertainty (or "state of knowledge" uncertainty); that is, incomplete understanding by scientists, and not statistical uncertainty (variability of data estimates, e.g., 95% confidence limits).[50, 51]

In acute situations, the public, policy makers, and the press look to health experts for definitive answers—certainty.[14, 16, 21, 26, 52, 53] When health experts cannot provide definitive answers, disagree among themselves (lack consensus), or send mixed or conflicting messages, lay audience uncertainty increases and people can become confused, anxious, fearful, distrustful, or angry.[7, 14, 19, 30, 37, 49] Uncertainty and lack of consensus among scientists, and the subsequent effects of these on lay audiences, can be reduced in many acute situations through further research and knowledge synthesis by scientists. This can happen fairly quickly, for example, when potential or actual infectious disease or other outbreak situations are resolved within a matter of hours or days.[54] In other situations, however, reducing uncertainty among lay audiences may take a long time to develop, or it may not occur at all.

## Communication Process and Message Delivery in Acute Situations

As with other situations, communicating scientific data to lay audiences in acute situations requires that the entire communication process be effective. These are high visibility situations with many potential pitfalls. Especially after an acute situation is recognized, there is an intense hunger among some lay audiences for frequent and up-to-date information.[7, 14, 17–19, 21, 30, 37]

Most people tend to use the expert heuristic to judge the believability of messages based on the perceived credibility of the source in acute situations (Chapters 2 and 3).[55] Relying on the expert heuristic is especially common for topics with which audiences are unfamiliar or have no comparable experience, which is often the case for acute situations involving infectious disease outbreaks or environmental chemical exposures. Thus, the importance of selecting the individual or organization that delivers messages (source) should not be underestimated (Chapter 2). They need to be viewed as highly credible and trusted, which is why, especially during the initial phase of the situation, a high-level scientist or other health professional (e.g., physician or doctorally trained scientist) from a well-respected government agency or research institution is usually the best choice as a communication source.[4, 7] This does not mean, however, that scientists or their respective organizations should not explain the rationale for their recommendations or decisions. Lay audiences want to understand how decisions were reached by experts and to believe that they are empowered and have some role in the process.

There are distinct audiences for communication in acute situations. General public audiences usually can be segmented into three broad groups[30]: (a) those directly exposed, affected, or at risk ("victims"); (b) persons who are physically close to, or involved with, those directly affected (e.g., relatives, friends, neighbors); and (c) others for whom the situation or issue is salient. This last group can range from community members to international audiences. The interest and involvement of policy makers is proportional to whether they perceive themselves as having some role or responsibility for addressing the situation.[56, 57]

Many acute situations generate news media interest,[4, 7, 14, 16, 19–21, 58] and policy-maker interest and involvement increases when news media coverage is frequent.[56, 59, 60] The news media can play a valuable role in disseminating public health messages to large numbers of people.[4, 7, 20, 21, 31, 37] This underscores the importance of developing good relationships with journalists, such as regularly providing them with updates about situations and responding to their requests for further information. Failing to communicate frequently and accurately with the press during such situations can result in media hype, risk amplification, distrust of information sources, and less-optimal decision making by the public and policy makers.[20, 61, 62]

Public health agency partners and other stakeholders (intermediaries) are also important audiences for communication.[7, 23, 30, 37, 63] They may include other government agencies, voluntary or private organizations, health care providers, or law enforcement groups. Stakeholders have an important role separate from that of government agencies for communicating with some lay audiences[63] making it important for health agencies to communicate regularly in acute situations with appropriate partners to minimize the chances of creating mixed messages and confusing audiences.

Table 6.3, adopted from research and practice in crisis communication, describes communication planning based on Pre-Crisis (Event), Crisis, and Post-Crisis phases and is applicable to many acute public health situations. A key aspect of communication planning is that it is critical to have a clear chain of command for communications so that organizations and the individuals within them understand their roles and what they should (and should not) be doing.

Turning to more specific communication practice suggestions, Table 6.4 provides a list of the types of questions that lay audiences can have in acute situations and that may need to be addressed by communicators.[4, 7, 14, 17, 21, 31, 37] Message content and delivery recommendations include

- providing accurate information about the situation, decisions being made, and actions being taken
- using simple and nontechnical language
- using consistent messages

**Table 6.3 Acute public health situations: Communication phases and objectives**

| Phase | Objectives |
| --- | --- |
| *Pre-Crisis*[a] | 1. Be prepared |
| | 2. Foster alliances |
| | 3. Develop consensus recommendations |
| | 4. Test messages |
| *Crisis* (a) Initial | 1. Acknowledge event and uncertainty |
| | 2. Explain and inform audiences, in simple terms, about risk(s) |
| | 3. Establish organizational/spokesperson credibility |
| | 4. Provide emergency courses of action (i.e., how and where to get more information) |
| | 5. Commit to stakeholders and public continued communication |
| *Crisis* (b) Maintenance | 1. Help people more accurately understand their own risks |
| | 2. Provide background and encompassing information to those who need it (e.g., how it happened, whether it has happened before, how to prevent in the future, will recovery occur or whether there will be long-term effects) |
| | 3. Gain understanding and support for response and recovery plans |
| | 4. Listen to stakeholder and audience feedback and correct misinformation |
| | 5. Explain emergency recommendations |
| | 6. Empower risk/benefit decision making |
| *Post-Crisis* (Resolution and evaluation) | 1. Evaluate communication plan performance |
| | 2. Document lessons learned |
| | 3. Determine specific actions to improve crisis systems or the crisis plan |
| | 4. Consider ways to better educate the public response in the event of future similar emergencies |
| | 5. Honestly examine problems and mishaps and then reinforce what worked in the recovery and response efforts |
| | 6. Encourage support for policies or resource allocation to promote effective responses to future acute situations |
| | 7. Promote activities and capabilities of the organization |

*Note*: [a]Crisis and event are often used interchangeably to describe communication phases.

*Source*: Fearn-Banks K. *Crisis Communications: A Casebook Approach*. Mahwah, N.J.: Lawrence Erlbaum; 2002. Coombs WT. *Ongoing Crisis Communication: Planning, Managing, and Responding*. 2nd ed. Thousand Oaks, Calif.: Sage; 2007. Reynolds B, Galdo JH, Sokler L. *Crisis and Emergency Risk Communication*. Atlanta, Ga.: Centers for Disease Control and Prevention; 2002. Seeger MW, Sellnow TL, Ullmer RR. *Communication and Organizational Crisis*. Westport, Conn.: Praeger; 2003.

- providing messages rapidly and regularly
- demonstrating empathy, caring, honesty, openness, commitment, and dedication
- acknowledging the uncertainty of the situation and audience fears or concerns
- correcting misinformation quickly
- not being overly reassuring.

**Table 6.4 Questions lay audiences may have in acute public
health situations**

1. What is the problem and how serious is it (what is happening)?
2. Are my family and I (or community members, friends) safe?
3. Is there a chance that I, or those who matter to me, could be affected?
4. What should I (or others) do to protect myself (themselves)?
5. Who or what caused this problem (how or why did this happen)?
6. What does this information mean (interpretation)?
7. What can we expect will happen?
8. Can the problem be fixed?
9. What is being done to address the problem and why?
10. How are those who are affected getting help?
11. Is the problem being contained (e.g., is the intervention or action working)?
12. When did you begin working on this problem (when were you notified about it, when did you determine that there might be a problem)?
13. Did you have any forewarning that this might happen?
14. Why wasn't this prevented from happening?
15. What else can go wrong? ("worst-case" or "what-if" scenarios)
16. Who is in charge?
17. What is not yet known?
18. What bad (or good) things aren't you telling us?
19. Who can I turn to, or where can I go, to get more information?
20. When will you be providing us with more information?
20. How much will it cost to fix this problem?[a]
21. Who is or will be responsible for paying to fix this problem or compensate those affected for their losses?[a]

*Note*: [a]Primarily from policy makers.
*Source*: Refs (87, 88).

Unlike in some other public health communication activities, developing specific messages for different audiences is not recommended in acute situations. It is essential that the same messages (modified for lower literacy audiences as necessary)[23] be used consistently across audiences to minimize the chance for misunderstanding or accusations of a "cover up."[4] Using multiple communication channels for messages helps to meet the great need for information of different audiences.[7, 30, 37] Internet Web sites can be an especially helpful way to provide more detailed information,[64] such as about scientific processes and data interpretation (e.g., through frequently asked questions (FAQs), fact sheets, or more detailed background papers). Email listservs can be an effective tool to communicate consistent messages to large numbers of people quickly, and to provide regular updates.

Learning more about intended audiences (planning and testing phases of the OPT-In framework, Chapter 5) through formal formative research or usability testing or through informal interviews and discussions, is important in acute situations, especially for those situations likely to be longer lasting, potentially involving large numbers of people, or with a high level of scientific uncertainty. Such research can uncover common audience beliefs, mental models, and preferred communication channels, which can lead to developing improved messages and message delivery.[28]

## Acute Public Health Situation Categories

To help provide more guidance to readers about the selection and presentation of data to communicate to lay audiences in acute situations, it is useful to consider acute public health situations as being within one of two categories: those with lower controversy potential and those with higher controversy potential.

*Lower controversy potential situations* typically involve localized infectious disease outbreaks, natural disasters, or acute chemical exposures, all of which tend to have lower levels of scientific uncertainty.[38, 54, 65] Public health agencies are experienced, for example, in rapidly identifying and ameliorating certain infectious agents that commonly cause certain types of foodborne or water-borne outbreaks.[54]

Such situations typically have several distinguishing characteristics. There is a well-defined and identifiable health outcome for which there is strong scientific consensus that it exists; the outcome is occurring at a higher rate than expected, there is an identifiable cause or agent with a plausible and strong cause-and-effect relationship, and there is a relatively short time period (i.e., within a few days) over which the exposure, outcome, and cause-and-effect relationship are recognized. If a public health intervention or measure is warranted, it falls within acceptable normative beliefs of the public and policy makers based on the potential seriousness or magnitude of the situation or past history of intervention success. In many instances, there may be no organization or individuals perceived as being accountable. Lower controversy potential situations tend to pose fewer challenges concerning communicating data to lay audiences.

*Higher controversy potential situations* are the second major acute public health situation category, and they are basically of three types: (a) an extended outbreak, (b) a scientific consensus at odds with an audience's strongly held beliefs (often because of a changed consensus among scientists), or (c) higher levels of scientific uncertainty exist and adequate or widely accepted resolutions may not occur (Figure 6.1).

Extended outbreak situations often, although not always, result from infectious disease causes. They can occur because of a delay in identifying a definitive cause.[4, 7] Scientists may be confident, for example, that there is

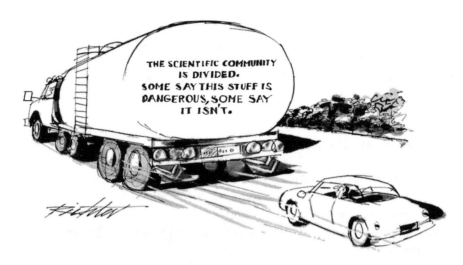

**Figure 6.1** Source: *The New Yorker* magazine.

an infectious or other causal agent (e.g., a chemical exposure or a newly recognized microbial agent, manifestation, or syndrome) but have yet to successfully identify it.[9, 31, 66] More serious health effects such as death, or a dreaded disease or condition; having a large number of people affected or potentially affected; or if the situation has a large geographic scope (multistate or international)[67] will increase controversy potential. Not surprisingly, such situations are popular with journalists who can report on a "mystery" (something new and potentially dangerous) as it unfolds,[68, 69] and it explains why journalists and some other lay audiences want more details about scientific methods, analytic approaches (including data measures), the longer a situation lasts.

Another type of higher controversy potential situation occurs when scientists reach consensus, but their explanations, conclusions, or recommendations are unacceptable to lay audiences, influential organizations, or powerful business interests.[52, 70–72] Such situations are more common for environmental issues, product exposures, or scientific bombshells. Specific examples include psychological explanations for health problems such as anxiety or mass psychogenic illness[8, 73]; negative findings for a suspected problem, exposure, or cause-and-effect relationship between an environmental, occupational, or product exposure and a specific health outcome (e.g., cancer clusters)[72, 74, 75]; major changes in recommendations about health risk behaviors or disease screening[5, 24, 76]; quarantine recommendations; or organizational culpability.[71]

Such situations are difficult from a communication perspective because messages may contradict previous consensus recommendations from scientists (experts), challenge strongly held lay audience beliefs, be at odds with cultural norms, or have potentially severe adverse economic or legal impacts (e.g., removing products from the market or lawsuits). Scientists or their organizations may be challenged about their methodology, data quality, findings, conclusions, or even their professional or personal credibility or motivations.[49, 52]

Situations that involve high levels of scientific uncertainty, almost by definition, have higher controversy potential for lay audiences. From both a scientific and a lay perspective, such situations often fail to result in adequate or widely acceptable resolutions. They usually involve high levels of anxiety or fear among audiences, and often are long-lasting, continuing for months or years, and require extensive and long-term communication efforts with lay audiences.[1, 24, 26] They most likely are the result of

---

**Box 6.3** A higher controversy potential situation: The ban on silicone breast implants

The banning of silicone breast implants demonstrates some of the communication and other challenges involved in attempting to communicate scientific information to lay audiences in a higher scientific uncertainty and higher controversy potential. Women in the United States had access to silicone breast implants, either for cosmetic or reconstructive purposes (e.g., postmastectomy), beginning in the 1970s. Dow Corning was the major U.S. manufacturer of such implants, and use was unregulated before the early 1990s. When the Food and Drug Administration (FDA) banned the implants in 1992, an estimated 1–2 million women were using them.

There had been reports over several years from women with silicone implants complaining of connective-tissue type disorders, such as rheumatoid arthritis or lupus erythematosis; some people were concerned that the implants were the cause of their health problems. Initially, there was some scientific uncertainty about the strength of evidence supporting a cause-and-effect relationship, although the vast majority of studies suggested the absence of an association. (Further research has failed to establish a link between silicone breast implants and connective-tissue disease.)

Contrary to the usual route by which medical devices are approved for use by the public, which requires the manufacturer to show that a product works effectively as claimed, the FDA required manufacturers of silicone

*(continued)*

**Box 6.3** (*continued*)

implants to prove their product was safe. The FDA ultimately decided to ban silicone breast implants because manufacturers could not prove their safety, women were becoming suspicious that the implants were making them ill, and public opinion at the time generally mistrusted the intentions of large corporations such as Dow Corning.

Immediately after the ban went into place, lawyers working for women with implants and the news media widely publicized the FDA decision. Media reports covered the ban and women's health concerns—a few stories even mentioned women who attempted to cut out their own breast implants—but said little about the lack of scientific evidence of a cause-and-effect relationship. Some lawsuits were successful, with information in court from epidemiologists about research trumped by personal testimonials from individual women with connective-tissue disorders. Since the ban, Dow Corning no longer manufactures silicone breast implants. Many women still believe they have been harmed by silicone implants, and lawsuits are ongoing.

Source: Brownson RC, Petitti DB. *Applied Epidemiology: Theory to Practice*. 2nd ed. New York, N.Y.: Oxford University Press; 2006. Sanchez-Guerrero J, Colditz GA, Karlson EW, Hunter DJ, Speizer FE, Liang MH. Silicone breast implants and the risk of connective-tissue diseases and symptoms. *N Engl J Med*. 1995;332(25): 1666–1670. Tugwell P, Wells G, Peterson J, et al. Do silicone breast implants cause rheumatologic disorders? A systematic review for a court-appointed national science panel. *Arthritis Rheum*. 2001;44(11):2477–2484.

environmental, occupational, or product safety or consumer protection issues (Box 6.3).[24, 28, 35, 37, 74]

Scientific uncertainty may exist for one or more aspects of the situation, which may include exposure (e.g., whether it occurred, who was exposed, what constitutes a hazardous level), health outcome (occurrence, definition), cause and effect (whether there is an association between an exposure and an outcome, level of risk), recommendations, or interventions. In some cases, if a potentially adverse health outcome is possible, it may not happen until the distant future (e.g., cancer or infertility). In other situations, adverse health outcomes have occurred but there is no readily identifiable causative agent (e.g., disease clusters, autism).[75]

In comparison to lower controversy potential situations, higher controversy situations require more extensive communication efforts, including communicating about data, with lay audiences. These may include detailed explanations about investigations, causative agents, and descriptions of how scientists reached their conclusions or on what they based their recommendations.[7, 26, 33, 34, 45, 48, 77, 78] They can require extensive explanations of unfamiliar and complex scientific and mathematical terms and concepts.[12, 14, 16–21, 26, 37, 41, 45, 48, 52]

In higher scientific uncertainty and higher controversy potential situations, lay audiences may not be able to rely upon the expert heuristic because scientists do not have definitive answers. Complicating communication is that most lay audiences do not understand scientific or mathematical terms, concepts, or approaches, especially when it comes to probability data (Chapters 1 and 3). Mixed messages from scientists or organizations may occur (e.g., some scientists state that there is a serious risk while others state there is minimal or no risk), which can increase confusion and fear, especially among persons who have difficulty with ambiguity.[26, 53] Lay audiences, then, tend to reach conclusions based on their preexisting beliefs, values, worldviews, and previous experiences (Chapter 3).[42, 52] The news media can compound the problem with hype, emphasizing the scary nature of health outcomes through interviews with concerned individuals, the controversy among scientists, or hints of a cover-up, which can result in social amplification of risk.[20, 21, 61, 62, 79]

Ongoing efforts by scientists, public health practitioners, and others to increase trust by actively engaging community members, listening to their concerns, acknowledging emotions, being empathetic, and empowering audiences to be part of the decision-making process are especially important in this category of acute situations (see Tables 6.3 and 6.4).[4, 7, 12, 18, 21, 24, 26, 37, 39, 41, 80–82]

The two acute public health situation categories described above should not be considered static. A situation may move from higher to lower controversy potential based on more definitive research findings, or a situation initially assessed as a run-of-the-mill local infectious disease outbreak may be found to be much larger in scope or involve an unexpected agent or variation.[83] But these categories can provide a practical scheme for considering communication in acute situations within a larger context and help when it comes to selecting and presenting data to lay audiences.

## Data Selection in Acute Public Health Situations

The stages of the OPT-In framework (organize, plan, test, and integrate) discussed in Chapter 5 are applicable to acute public health situations. From the perspective of selecting and presenting data to lay audiences, however, developing storylines, determining the purpose for communication, and understanding audiences are most relevant and are highlighted in the rest of this chapter.

Storyline

There are many potential storylines for acute public health situations, and they can vary greatly, depending on the level of scientific knowledge and consensus about the potential health outcome or exposure, controversy potential, and length of time over which situations occur. Here are a few examples of science-based storylines:

- Scientists believe that people who take action *A* reduce their chance of developing health condition *B*.
- The main reasons why this situation developed are *X* and *Y*.
- Scientists cannot determine at this time whether there is an excess health risk associated with exposure to chemical *A*.

When considering selecting and presenting data to lay audiences in an acute situation, the first determination is whether data-containing messages are needed to support the storyline. In many acute situations, there is no need to communicate data, particularly if messages are more action- or recommendation-oriented (e.g., do these things; don't do those things). However, data-containing messages can help to communicate storylines in many such situations, particularly for description or explanation.[3, 7, 84–88]

Purpose

Selecting data to present to lay audiences depends on the communication purpose. As discussed elsewhere in this book, purpose can be categorized as being designed to increase knowledge, instruct, facilitate decision making, or persuade. Instructing audiences is common in acute situations, such as about specific actions to take to prevent injury in the event of a natural disaster. Data are not needed when instruction is the communication purpose.

Data, however, can be helpful when used for one of the other three purposes. Trying to increase knowledge without regard to facilitating decision making or attempting to persuade audiences is a common communication purpose in these types of situations. It usually takes the form of letting audiences know the current status of the situation, the events taking place, and what health departments or other organizations are doing to address it. Data used for this purpose often consist of regularly reporting the magnitude of the problem, especially the number of people affected or potentially affected, for example, "As of September 15th, there have been 16 confirmed cases of Norwalk virus among persons who camped at Smith Park." Facilitating informed decision making sometimes is the communication purpose, especially for situations with higher level of scientific uncertainty and higher controversy potential.[26, 89] Data may help lay audiences weigh the risks and benefits of certain actions, such as whether to continue the use of a consumer product.

Persuasion is also a common purpose in acute situations, and data can be used in many ways to provide evidentiary matter. Data can, for instance, help explain why scientists believe in the presence of a cause-and-effect relationship, their rationale for action, or the effectiveness of an intervention (evaluation).[26, 42] Conversely, data can be used for persuasion in the reverse direction, in other words to reassure lay audiences that an exposure is not hazardous, no cause-and-effect relationship exists, or no action is needed.[26, 42]

As discussed in Chapter 3, data selection for persuasion in acute as well as other types of situations depends on whether they are being used to maximize or minimize levels of concern among lay audiences, recognizing that the choice of relative or absolute risk estimates can make different contributions as to whether risk is likely to be perceived as being higher or lower.[90]

## Audience Analysis

Understanding audiences is a key aspect of communicating in acute situations. Because of the high level of interest and limited scientific and quantitative literacy of lay audiences (Chapter 3), it is essential to carefully define and describe terms and concepts.[4, 7, 45, 80] Some acute situations where data need to be presented involve complex science and mathematics, especially probability (risk) data, which are difficult for lay audiences to comprehend (Chapter 3),[26, 39] especially in higher controversy potential situations. Presenting statistical uncertainty data, for instance, may result in some lay audiences, especially persons with lower levels of quantitative or document literacy (Chapter 3), having lower levels of trust for scientists because they perceive them to be demonstrating vagueness.[91, 92]

More extensive, clear, and complete communication efforts may be needed to help lay audiences understand how scientists study a situation, how they reached their conclusions (e.g., describing scientific or statistical methods), or the limits of science to resolve the issue at hand.[93] Examples or analogies that illustrate what a scientific or statistical term means—or does not mean—can help increase understanding and avoid misconceptions.[26, 45, 48, 94, 95] Persons with low scientific and quantitative literacy, however, are capable of increasing their understanding of complex concepts and phenomena when it is salient to them and information is communicated well (Chapter 2).[49, 52, 96]

Communicators sometimes consider using risk data comparisons as an approach for increasing understanding among lay audiences. There has been much research on the way lay audiences understand risk comparison data in acute situations when they are provided as contextual information to help with data interpretation.[32, 43, 97–101] However, because lay audiences make judgments about what constitutes risk across multiple dimensions besides scientific data,[52] the choice of comparison data needs to be carefully considered.[26, 43, 45, 101]

If risk comparison data are used, they must be appropriate to the situation[37, 101–104]; comparisons should not be seen as trivial or unimportant by audiences, such as the risk of cancer associated with eating small amounts of peanut butter.[45] Comparisons with involuntary risk factors can be used if they involve a health risk associated with an exposure familiar to audiences, such as the disease risk associated with the therapeutic use of x-rays, being struck by a meteor, or dying from an animal bite (e.g., "Scientists estimate that the chance of an individual developing condition $Y$ based on exposure to chemical $Z$ is less than one in a million, which is similar to the risk of dying from a spider bite"). Comparing an involuntary with a voluntary risk factor, such as cigarette smoking or alcohol use, may not be a good idea for some audiences, as some people make a clear distinction between risks they voluntarily choose versus those imposed on them.[43, 45, 97]

## Types of Data Measures to Use in Communication

As shown in Table 6.4, lay audiences have many questions and concerns when acute public situations occur. Although most are not data-related, the selection and presentation of data can help to address some of these concerns.[105, 106] These lay audience concerns, when considered in conjunction with the purpose for communication and the roles that data can play, provide guidance for selecting data to communicate (Table 6.5). These concerns of audiences addressable using data are interrelated and build upon each other; for example, "what is being done about it and why" requires at least some answers (or hypotheses) for previous concerns. But communicators may not need to address all five concerns, let alone use data to do so, in every situation. As shown in Table 6.5, only a limited number of data measures are likely to be needed to communicate to lay audiences in most acute situations.

*What's happening* refers to collecting the basic information needed to inform audiences about the situation for the purpose of increasing knowledge. Descriptive data that can answer the questions of what, who, where, and when, that is, the basic epidemiologic measures of person, place, and time,[107] are usually sufficient. Frequencies, percentages, or in some instances, rates, should suffice, especially for most infectious disease outbreaks. By definition, because outbreaks involve an increase over the expected or background rate (in many instances, the background rate is zero), trends can help

**Table 6.5 Major considerations when selecting data to present to lay audiences in acute public health situations**

| Audience concern | Communication purpose | Role for data | • Data measures |
|---|---|---|---|
| What is happening? | • Increase knowledge | Description (what, who, where, when) | • Frequencies (counts)<br>• Percentages<br>• Rates |
| How and why is it happening? | • Increase knowledge<br>• Persuasion | Explanation (cause and effect) | • Frequencies<br>• Probability (risk) |
| What does it mean? (interpretation) | • Persuasion<br>• Facilitate informed decision making | Review and synthesis<br>Context<br>Statistical uncertainty | • Frequencies<br>• Percentages<br>• Rates<br>• Probability (risk)<br>• Reference or population standards<br>• Confidence intervals or data ranges |
| What is being done about it and why? (rationale for action) | • Persuasion<br>• Facilitate informed decision making | Review and synthesis | • Probability (risk)<br>• Percentage (especially relative percentage) |
| Is the action working? (evaluation) | • Increase knowledge<br>• Persuasion<br>• Facilitate informed decision making | Evaluation | • Frequencies<br>• Rates<br>• Probability (risk change)<br>• Percentage (especially percentage change) |

*Source*: Cohn V, Cope L. *News and Numbers: A Guide to Reporting Statistical Claims and Controversies in Health and Other Fields.* 2nd ed. Ames, Iowa: Iowa State Press; 2001. Nelson DE, Brownson RC, Remington PL, Parvanta C, eds. *Communicating Public Health Information Effectively: A Guide for Practitioners.* Washington, D.C.: American Public Health Association; 2002. Reynolds B. *Crisis and Emergency Risk Communication: By Leaders for Leaders.* Atlanta, Ga.: Centers for Disease Control and Prevention; 2004.

provide context for lay audiences to understand why public health professionals believe that there may be a problem.[108, 109]

Simple descriptive findings such as frequencies that address the concern about what's happening are probably the only necessary data to communicate to lay audiences in many acute situations.[3, 7, 106, 110] The need to communicate additional types of data to address the remaining audience concerns will increase proportionately based on the presence and number of factors listed in Table 6.2 (e.g., dreaded disease, identifiable persons, media coverage) and level of scientific uncertainty.

The second concern that data can help answer is *how and why it is happening.* Data for this concern are explanatory in nature, with the goal of uncovering cause-and-effect relationships. Research, at least initially, typically involves "shoe leather" epidemiology, that is, rapid investigations by health department epidemiologists.[54] The communication purpose may be to increase knowledge or for persuasion. Depending on how a situation unfolds over time, communicating about cause-and-effect relationships may be preliminary (e.g., hypotheses or best guesses) or more definitive (e.g., consumption of food X at restaurant Y was the likely cause of the Salmonella outbreak; there is no relationship between community groundwater contamination from chemical A and birth defect B).

Although simple descriptive data, such as frequencies, may be used, more often probability (risk) data are used to ascertain cause-and-effect relationships, especially relative risks (e.g., odds ratios, rate ratios).[91, 111] Note that if there are delays in identifying the presence or absence of cause-and-effect relationships, if expected cause-and-effect relationships are not borne out (e.g., disease clusters), or if the level of scientific uncertainty remains high over time, then the complexity of data analyses, and subsequently the types of data that need to be translated to lay audiences to help explain how and why, will likely be more complex.

The next concern that data can help address is *what does it mean*, or interpretation. This involves synthesizing the descriptive and cause-and-effect data used to answer the concerns of "what is happening" and "how and why is it happening" with additional information (e.g., past experiences or prior knowledge based on the scientific literature among scientists investigating the problem). The purpose of communicating about data for this audience concern is primarily for persuasion or to facilitate informed decision making, and several data measures may be helpful for interpretation (Table 6.5). Data can be used to let audiences know (a) if public health professionals believe if a problem does or does not exist, (b) what population groups are or are not at increased risk for an adverse health condition or outcome, (c) the magnitude of the problem, or (d) contextual information for assessing the situation.

Interpretation is straightforward in many instances, especially for lower controversy potential situations resulting from infectious disease outbreaks. Determining whether a problem exists, what populations are at increased risk, the magnitude of risk, and the context become obvious fairly quickly, as the expected or background number of cases or rates is low, a specific cause is found, and those exposed or at greatest risk are identified. Although interpreting findings for lay audiences is facilitated by using different types of information, frequencies of the number of affected individuals are probably all that is needed in most situations.

At the opposite end of the spectrum, interpretation is no simple matter in acute situations involving many environmental, occupational, or consumer product exposures, or with scientific "bombshells" (i.e., higher controversy potential situations). There are many examples of pitfalls that scientists can face when attempting to communicate their interpretations with lay audiences.[16, 17, 24, 26, 43, 81] Such situations usually require extensive communication efforts to present and explain methodology, analyses, and scientific and mathematical concepts.

Difficulties arise because it may not be evident that there is a health-related problem present, whether a cause-and-effect relationship exists, or the level of risk. In some situations, level of risk can be estimated but there is no consensus among scientists about the meaning of the magnitude health risk, or answers to the challenge of communicating probability data involving very large or very small numbers (e.g., 3 in 100,000) to lay audiences (Chapter 3).[28, 40, 65, 93, 112–114] A further complication is that because some research is based on population probabilities, it is difficult or impossible to ascertain which specific individuals are at higher risk.

If scientists conclude that the probability of an adverse health outcome, if present, is likely to be minimal, an absolute risk estimate, rather than a relative risk estimate, is a better choice for helping frame a minimal risk message to lay audiences (Chapter 4). Also as mentioned in Chapter 4, absolute risk data can be expressed using different formats such as "Only four persons out of a million are likely to develop the disease based on this exposure"; "Among persons exposed at the highest levels, we estimate that the increased risk of long-term health effects is less than 1%," but such data need to be explained clearly to help ensure audience comprehension.

The next major concern of lay audiences that data can help answer is *what is being done about it and why*, or the rationale for action. Rationale is based on reviewing and synthesizing prior research and experiences in the context of the current situation. In many acute situations, especially those with lower controversy potential, it is not necessary for public health professionals to communicate data to audiences to explain the rationale for their actions or recommendations; most lay audiences, especially initially, will rely on the expert heuristic and assume that actions taken or recommended are based on a solid science.

Myriad public health actions and communication messages to lay audiences about them are possible depending on the situation (e.g., closing a body of water to swimming, instituting a mandatory vaccination policy, recommending screening by health care providers, conducting a trace-back study of a specific product or lot, or taking no action). Conversely, communication may involve providing messages to the public, policy makers, or press to discourage actions already underway or under consideration.

Some public health actions may be viewed with skepticism by lay audiences, hence the value of communicating data to support them; for such communications, the primary purpose for communicating data is for persuasion (the rationale is sound) or to facilitate informed decision making. Although different measures may be used depending on the situation, the most common data for demonstrating the rationale for action are probability data, especially relative risk or relative percentage point changes (usually reductions) expected to occur, or occurring, because of the action, for example, "this vaccination should reduce the chance of developing illness by more than 99%."

The last concern for which data can be used to address lay audience concerns is, Is the action working? This is a question that evaluation research data can help answer. Depending upon the audience and their level of involvement with the situation, the purpose for data communication may be to increase knowledge, persuade, or facilitate informed decision making. Data used for evaluation in acute, as well as in other situations, are designed to demonstrate whether a change occurred as a result of the action taken or the intervention occurring. Data measures used will typically be the same as those used for describing what happened or the rationale for action, such as changes in frequencies (e.g., the number of cases of disease), percentages, rates, or probability (risk).

Change can be presented in relative or absolute terms, for example, a relative percent decrease in frequency or a decrease in the absolute risk of developing a health condition. Because the magnitude of relative and absolute differences often differ greatly (Chapter 3), the choice of which data measure to use, or a decision to use both relative and absolute data differences, depends on the purpose of communication, ethical considerations, and audience characteristics (e.g., cognitive processing limits, level of involvement, quantitative literacy).

## Data Presentation in Acute Public Health Situations

Once decisions have been made about what data should be communicated to lay audiences, it is time to consider the modalities for presenting them. In this section we review these options and provide recommendations for presenting data in acute lower and higher controversy potential public health situations.

### General Considerations

Public health data can be presented verbally, visually, or through some combination of the two (Chapter 4). There are several general recommendations discussed in Chapter 4 that apply to presentations in acute situations, especially including integrating words, numbers, and symbols. For visual modalities, it is essential to use titles, labels, legends, and other contextual cues, including text. Visual data comparisons are important cues because they provide important contextual information to assist with audience understanding; they are especially relied upon by people with little or no familiarity with the specific issue at hand, or when the mathematical or scientific information is complex,[55, 115, 116] both of which often happen in acute situations. (The term data comparison, as used here, does not refer to comparison of involuntary with voluntary risk data discussed earlier in this chapter.)

For acute situations, recommended data comparisons for acute situations include (a) trends over time, (b) geographic area differences, or (c) to established reference standards (e.g., maximum acceptable levels) previously published by reputable scientific organizations or government agencies. (Figure 6.2, note the dark arrow in the middle of the figure that contains the EPA recommended limit).[37, 45, 102–104, 109] Comparisons can be shown in different ways (Chapter 4), for example, trend lines for other populations such as national or state estimates, lines or arrows demonstrating referent levels, comparison bars in a bar chart, or using different colors or shading for different geographic regions on maps. Trend data are generally well understood by both lay and scientific audiences and are especially valuable in acute situations because they can have roles in description, explanation, and evaluation.

There are several data presentation modalities that are less commonly used by public health scientists and practitioners in acute situations. Narratives, which are especially helpful to gain audience attention or raise awareness about a particular problem, rarely are appropriate, as attention and awareness levels are usually already high among lay audiences. Although pie charts are easy for lay audiences to grasp (Chapter 4), their use is usually limited to helping people judge the magnitude of proportions as a part of a whole (i.e., to 100%), which is rarely relevant in most acute situations. Although pie charts can sometimes be used for data comparisons, such comparisons can better be demonstrated using other modalities, especially bar charts.

Turning now to presentation choices more commonly used, verbal presentations of data can be an effective option and may be all that are necessary in lower controversy potential situations.[3, 7, 85–88] One or two numbers can be included as part of written text or spoken words designed for lay audiences; for example, "6 people were hospitalized with severe respiratory difficulties today after they were exposed to toxic levels of sulfuric acid at company *Z* after an explosion."

Verbal qualifiers without numbers (e.g., "greater risk," "rare," "many people were affected") are especially helpful for interpreting for lay audiences what data mean. Examples include quantifying specific exposures or populations at higher risk, "prior research has shown that this strain of *E. coli* is more likely to result in severe illness than other strains," or "persons aged 65 years or older are at the greatest risk of heart-related illnesses."[48] Verbal qualifiers also

## Cancer Deaths from Lifetime Radon Exposure

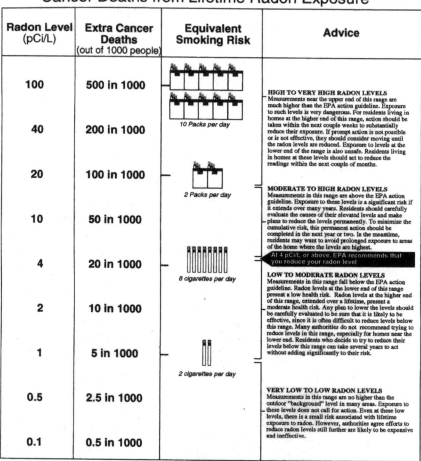

**Figure 6.2** Use of a reference standard in a table to provide a contextual clue about risk data. (Source: Lipkus IM, Hollands JG. Visual communication of risk. *Monogr J Natl Cancer Inst.* 1999;25:149–162.)

can describe what is being done and why (rationale for action) or for evaluation: "discontinuing the use of chemical *Z* in the production process drastically reduced the number of individuals with severe allergic reactions."

Metaphors are sometimes used in acute situations and typically are in the form of data analogies that make comparisons with topics and numbers likely to be familiar to lay audiences (e.g., "the 1 in ____ risk of developing serious gastrointestinal bleeding discovered among users of medication *P* is similar to that of persons taking a daily aspirin tablet"). As discussed previously, data risk comparisons can be tricky in acute situations, especially if the comparison is to involuntarily assumed risks.

Turning to visual modalities, tables, which are used to present a larger number of numbers, are usually not a common choice. If used at all, they are more likely to be used in longer lasting acute situations, such as a short list of the number of people experiencing a health condition or exposure by state or county.[117] Bar charts are the most common and versatile choice for visually presenting data in acute situations, as they can demonstrate overall or comparative magnitudes for frequencies, percentages, or probability (risk) data (Chapter 4).[91, 109, 118] They can also be used to demonstrate trends although line graphs are a better choice for this use. Bar charts can be used for description, explanation, or evaluation (Figure 6.3) and also contain comparison data, such as including reference standards or national population numbers.

As discussed in Chapter 4, line graphs are the most effective way to demonstrate trends.[108, 109, 117, 119] Similar to bar charts, they can be used for description, explanation, or evaluation in acute situations and can allow audiences to compare data from the acute situation to a reference standard or some type of population data.[109] Line graphs are especially helpful for visualizing changes in disease frequencies or rates before and after interventions or actions occur (evaluation).

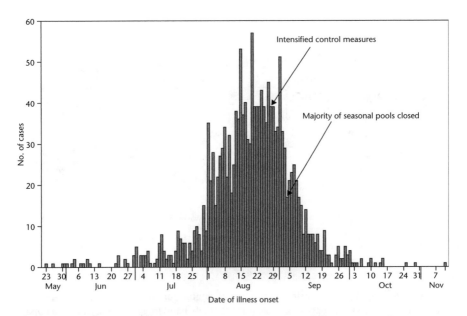

**Figure 6.3** Bar chart demonstrating the impact of implementing intensive control measures for controlling a large cryptosporidium outbreak in Utah during 2007. (Source: Rolfs RT, Beach MJ, Hlavsa MC, Calanan RM. Community cryptosporidiosis outbreak—Utah, 2007. *MMWR*. 2008;57:989–993.)

Maps or diagrams can be used with lay audiences in some acute situations for description or explanation.[120, 121] Maps can demonstrate where a situation is occurring (Figure 6.4) and can provide context by visually demonstrating geographic comparisons. Diagrams, such as of a particular facility in which an outbreak occurred, can be helpful for cause-and-effect explanations in some instances, for example, showing where certain exposures physically occurred within a facility or area (Figure 6.5).[120]

Icons and visual scales (Chapter 4) can be considered for use in some higher controversy potential situations. Icons are usually used to help communicate probability (risk) data to lay audiences, especially absolute risk data. Risk scales can show relative or absolute magnitude of risk along a data continuum in ascending or descending order (e.g., from 0.001 to 1,000) (Chapter 4) (Figure 6.6).[37, 91, 99, 122–125] These presentation options are more commonly used in environmental, occupational, or consumer product situations, such as attempting to help increase audience knowledge and understanding of low probability data. These formats are not readily intuitive and require more explanation to lay audiences than do other visual modalities (e.g., in clinical or small group settings), and may not be feasible in situations with limited or no research about health risks.

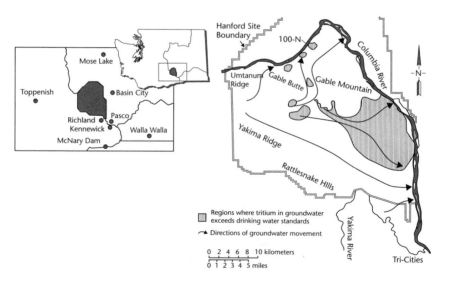

**Figure 6.4** Maps demonstrating groundwater contamination from tritium associated with Hanford (WA) nuclear site. Note that the left-hand map includes an inset map to help orient viewers to the relevant geographic region in Washington state. (Source: Lundgren RE, McMakin AH. *Risk Communication: A Handbook for Communicating Environmental, Safety, and Health Risks* 3rd Ed. Columbus, Ohio: Battelle Press; 2004:222–223. Pacific Northwest National Laboratory.)

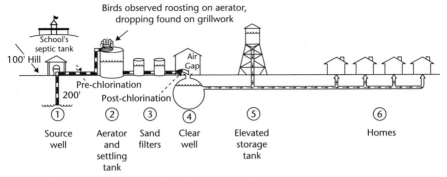

Birds observed roosting on aerator, dropping found on grillwork

School's septic tank

100' Hill

Pre-chlorination

200'

Post-chlorination

Air Gap

① Source well
② Aerator and settling tank
③ Sand filters
④ Clear well
⑤ Elevated storage tank
⑥ Homes

1. No evidence of contamination with coliform bacteria (based on laboratory testing of specimens)
2. No specimens collected for testing
3. Laboratory-confirmed contamination
4. Laboratory-confirmed contamination
5. No evidence of contamination
6. Laboratory-confirmed contamination

**Figure 6.5** Diagram showing process by which a community's water supply was contaminated by *Campylobacter Jejuni*. (Source: Sacks JJ, Lieb S, Baldy LM, et al. Epidemic campylobacteriosis associated with a community water supply. *Am J Public Health*. 1986;76:424–429. p. 425.)

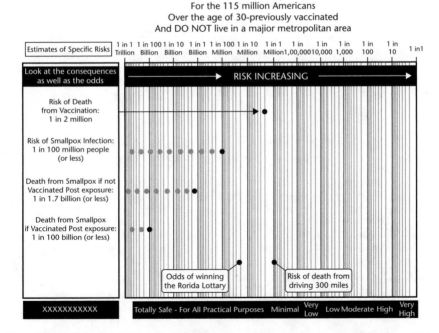

**Figure 6.6** Use of a risk ladder to demonstrate absolute risks associated with smallpox and smallpox vaccination. (Source: Paling J. Strategies to help patients understand risks. *BMJ*. 2003;327:745–748:745.)

245

There are a couple of final points to consider. Depending on the audience concern being addressed, data can be presented using two or more formats simultaneously, such as by presenting one or two numbers (*what's happening*) in conjunction with verbal qualifiers (*what does it mean*). Also, the longer an acute situation continues, the more likely it is that scientists and public health practitioners will need to use different types of data presentations with lay audiences to help describe or explain current status or recent developments.

## Presentation Recommendations: Lower Controversy Potential Situations

Data presentation to lay audiences for lower controversy potential situations is usually relatively straightforward (Table 6.6). One or two numbers, verbal qualifiers, or both will often suffice.[3, 7] Frequencies of the affected number of individuals ("Ten people developed severe headaches and nausea and two people became unconscious while attending an ice hockey game at the city arena last night") are commonly the only type of data needed. Visual modalities are often unnecessary; if used, bar charts to demonstrate frequency or relative risk magnitudes, or simple maps showing the location of affected geographic areas (e.g., towns or neighborhoods), are good choices.

Box 6.4 illustrates the use of data in a typical lower controversy situation (in this instance, an infectious disease outbreak). From a data perspective, it is evident that most of the information provided to lay audiences did not involve data. Note, however, the inclusion of contextual text cues and interpretation of findings based on the investigation.

**Table 6.6 Data format options in lower and higher controversy potential situations**

| Data format option | Lower controversy potential situations | Higher controversy potential situations |
| --- | :---: | :---: |
| One or two numbers | √ | √ |
| Verbal qualifier | √ | √ |
| Metaphor | | √ |
| Table | | √ |
| Bar chart | √ | √ |
| Line graph | √ | √ |
| Map or diagram | √ | √ |
| Icons | | √ |
| Visual scale | | √ |

*Note*: These are general guidelines, as choices can vary widely by specific situation and length of time it lasts, and multiple formats may be appropriate.

**Box 6.4** Communicating about data in a lower controversy potential situation: An *E. coli* 0157 outbreak in Oregon

The Oregon Health Division identified an outbreak of *E. coli* 0157 disease among persons who attended a gathering at a residential religious camp in Yamhill county in May 2005. The investigation ultimately found 12 laboratory-confirmed *E. coli* 0157 cases. This bacteria causes severe diarrhea (often bloody) and abdominal cramps, but can be more serious in a small percentage of people who can develop kidney failure. Infection can be contracted through a variety of means, ranging from eating undercooked beef to swimming in contaminated water, and is easily spread by person-to-person contact.

The Health Division issued a press release on May 27, 2005, about the outbreak and the investigation (see below), which covered several key points and recommendations. Note that only limited amounts of data were included in the press release. One statement mentions the number of people potentially at risk for the illness (120); one data-containing element is that about 5% of infected persons develop kidney complications; and finally, time trend data provide context, noting that about 117 cases of *E. coli* 0157 occurred in the state annually over the past 5 years.

**Oregon DHS news release**

**May 27, 2005**

*Public health officials investigate Yamhill E.Coli 0157 outbreak*

A cluster of E.coli 0157 illnesses among people who attended a gathering at Camp Yamhill in northwest Yamhill County is being investigated by state and county public health officials.

As many as 120 people who attended a gathering there between May 17 and 20 may be at risk of illness, said Mel Kohn, M.D., state epidemiologist in the Oregon Department of Human Services (DHS).

"We are actively investigating this outbreak," said Kohn. "We will continue to inform the public as we determine extent of illness and ultimately the source of infection."

Anyone attending the camp on May 16 or after and who has diarrhea should contact their local health department; if they have bloody diarrhea they should seek medical care. People with diarrhea should drink plenty of fluids, Kohn advised.

Symptoms of E.coli infection include diarrhea, often bloody, and cramps. About 5 percent of cases develop kidney problems. Children are particularly at risk of kidney complications from E.coli 0157, which can lead to kidney failure and death, Kohn said.

E.Coli is easily spread from person to person. Frequent handwashing, especially after using the toilet, can prevent spread.

*(continued)*

247

**Box 6.4** (continued)

DHS and six county health departments—Clackamas, Lane, Marion, Multnomah, Polk and Yamhill—are actively investigating the outbreak.

The camp has voluntarily closed until the source of the illness is identified, Kohn said.

An average of 117 E.coli O157 cases have been reported each year in Oregon over the past five years. Common ways of acquiring the infection include eating undercooked ground beef, touching infected animals, drinking unpasteurized milk, juice or contaminated water, swimming in contaminated water and contracting the illness from another person.

Source: Oregon Department of Human Services. *DHS News Release: Public Health Officials Investigate Yamhill E. coli 0157 Outbreak.* Portland, Or.; 2005. Lore Lee and June Bancroft. Personal communication. Oregon Health Division, July 12, 2006.

## Presentation Recommendations: Higher Controversy Potential Situations

Given the heterogeneity of higher controversy potential situations, there are many data presentation options that range from simple to complex. An extended outbreak that lasts for several weeks may only require regularly providing updates of one or two numbers, such as the number of persons diagnosed with a disease.

Conversely, certain situations, especially those involving environmental, occupational, consumer product issues, and actual or potential exposures, may involve attempting to communicate about complex scientific or statistical concepts. In addition to using verbal options to communicate about data (one or two numbers; verbal qualifiers), any, and sometimes all, of the presentation options listed in Table 6.6 may be used over the course of time.

Box 6.5 provides a case study on data presentation to lay audiences for the SARS disease outbreak in 2003.[9, 126, 127] It is an example of an extended multinational infectious disease outbreak that garnered worldwide media attention. Scientists in many countries worked diligently to determine the causal agent and institute protective measures. Note that most data included in the updates from the World Health Organization (WHO) and the CDC were frequencies: the number of persons with SARS (new or cumulative number of cases), the number of deaths, and the number of countries involved. A few data in the form of percentages (e.g., percentage of cases who were health workers) were also included.

**Box 6.5** Data communication in a higher controversy potential situation: 2003 worldwide SARS extended outbreak

Severe Acute Respiratory Syndrome (SARS) is a respiratory disease (often in the form of pneumonia) caused by a previously unrecognized virus. SARS first appeared in China in November 2002 and was recognized as a global health threat in March 2003. Over the course of the outbreak, it was evident early on that the illness was contagious and that some type of microbial agent was the likely cause, although it took several weeks before the actual virus was identified. By the time the outbreak was over in July 2003, nearly 8,100 persons were considered to have had probable cases of SARS, 774 of which died. Cases were reported from more than 30 countries in 6 continents, with most cases occurring in a few Asian countries (China, Viet Nam, Singapore, and Taiwan). About 20% of persons with SARS were health care workers.

The World Health Organization (WHO) took a major lead in communication efforts concerning SARS as there was enormous interest worldwide throughout the course of this large and extended outbreak. Such efforts involved coordinating communication with major health agencies and organizations in other countries, including the CDC in the United States. Frequent updates and current communication products were regularly provided to the news media and others by WHO, CDC, and health organizations in other countries through several formats. These included press releases, press conferences, telebriefings, fact sheets, daily summary tables of suspect and probable cases (by WHO), Morbidity and Mortality Weekly Reports (by CDC), and frequently asked question (FAQ) sheets. From March 15 through July 5, 2003, the WHO alone published 96 SARS updates. WHO and CDC Web sites were especially important communication channels and repositories of information by health care providers for the public, policy makers, and the press who were looking for more information.

Communication messages by WHO and CDC covered many different aspects of the outbreak, such as which countries were affected, progress in identifying the causative agent, diagnosis and treatment, steps taken to control the outbreak, prevention, and travel advisories. However, data, in the form of simple frequencies, were a regular component of most of the information updates. WHO and CDC routinely stated the number of suspected or probable cases of SARS, the countries in which they occurred, and the number of deaths. To help provide context, both the number of new SARS cases since the previous report and the number of cumulative cases since the start of the outbreak were usually included. Below are several excellent examples that illustrate the effective reporting of simple but consistent SARS data over time.

*(continued)*

249

**Box 6.5** (continued)

**March 16, 2003 (WHO Update 1):** As of 15 March 2003, reports of over 150 cases of Severe Acute Respiratory Syndrome (SARS) have been received by the World Health Organization since 26 February 2003...As of 15 March the majority of cases have occurred in people who have had very close contact with other cases, and over 90% of cases have occurred among health care workers.

**March 24, 2003 (WHO Update 8):** Reports from health authorities in 13 countries, compiled today, indicate a cumulative total of 456 cases of SARS and 17 deaths. This compares with reports a week ago (17 March) of 150 cases in 7 countries.

**April 24, 2003 (Telebriefing by CDC Director Julie Gerberding):** I'm here to provide an update on SARS, the Severe Acute Respiratory Syndrome, and to follow up on some of the information that was presented in today's MMWR, the *Morbidity and Mortality Weekly Report*, that CDC has published. WHO is reporting 4,402 cases of SARS; 263 deaths in 26 countries overall. In the United States, we are tabulating 247 cases of SARS, 39 of these are probable.

**June 18, 2003 (WHO Update 83):** Tomorrow will mark the 100th day since WHO first alerted the world, on 12 March, to the SARS threat. From the 55 cases recognized on that day, alarmingly concentrated in hospitals in Hong Kong, Hanoi, and Singapore, the outbreak within a month went on to cause some 3,000 cases and more than 100 deaths in 20 countries on all continents...Although the causative agent was conclusively identified on 17 April, the disease had no vaccine, no effective treatment, an overall case fatality of 15%, and many unexplained features...During the peak of the global outbreak, near the start of May, more than 200 new cases were being reported each day. Detection of new infections subsequently slowed, passing 8,000 on 22 May.

Source: Centers for Disease Control and Prevention. *Severe Acute Respiratory Syndrome (SARS)*. Atlanta, Ga.: Centers for Disease Control and Prevention; 2007. World Health Organization. *Severe Acute Respiratory Syndrome (SARS)*. Geneva, Switzerland: World Health Organization; 2007.

Different (and more complex) data presentation modalities may be appropriate for other types of situations. For example, if scientists determine that if a cause and effect exists but the level of risk is minimal, data presentation to lay audiences may involve using bar charts or risk scales to try to explain probability using absolute risk estimates.

The case study in Box 6.6 is an example of communicating data in another type of higher controversy potential situation for a noninfectious disease

**Box 6.6** Data communication in a higher controversy potential situation: Bjork-Shiley heart valve notification

Research in the late 1980s demonstrated that persons who had received a Bjork-Shiley mitral heart valve were at increased risk of experiencing sudden failure (fracture) of the device. The effects of valve failure can be catastrophic, including potentially causing heart failure, respiratory difficulty, irregular heartbeat, shock, cardiac arrest, or sudden death, and prompt diagnosis and treatment is essential. A congressional hearing was held in 1990 about the problem with the valves. Ironically, although the potential effects of failure were serious, the risk of valve failure was lower than the risk associated with elective surgical replacement. Later in 1990, the Food and Drug Administration (FDA) was informed by the manufacturer that it planned to develop a patient notification program for the 23,000 persons estimated to have the surgically implanted valves.

Working closely with the FDA, Shiley Incorporated developed a notification letter for patients and physicians. Focus group research was conducted with patients and risk communication experts to improve the message content; the letter ultimately contained information that described the valve problem, the associated risks, recommended actions, and a personal appeal. Absolute risk estimates were included in the letter, stating that the annual risk of valve failure ranged from about 2 valves per 10,000 to about 29 per 10,000, depending on the size of the valve and date of manufacture. The letter also pointed out the much greater risk (about 5 out of 100) associated with elective reoperation to replace the valve.

Follow-up evaluation found that about 90% of patients who received the letter understood the material, 55% felt relief rather than irritation upon reading the material, and 72% reported being satisfied with the notification program and believed the program was appropriate. Although the majority of those who received the notification letter reported understanding it, as is often the case in such situations, not everyone was satisfied. Further evaluation research resulted in modifications to the letter, as additional research about the risk estimates associated with valve use became available and communicators recognized that the initial letter did not adequately explain the symptoms associated with valve failure or the need for persons to have an emergency plan to locate an appropriate hospital with open-heart surgery capacity. In addition, several lawsuits were filed against the manufacturer.

Source: Food and Drug Administration. *Shiley C-C Heart Valve Alert.* Washington, D.C.: FDA Consumer; 1990. Farley D. Shiley saga leads to improved communication. *FDA Consumer* 1994;28(1):12–17. Department of Health and Human Services. *Recommendations to Improve Health Risk Communication: A Report on Case Studies in Health Risk Communication.* Washington, D.C.: Department of Health and Human Services, Environmental Policy Committee, Subcommittee on Risk Communication and Education; 1994.

**Box 6.7** Communicating data in a higher controversy potential situation: Environmental exposure associated with a resource recovery (industrial recycling) plant in New York

A resource recovery plant in Hempstead, New York, had been closed because of economic reasons and because the technology used produced unpleasant odors noticeable in the community. In 1981, state and local officials were attempting to determine if the plant could safely reopen; however, many community members believed it had been closed because the U.S. Environmental Protection Agency had discovered that the plant was emitting dioxin compounds. The owners of the facility contacted two professors at Cornell University to try to explain potential risks; however, when their findings were reported to the community in a local high school gymnasium, residents left angry and confused. A citizens' advisory committee (CAC), with funding support from the New York City Department of Sanitation, was appointed by a county executive to oversee a health risk assessment. This committee had broad support from the public (trust), who had had input into the selection of health experts. Members of the CAC endorsed the fairness and thoroughness of the process and expressed their support to news reporters.

The scientific findings from the risk assessment were communicated effectively to community members in several ways. Two physicians from Mt. Sinai Medical Center, who were members of the CAC, reported that the overall health effects of the plant would be minimal and nondetectable (verbal qualifiers), which was far easier for lay audiences to understand than that the quantitative risks were "in the range of 0.24 to $5.9 \times 10^{-6}$." To help provide context to help lay audiences understand what the overall risk numbers meant, the public was informed that the added average risk for county residents was 0.11 every 70 years or about one additional case of cancer every 600 years.

Meaningful specific data comparisons were also provided. The press reported that the maximum health risk from the resource recovery facility of 1.7 in a million was less than the risk of 2.4 in a million that the public was exposed to by drinking and showering each day using the local chlorinated public water supply. In addition, estimated maximal polychlorinated biphenyl (PCB) exposure in the community resulting from the resource facility was compared with average PCB levels found in kitchens from a study in New York State, and it was reported that existing PCB levels in these kitchens were about 10,000 times higher.

Source: Ref. (82).

situation (a problem with a medical consumer product). Although the magnitude of health risk associated with the Bjork-Shiley heart valve was clearly evident to scientists (i.e., low scientific uncertainty), communicating about the risks and benefits of the valve, and valve removal, to lay audiences was difficult. Much formative research was conducted prior to the Shiley Corporation sending notification letters to the public[128–130] ; additional research resulted in further changes to additional correspondence with lay and physician audiences.[129] Absolute risk data were included in the letter to describe the level (and range) of risk of valve rupture, with comparison data provided about risk associated with having surgery to replace the heart valves.

Finally, Box 6.7 provides an example of communicating data well in a higher controversy potential situation involving an environmental exposure in New York State.[1] This situation lasted over a few years, showing how long such situations can continue over time; particularly noteworthy was the inclusion of the citizens' advisory committee, which acted to increase trust. From a data perspective, communication materials at various times included verbal qualifiers, comparative data on health risks from polychlorinated biphenyl (PCB) exposure in kitchens or in the public water supply (involuntary health risk), and the small number of estimated excess cancer deaths over time. These data helped greatly with interpretation, demonstrating to lay audiences the low magnitude of health risk to which they were subjected.

---

**The bottom line**

Acute public health situations can be categorized based upon their potential for controversy

Acute public health situations, particularly those with higher controversy potential, may generate intense lay audience interest, which may make audience members more motivated to understand data

Major challenges influencing audiences' understanding of data are intense emotion, involuntary risk, and trust or distrust

Lower controversy potential situations may require no or minimal communication involving data, whereas higher controversy potential situations may require extensive data communication efforts

Data presentation modalities in acute situations can range from verbally providing one or two numbers to using more complex icon displays of absolute risk data

## Conclusion

Acute public health situations occur for a wide variety of reasons and generate a lot of lay audience attention. Communicating data in these types of situations ranges the gamut from very simple (no data or only one or two numbers) to the most difficult that public health practitioners or scientists will face (complex probability findings). Particularly in higher controversy potential situations, there may be skepticism and intense scrutiny concerning science, including data, and methods, as well as scientists or the public health organizations they represent.

A critical component of communication in many acute situations is media relations. News media representatives play a key role in communicating information, including data, to the public and to policy makers. This means that representatives of public health agencies and other organizations involved in acute situations need to work proactively and on an ongoing basis to meet the needs of news media representatives, and regularly provide them with accurate and up-to-date information updates.

## Further Reading

### Crisis Communication

Coombs WT. *Ongoing Crisis Communication: Planning, Managing, and Responding.* 2nd ed. Thousand Oaks, Calif.: Sage; 2007.

Fearn-Banks K. *Crisis Communications: A Casebook Approach.* 3rd ed. Mahwah, N.J.: Erlbaum, 2007.

Reynolds B, Galdo JH, Sokler L. *Crisis and Emergency Risk Communication.* Atlanta, Ga.: Centers for Disease Control and Prevention; 2002.

Seeger MW, Sellnow MW, Ullmer RL. *Crisis Communication and the Public Health.* Cresskill, N.J.: Hampton Press, 2007.

### Risk Communication

Bennett P, Calman K. eds. *Risk Communication and Public Health.* New York: Oxford; 1999.

Glik DC. Risk communication for public health emergencies. *Annu Rev Public Health.* 2007;28:33–54.

Goldstein BD. Advances in risk assessment and communication. *Annu Rev Public Health.* 2005;26:141–163.

Lundgren RE, McMakin A. *Risk Communication: A Handbook for Communicating Environmental, Safety, and Health Risks.* 3rd ed. Columbus, Ohio: Battelle; 2004.

## Risk Perception

Fischhoff B. Risk perception and communication unplugged: Twenty years of process. *Risk Anal.* 1995;13:137–145.

Fischhoff B, Bostrom A, Quadrel MJ. Risk perception and communication. *Annu Rev Public Health.* 1993;14:183–203.

Klein WMP, Stefanek ME. Cancer risk elicitation and communication: Lessons from the psychology of risk perception. *CA Cancer J Clin.* 2007;56:147–167.

Slovic P. ed. *The Perception of Risk.* Sterling, Va.: Earthscan; 2000.

## References

1. Keeney RL, von Winterfeldt D. Improving risk communication. *Risk Anal.* 1986;6(4):417–424.
2. Nicholson PJ. Communicating occupational and environmental issues. *Occupational Medicine.* 2000;50:226–230.
3. Reynolds RA, Reynolds JL. Evidence. In: Dillard JP, Pfau M, eds. *The Persuasion Handbook: Developments in Theory and Practice.* Thousand Oaks, Calif.: Sage; 2002:427–444.
4. Reynolds BA, Galdo JH, Sokler L. *Crisis and Emergency Risk Communication.* Atlanta, Ga.: Centers for Disease Control and Prevention; 2002.
5. U.S. Department of Health Education and Welfare. *Smoking and Health: Report of the Advisory Committee to the Surgeon General of the Public Health Service.* Washington, D.C.: U.S. Department of Health, Education, and Welfare; 1964.
6. Writing Group for the Women's Health Initiative. Risks and benefits of estrogen plus progestin in healthy postmenopausal women: Principle results from the Women's Health Initiative randomized controlled trial. *JAMA.* 2002;288: 321–333.
7. General Accountability Office. Strengthening the use of risk management principles in homeland security. Paper presented at highlights of a forum convened by the comptroller of the United States. Washington, D.C.; April 2008.
8. Brodsky CM. The psychiatric epidemic in the American workplace. *Occup Med.* 1988;3:653–662.
9. Brookes T, Khan OA. *Behind the Mask: How the World Survived SARS, the First Epidemic of the Twenty-First Century.* Washington, D.C.: American Public Health Association; 2005.
10. Powell M, Dunwoody S, Griffin R, Neuwirth K. Exploring lay uncertainty about an environmental health risk. *Public Understand Sci.* 2007;16:323–343.
11. Reynolds B. Response to best practices. *J Appl Commun Res.* 2006;34:249–252.
12. Sandman PM. Crisis communication best practices: Some quibbles and additions. *J Appl Commun Res.* 2006;34:257–262.
13. Young N, Matthews R. Experts' understanding of the public: Knowledge control in a risk controversy. *Public Understand Sci.* 2007;165:123–144.
14. Coombs WT. *Ongoing Crisis Communication: Planning, Managing, and Responding.* 2nd ed. Thousand Oaks, Calif.: Sage; 2007.
15. Millar DP, Heath RL. *Responding to Crisis: A Rhetorical Approach to Crisis Communication.* Mahwah, N.J.: Lawrence Erlbaum; 2004.

16. Ullmer R, Sellnow TL, Seeger MW. *Effective Crisis Communication: Moving from Crisis to Opportunity.* Thousand Oaks, Calif.: Sage; 2006.

17. Fearn-Banks K. *Crisis Communications: A Casebook Approach.* 3rd ed. Mahwah, N.J.: Lawrence Erlbaum; 2007.

18. Covello VT. Best practices in public health risk and crisis communication. *J Health Commun.* 2003;8:5–8.

19. Glik DC. Risk communication for public health emergencies. *Annu Rev Public Health.* 2007;28:33–54.

20. Johnson JA, Ledlow GR, Cwiek MA, eds. Community Preparedness and Response to Terrorism. *Volume III: Communication and the Media.* Westport, Conn.: Greenwood; 2005.

21. Seeger MS, Sellnow MW, Ullmer RL. *Crisis Communication and the Public Health.* Cresskill, N.J.: Hampton Press; 2007.

22. Seeger MW. Best practices in crisis communication: an expert panel process. *J Appl Commun Res.* 2006;34:232–244.

23. Vanderford ML, Nastoff T, Telfer JL, Bonzo SE. Emergency communication challenges in response to Hurricane Katrina: Lessons from the Centers for Disease Control and Prevention. *J Appl Commun Res.* 2007;35:9–25.

24. Bennett P, Calman K, eds. *Risk Communication and Public Health.* New York, N.Y.: Oxford University Press; 1999.

25. Leiss WPD. *Mad Cows and Mother's Milk: The Perils of Poor Risk Communication.* Montreal, Canada: McGill-Queen's University Press; 2005.

26. National Research Council. *Improving Risk Communication.* Washington, D.C.: National Academy Press; 1989.

27. Friedman SM, Dunwoody S, Rogers CL, eds. *Communicating Uncertainty: Media Coverage of New and Controversial Science.* Mahwah, N.J.: Lawrence Erlbaum; 1999.

28. Morgan MG, Fischhoff B, Bostrom A, Atman CJ. *Risk Communication: A Mental Models Approach.* Cambridge, UK: Cambridge University Press; 2002.

29. Nelkin D. *Selling Science: How the Press Covers Science and Technology.* New York, N.Y.: W. H. Freeman; 1995.

30. Reynolds B, Galdo JH, Sokler L. *Crisis and Emergency Risk Communication.* Atlanta, Ga.: Centers for Disease Control and Prevention; 2002.

31. Seeger MW, Sellnow TL, Ullmer RR. *Communication and Organizational Crisis.* Westport, Conn.: Praeger; 2003.

32. Berry D. *Risk, Communication, and Health Psychology.* Berkshire, UK: Open University Press; 2004.

33. Goldstein BD. Advances in risk assessment and communication. *Annu Rev Public Health.* 2005;26:141–163.

34. Kasperson JX, Kasperson RE. *The Social Contours of Risk. Vol I: Publics, Risk Communication and the Social Amplification of Risk.* Sterling, Va.: Earthscan; 2005.

35. Tinker T, Vaughn E. Risk Communication. In: Nelson DE, Brownson RC, Remington PL, Parvanta C, eds. *Communicating Health Information Effectively: A Guide for Practitioners.* Washington, D.C.: American Public Health Association; 2002:185–203.

36. Willis J, Okunade AA. *Reporting on Risks: The Practice and Ethics of Health and Safety Communication.* Westport, Conn.: Praeger; 1997.

37. Lundgren RE, McMakin AH. *Risk Communication: A Handbook for Communicating Environmental, Safety, and Health Risks.* 3rd ed. Columbus, Ohio: Battelle; 2004.

38. Covello VT, Peters RG, Wojtecki JG, Hyde RC. Risk communication, the West Nile Virus epidemic, and bioterrorism: Responding to communication challenges posed by the intentional or unintentional release of a pathogen in an urban setting. *J Urban Health.* 2001;78:382–391.
39. Fischhoff B, Bostrom A, Quadrel MJ. Risk perception and communication. *Annu Rev Public Health.* 1993;14:183–203.
40. Koenig BA, Silverberg HL. Understanding probabilistic risk in predisposition genetic testing for Alzheimer disease. *Genet Test.* 1999;3(1):55–63.
41. Renn O. Perceptions of risks. *Toxicol Lett.* 2004(149):405–413.
42. Slovic P, ed. *The Perception of Risk.* Sterling, Va.: Earthscan; 2000.
43. Slovic P, Fischhoff B, Lichtenstein S. Rating the risks. In: Slovic P, ed. *The Perception of Risk.* Sterling, Va.: Earthscan; 2000:104–120.
44. Graham DJ, Campen D, Hui R, et al. Risk of acute myocardial infarction and sudden cardiac death in patients treated with cyclo-oxygenase 2 selective and non-selective non-steroidal anti-inflammatory drugs: Nested case-control study. *Lancet.* 2005;365(9458):475–481.
45. Bier VM. On the state of the art: Risk communication to the public. *Reliab Eng Syst Saf.* 2001(71):139–150.
46. McComas KA, Trumbo CW, Besley JC. Public meetings about suspected cancer clusters: The impact of voice, interactional justice, and risk perception on attendees' attitudes in six communities. *J Health Commun.* 2007;12:527–549.
47. Meredith LS, Eisenman DP, Rhodes H, Ryan G, Long A. Trust influences response to public health messages during a bioterrorist event. *J Health Commun.* 2007;12:217–232.
48. Bier VM. On the state of the art: Risk communication to decision-makers. *Reliab Eng Syst Saf.* 2001;71:151–157.
49. Nelkin D. Communicating technological risk: The social construction of risk perception. *Annu Rev Public Health.* 1989;10:95–113.
50. Bier VM. On the state of the art: Risk communication to decision-makers. *Reliab Eng Syst Saf.* 2001;71:151–157.
51. Bier VM. On the state of the art: Risk communication to the public. *Reliab Eng Syst Saf.* 2001;71:139–150.
52. Garvin T. Analytical paradigms: The epistemological distances between scientists, policy makers, and the public. *Risk Anal.* 2001;21(3):443–455.
53. Merskin D. Media dependency theory: Origins and directions. In: Demers D, Viswanath K, eds. *Mass Media, Social Control, and Social Change.* Ames, Iowa: Iowa State University Press; 1999:77–98.
54. Gregg MB, ed. *Field Epidemiology.* 3rd ed. New York, N.Y.: Oxford University Press; 2008.
55. Hastie R, Dawes RM. *Rational Choice in an Uncertain World: The Psychology of Judgment and Decision Making.* Thousand Oaks, Calif.: Sage; 2001.
56. Croteau D, Hoynes W. *Media/Society.* 3rd ed. Thousand Oaks, Calif.: Sage; 2003.
57. McDonough JE. *Experiencing Politics: A Legislator's Stories of Government and Health Care.* Berkeley, Calif.: University of California Press; 2000.
58. Robinson SJ, Newstetter WC. Uncertain science and certain deadlines: CDC responses to the media during the anthrax attacks of 2001. *J Health Commun.* 2003;(8 Suppl):17–34.
59. Dearing JW, Rogers EM. *Agenda-Setting.* Thousand Oaks, Calif.: Sage; 1996.
60. Scheufele DA, Tewksbury D. Framing, agenda setting, and priming: The evolution of three media effects models. *J Commun.* 2007;57:9–20.

61. Pidgeon N, Kasperson RE, eds. *The Social Amplification of Risk*. New York, N.Y.: Cambridge University Press; 2003.
62. Vasterman P, Yzermans CJ, Dirkzwager AJ. The role of the media and media hypes in the aftermath of disasters. *Epidemiol Rev.* 2005;27:107–114.
63. Remington PL, Ahrens D. Communicating public health information to private and voluntary health organizations. In: Nelson DE, Brownson RC, Remington PL, Parvanta C, eds. *Communicating Public Health Information Effectively: A Guide for Practitioners*. Washington, D.C.: American Public Health Association; 2002:115–126.
64. Procopio CH, Procopio ST. Do you know what it means to miss New Orleans? Internet communication, geographic community, and social capital in crisis. *J Appl Commun Res.* 2007;35:67–97.
65. Slovic P. Perception of risk. *Science.* 1987;236(4799):280–285.
66. Okudera T, Morita H, Iwashita T, et al. Unexpected nerve gas exposure in the city of matsumoto: Report of rescue activity in the first sarin gas terrorism. *Am J Emerg Med.* 1997;5:618–624.
67. Van Beneden CA, Keene WE, Strang RA, et al. Multinational outbreak of *Salmonella enterica* serotype Newport infections due to contaminated alfalfa sprouts. *JAMA.* 1999;281(2):158–162.
68. Markel H. Public health and the public's fascination with epidemics: Contagious narratives. *JAMA.* 2007;20:2292–2294.
69. Roueche B. A good, safe tan. *New Yorker.* 1991;67:69–73.
70. May T. Public communication, risk perception, and the viability of preventive vaccination against communicable diseases. *Bioethics.* 2005;31:425–433.
71. Waxman HA. The lessons of Vioxx—drug safety and sales. *N Engl J Med.* 2005;352(25):2576–2578.
72. Baker JP. Mercury, vaccines, and autism: One controversy, three histories. *Am J Public Health.* 2008;98(2):244–253.
73. Jones TF, Craig AS, Hoy D, et al. Mass psychogenic illness attributed to toxic exposure at a high school. *N Engl J Med.* 2000;342(2):96–100.
74. Angell M. *Science on Trial: The Clash of Medical Evidence and the Law in the Breast Implant Case*. New York, N.Y.: Norton; 1997.
75. Brownson RC, Petitti DB, eds. *Applied Epidemiology: Theory to Practice*. 2nd ed. New York, N.Y.: Oxford University Press; 2006.
76. National Institutes of Health. *Breast Cancer Screening for Women Ages 40–49*. Bethesda, Md.: National Institutes of Health; 1997.
77. Institute of Medicine. *Exposure of the American people to Iodine-131 from Nevada Nuclear-Bomb Tests. Review of the National Cancer Institute Report and Public Health Implications*. Washington, D.C.: IOM; 1999.
78. Reynolds RA, Reynolds JL. Evidence. In: Dillard JP, Pfau M, eds. *Persuasion Research Handbook: Developments in Theory and Practice*. Thousand Oaks, Calif.: Sage; 2002:427–444.
79. Slovic P, ed. *The Perception of Risk*. London; Sterling, Va.: Earthscan; 2000.
80. Reynolds B. *Crisis and Emergency Risk Communication: By Leaders for Leaders*. Atlanta, Ga.: Centers for Disease Control and Prevention; 2004.
81. Sandman PM. Bioterrorism risk communication policy. *J Health Commun.* 2003;8(Suppl 1):146–147; discussion 148–151.
82. Tinker T, Vaughn E. Risk communication. In: Nelson DE, Brownson RC, Remington P, Parvanta C, eds. *Communicating Public Health Information Effectively*. Washington, D.C.: American Public Health Association; 2002:185–203.

83. Henretig FM, Cieslak TJ, Madsen JM, et al. The emergency department response to incidents of biological and chemical terrorism. In: Fleisher GR, Ludwig S, eds. *Pediatric Emergency Medicine*. 4th ed. Philadelphia, Pa.: Lippincott, Williams, & Wilkins; 2000.

84. Hibbard JH, & Peters, E. Supporting informed consumer health care decisions: Data presentation approaches that facilitate the use of information in choice. *Annu Rev Public Health*. 2003;24:413–433.

85. Parrott R, Silk K, Dorgan K, Condit C, Harris T. Risk communication and judgments of statistical evidentiary appeals. When a picture is not worth a thousand words. *Hum Commun Res*. 2005;32:423–452.

86. Reinard JC. The persuasive effects of testimonial assertion evidence. In: Allen M, Preiss RW, eds. *Persuasion: Advances through Meta-Analysis*. Cresskill, N.J.: Hampton Press; 1998.

87. Peters E, Hibbard J, Slovic P, Dieckmann N. Numeracy skill and the communication, comprehension, and use of risk–benefit information. *Health Aff (Millwood)*. 2007;26(3):741–748.

88. Peters E, Dieckmann N, Dixon A, Hibbard JH, Mertz CK. Less is more in presenting quality information to consumers. *Med Care Res Rev*. 2007;64(2):169–190.

89. Lum M, Parvanta C, Maibach E, Arkin E, Nelson DE. General public: Communicating to inform. In: Nelson DE, Brownson RC, Remington PL, Parvanta C, eds. *Communicating Public Health Information Effectively: A Guide for Practitioners*. Washington, D.C.: American Public Health Association; 2002:47–57.

90. Edwards A, Elwyn G. Understanding risk and lessons for clinical risk communication about treatment preferences. *Qual Health Care*. 2001;10(Suppl 1):i9–i13.

91. Schapira MM, Nattinger AB, McHorney CA. Frequency or probability? A qualitative study of risk communication formats used in health care. *Med Decis Making*. 2001;21(6):459–467.

92. Frewer L. The public and effective risk communication. *Toxicol Lett*. 2004;149(1–3):391–397.

93. Fischhoff B. Risk perception and communication unplugged: Twenty years of process. *Risk Anal*. 1995;13:137–145.

94. Rowan KE. Strategies for explaining complex science news. *J Educator*. 1990;45(2):25–31.

95. Rowan KE. When simple language fails: presenting difficult science to the public. *J Tech Writ Commun*. 1991;21:369–382.

96. Turney J. Public understanding of science. *Lancet*. 1996;347(9008):1087–1090.

97. Johnson BB. Are some risk comparisons more effective under conflict? A replication and extension of Roth et al. *Risk Anal*. 2003;23:767–780.

98. Klein WMP, Stefanek ME. Cancer risk elicitation and communication: Lessons from the psychology of risk perception. *CA Cancer J Clin*. 2007;56:147–167.

99. Lipkus IM, Crawford Y, Fenn K, et al. Testing different formats for communicating colorectal cancer risk. *J Health Commun*. 1999;4(4):311–324.

100. McComas KA. Defining moments in risk communication research: 1996–2005. *J Health Commun*. 2006;11(1):75–91.

101. Visschers VHM, Meertens RM, Passchier WF, De Vries NK. How does the public evaluate risk information? The impact of associations with other risks. *Risk Anal*. 2007;27:715–727.

102. Hux JE, Naylor CD. Communicating the benefits of chronic preventive therapy: Does the format of efficacy data determine patients' acceptance of treatment? *Med Decis Making*. 1995;15(2):152–157.

103. Phillips KA, Glendon G, Knight JA. Putting the risk of breast cancer in perspective. *N Engl J Med.* 1999;340(2):141–144.

104. Stone ER, Yates JF, Parker AM. Risk communication: Absolute versus relative expressions of low-probability risks. *Org Behav Hum Decis Process.* 1994;60:387–408.

105. Nelson DE. Translating public health data. In: Nelson DE, Brownson RC, Remington PL, Parvanta C, eds. *Communicating Public Health Information Effectively: A Guide for Practitioners.* Washington, D.C.: American Public Health Association; 2002:33–45.

106. Cohn V, Cope L. *News and Numbers: A Guide to Reporting Statistical Claims and Controversies in Health and Other Fields.* 2nd ed. Ames, Iowa: Iowa State Press; 2001.

107. Morton RF, Hebel JR, McCarter RJ. *A Study Guide to Epidemiology and Biostatistics.* 5th ed. Boston, Mass.: Jones and Bartlett; 2004.

108. Macdonald-Ross M. How numbers are shown: A review of research on the presentation of quantitative data in texts. *AV Commun Rev.* 1977;25:359–410.

109. Lipkus IM, Hollands JG. The visual communication of risk. *J Natl Cancer Inst Monogr.* 1999(25):149–163.

110. Gastel B. *Health Writer's Handbook.* Ames, Iowa: Iowa State University Press; 1998.

111. Gigerenzer G. *Calculated Risks: How to Know When Numbers Deceive You.* New York, N.Y.: Simon & Schuster; 2002.

112. Fischhoff B, Bostrom A, Quadrel MJ. Risk perception and communication. *Annu Rev Public Health.* 1993;14(14):183–203.

113. Redelmeier DA, Rozin P, Kahneman D. Understanding patients' decisions: Cognitive and emotional perspectives. *JAMA.* 1993;270(1):72–76.

114. Rothman AJ, Kiviniemi MT. Treating people with information: An analysis and review of approaches to communicating health risk information. *J Natl Cancer Inst Monogr.* 1999(25):44–51.

115. Kahneman D, Slovic P, Tversky A, eds. *Judgment under Uncertainty: Heuristics and Biases.* Cambridge, UK: Cambridge University Press; 1982.

116. Plous S. *The Psychology of Judgment and Decision-Making.* New York, N.Y.: McGraw-Hill; 1993.

117. Lipkus IM, Nelson DE. Visual communication. In: Nelson DE, Brownson RC, Remington PL, Parvanta C, eds. *Communicating Public Health Information Effectively: A Guide for Practitioners.* Washington, D.C.: American Public Health Association; 2002:155–172.

118. Spence I, Lewandowsky S. Displaying proportions and percentages. *Appl Cognit Psychol.* 1991;5:61–77.

119. Meyer J, Shinar D, Leiser D. Multiple factors that determine performance with tables and graphs. *Hum Factor.* 1997;39(2):268–286.

120. Holmes N. *Designer's Guide to Creating Charts and Diagrams.* New York, N.Y.: Watson-Guptill; 1991.

121. Slocum T, McMaster RB, Kessler FC, Howard HH. *Thematic Cartography and Geographic Visualization.* 2nd ed. Upper Saddle River, N.J.: Pearson Education; 2005.

122. Ancker JS, Senathirajah Y, Kukafka R, Starren JB. Design features of graphs in health risk communication: A systematic review. *J Am Med Inform Assoc.* 2006;13(6):608–618.

123. Feldman-Stewart D, Kocovski N, McConnell BA, Brundage MD, Mackillop WJ. Perception of quantitative information for treatment decisions. *Med Decis Making.* 2000;20(2):228–238.

124. Hoffman JR, Wilkes MS, Day FC, Bell DS, Higa JK. The roulette wheel: An aid to informed decision making. *PLoS Med.* 2006;3:e137.

125. Woloshin S, Schwartz LM, Byram SJ, Sox HC, Fischhoff B, Welch HG. Women's understanding of the mammography screening debate. *Arch Intern Med.* 2000;160(10):1434–1440.

126. Centers for Disease Control and Prevention. *Severe Acute Respiratory Syndrome (SARS).* Atlanta, Ga.: Centers for Disease Control and Prevention; 2007.

127. World Health Organization. *WHO Strategic Action Plan for Pandemic Influenza 2006–2007.* Geneva, Switzerland: World Health Organization.

128. Department of Health and Human Services. *Recommendations to Improve Health Risk Communication: A Report on Case Studies in Health Risk Communication.* Washington, D.C.: Department of Health and Human Services, Environmental Policy Committee, Subcommittee on Risk Communication and Education; 1994.

129. Farley D. Shiley saga leads to improved communication. *FDA Consumer.* 1994;28(1):12–17.

130. Food and Drug Administration. *Shiley C-C Heart Valve Alert.* Washington, D.C.: FDA Consumer; 1990.

# 7

## Communicating Data for Policy or Program Advocacy

> It must be a very good and rare day indeed when policy makers take
> their cues mainly from scientific knowledge.
>
> Brown, "Knowledge and power: Health services research
> as a political resource, *Health Services Research:*
> *Key to Health Policy*[1]

## Introduction

Policies and programs can have a major impact on the health of the public.[2–4]
Many studies have demonstrated improvements in public health resulting
from effective public health policies and programs (e.g., reduced lead exposure, receiving immunization, maintaining oral health, preventing alcohol
abuse and tobacco use, preventing motor vehicle injury, increased physical
activity, better nutrition, treatment for tuberculosis, and receipt of health care
services, to name just a few).[2, 5–11]

But policies and programs do not occur in a vacuum: extensive efforts by
committed individuals (advocates) and organizations are necessary.[12] For the
purposes of this book, we define advocacy as supporting or opposing specific
public or private policies or programs that directly or indirectly impact the
public's health.[3] It may involve laws, regulations, or resource allocation such
as funding or staffing of programs. As such, communication messages are
a critical aspect of advocacy. Advocacy can occur for a specific situation or
effort (e.g., in support or opposition to legislative bill, appropriation, regulation, or private organizational policy). It can also involve long-term efforts
to change or maintain policy or programs on a particular issue; indeed,
advocating for many specific public health policies or programs is usually a
long-term challenge.[3, 12–15] It not only may take many years—or decades, in

some instances—to be successful in instituting or establishing a change in a policy or program, but it may also require ongoing efforts to maintain a policy or program, especially when there is a powerful and committed opposition.

Advocacy has two aspects that contrast markedly with other types of public health situations. First, persuasion is the purpose for communicating information, including data, to lay audiences.[3, 16] As a result, ethical decisions are paramount in the selection or omission and presentation of public health data (Chapters 1 and 2).[17, 18] Second, except in situations involving ballot initiatives, policy makers are usually the primary audience, with the public and the press usually being secondary audiences.

Because persuasion is the purpose for communicating in advocacy situations, there can be a strong temptation to overstate or exaggerate to help build support for a position or belief.[19] This means that careful consideration needs to be given as to what type of data are selected and what presentation approaches to use to be most persuasive to lay audiences and yet be scientifically defensible. As with acute situations with higher controversy potential discussed in Chapter 6, scientists themselves, along with their methodology, results, interpretation, and conclusions, are likely to be challenged or questioned regardless of how strong they may be, in advocacy situations.

This chapter provides an overview of policy making, the communication process in advocacy situations, general considerations about the use of scientific data for advocacy, and selecting and presenting data most likely to be effective. Much of the information presented in this chapter is based on findings from public policy case studies,[20, 21] theories and models from political science and related fields,[14, 22–25] and from research in psychology and communication.[26, 27] Lessons from the political science and organizational research literature are applied to advocacy within private organizations, recognizing that decision making within private organizations is usually much more centralized and less formal (Chapter 2).[28]

Readers desiring more information about the many aspects of policy or program advocacy for public health purposes should review this literature (see Further Reading at the end of this chapter) or consult with advocacy experts. A final caveat to recognize is that, while there have been some studies of policy makers,[29–33] few formal studies on selecting and presenting health data to policy makers have been done,[34] as most advocacy efforts do not readily lend themselves to such research.

## Overview of Policy Making

Because many public health practitioners have limited or no experience in the policy-making world, and rarely receive formal training in this area, it is useful to consider the many aspects of policy making before considering, selecting, or presenting data for advocacy. Policy making, and decisions by policy makers about resource allocation for programs, can be viewed across multiple dimensions, for example, public or private policy making, roles of internal and external participants (actors), and the policy cycle.[19, 22, 23, 25] This section briefly highlights public policy theories and frameworks, public policy actors, the public policy cycle, and private policy making. Although described from a U.S. perspective, these policy-making principles and processes are similar to those found in many other countries.

## Public Policy Theories and Frameworks

There are several major theories and frameworks that describe or predict public policy making.[19, 22–25] Table 7.1 provides a short description of several of the most common. No one overarching theory or framework is considered to be best or most appropriate, as each provides a different way of understanding policy making.

As shown in both the punctuated equilibrium model and multiple streams framework for policy making, there are occasional, short-lived windows of opportunity during which policy makers attend to an issue and are much more likely to make decisions about policies or programs. This often occurs because of what are referred to as focusing events, that is, specific occurrences that garner media, public, and policy-maker attention. Focusing events usually involve adverse outcomes that are perceived as important and potentially preventable; the event itself may involve members of the public, or alternatively, prominent public persons such as well-known politicians, entertainers, or sports figures. Focusing events can become important times for advocacy; examples of several major public health-related focusing events are listed in Table 7.2.

### Public Policy Process and Actors

The public policy process depends on the system of government within a country. The United States and many other democracies have a multicentric policy system that relies upon several autonomous actors to form public policy, with government serving as a facilitator or a guardian of minimal standards.[13, 35, 36] At the federal, state, and local level in the United States, there are three distinct branches of government: legislative, executive, and judicial. In parliamentary systems, such as in Great Britain, the legislative and executive functions are combined.[13, 36]

The role of the legislature is to enact laws and allocate public financial resources; the legislative branch also has oversight responsibility over the executive branch.[25] The power of individual legislators depends on many different factors, such as political party affiliation (e.g., whether he or she is a

## Table 7.1 Major public policy-making theories and frameworks

| Name | Description |
| --- | --- |
| Rational Theory | Policy makers are presented with some type of problem (or goal). They gather all possible relevant information about the problem and potential solutions by consulting experts. After analyzing multiple options, they make the best choice that can achieve maximum social gain. This theory, although recognized as not how policy making actually occurs, is considered an idealized model |
| Disjointed Incrementalism ("Muddling Through") | Decisions by policy makers are made in relatively small increments in a piecemeal manner. This occurs when there are unstable or unpredictable situations, lack of consensus, or multiple actors with minimal power to influence the policy process. Policy makers' limited time and information results in bounded rationality when thinking about problems or potential solutions; this tends to lead them to build upon existing "solutions" rather than to create broad system-wide reforms |
| Multiple Streams Framework | The Multiple Streams Framework postulates that policy makers receive much random or chaotic information. Occasionally, a window of opportunity for change (e.g., new policy) occurs when three streams or processes work in parallel. First, policy makers believe that a problem exists that needs to be addressed (problem stream). Second, policy makers sense that because of the mood of the electorate, election results, or group mobilization, it is time for them to act (political stream). Third, there is an implementable policy that fits the problem, can gain adequate support, and is easily understandable (policy stream) |
| Punctuated Equilibrium Framework | The Punctuated Equilibrium Framework assumes that policy making involves incremental change over long periods of time, but that periodically there are brief periods of major policy changes. These major changes occur because advocates of policy change successfully create new policy images (reorientations) |
| Advocacy Coalition Framework | The Advocacy Coalition Framework postulates that there are discrete interest groups for a particular policy or issue (e.g., nutrition labeling, occupational health regulations). These groups have core values and beliefs and engage in debates about policy. Policy brokers with a stake in resolving the problem work to mediate competition between policy interest groups. This framework recognizes that policy making is an iterative process that may occur over many years and that a variety of system and environmental factors influence the process |

*Source*: McDonough JE. *Experiencing Politics: A Legislator's Stories of Government and Health Care*. Berkeley, Calif.: University of California Press; 2000. Spasoff RA. *Epidemiologic Methods for Health Policy*. New York, N.Y.: Oxford University Press; 1999. Birkland TA. *An Introduction to the Policy Process: Theories, Concepts, and Models of Public Policy Making*. Armonk, N.Y.: M.E. Sharpe; 2001. Kingdon JW. *Agendas, Alternatives, and Public Policies*. 2nd ed. New York, N.Y.: Longman; 2003. Lindblom CE, Woodhouse EJ. *The Policy-Making Process*. 3rd ed. Upper Saddle River, N.J.: Prentice-Hall; 2003. Longest B. *Health Policymaking in the United States*. Ann Arbor, Mich.: Health Administration Press; 2005. Oliver TR. The politics of public health policy. *Annu Rev Public Health*. 2006;27:195–233. Sabatier PA, ed. *Theories of the Political Process*. 2nd ed. Boulder, Colo.: Westview; 2007.

**Table 7.2 Selected major public health focusing events**

| Year | Focusing event | Issue |
|------|----------------|-------|
| 1948 | Excess mortality in Donora, Pennsylvania, associated with an air inversion | Air pollution |
| 1961 | Birth defects associated with thalidomide | Prescription drug safety; prenatal care |
| 1964 | U.S. Surgeon General's report on smoking | Tobacco |
| 1973 | Halting of the Tuskegee Study | Syphilis; racial discrimination |
| 1974 | First lady Betty Ford diagnosed with breast cancer | Breast cancer screening |
| 1979 | Three Mile Island nuclear accident in Pennsylvania | Radiation |
| 1982 | Cyanide contamination of Tylenol in Chicago area (Chapter 6) | Safety of nonprescription drugs |
| 1984 | Bhopal, India, chemical plant release of methyl isocyanate kills or injuries more than 100,000 people | Workplace and community safety |
| 1984 | 14-year-old Ryan White diagnosed with AIDS in Indiana | HIV treatment and prevention |
| 1996 | Bovine spongioform encephalopathy (Mad Cow Disease) and beef consumption in Great Britain | Food safety |
| 2001 | Anthrax deaths in Florida, Washington, DC, and Connecticut | Biological terrorism |

member of the majority party); committee positions; personal or professional relationships with other legislators, members of the executive branch, and representatives of outside organizations; and personal expertise or experience with specific issues.[14, 23, 24] Political party affiliation of legislators provides a clue as to their likely worldviews and ideology (Chapter 2).

The executive branch is responsible for interpreting and implementing what legislatures or judicial authorities mandate. Policy makers within the executive branch include elected officials or leaders (e.g., mayor, secretary of state) who can have a major agenda-setting role in determining what policies, issues, or programs to emphasize. However, executive branch policy makers also include appointed or civil servants ("permanent" employees, or bureaucrats) within administrative agencies.[22, 24, 25, 35, 37] Many policy decisions are made by individuals or boards within executive agencies; this is referred to as administrative policy making or rulemaking.[23, 25, 35, 37–39]

Members of the judiciary branch (judges) are responsible for deciding disputes about legislative or executive branch decisions, such as the constitutionality or interpretation of a legislative bill or rules made by executive branch agencies.[22] In addition, case law, based on judicial decisions in legal proceedings can also influence health policies. (Uses of data for advocacy purposes in judicial settings are not covered in this book.)

Members of the legislative, executive, and judicial branches are referred to as the official actors in policy making. However, there are several unofficial actors who have varying degrees of policy-making influence (Table 7.3).[22–24]

**Table 7.3  Official and unofficial actors involved in policy making**

| Public policy actors | Examples |
|---|---|
| *Official actors* | |
| Legislators | City council persons, state representatives |
| Elected and unelected executive branch officials | U.S. senators, governors, state treasurers, agency administrators |
| Judges | State Supreme Court Justices, administrative law judges |
| *Unofficial actors* | |
| Interest groups | National Association of Manufacturers, AFL-CIO, AARP, American Medical Association, Family Research Council |
| Political parties | Local, state, or national Republican or Democratic party organizations |
| General public | Beliefs and opinions of individuals within the public |
| News and entertainment media | Cable news networks, newspaper editors, selected movies, or television series |
| Independent research organizations (think tanks) | National Academy of Sciences, Heritage Foundation, Brookings Institute |

*Source*: Birkland TA. *An Introduction to the Policy Process: Theories, Concepts, and Models of Public Policy Making*. Armonk, N.Y.: M.E. Sharpe; 2001. Kingdon JW. *Agendas, Alternatives, and Public Policies*. 2nd ed. New York, N.Y.: Longman; 2003. Lindblom CE, Woodhouse EJ. *The Policy-Making Process*. 3rd ed. Upper Saddle River, N.J.: Prentice-Hall; 2003.

Interest groups, or lobbying interests, can be classified as economic (or private), public interest, or some other type (e.g., those with a specific ideological or moral emphasis).

The preferences of individual citizens can influence public policy makers.[14, 22] The most obvious role is at the ballot box, but there are times when a committed group of citizens mobilizes in support or opposition around a particular issue, policy, or program and communicates preferences vociferously to policy makers.

The news media play an important agenda-setting function, that is, influencing what are considered to be the most important current issues among the public and policy makers based on the selection, emphasis, and framing of news stories (Chapter 2).[40, 41] Because of this agenda-setting role, media advocacy, which refers to efforts to gain news media coverage (earned media) for a specific policy, issue, or program, is an important activity for advocates.[3, 15, 42] The entertainment media, through the production and airing of selected television shows or movies about certain topics with a definitive slant, can sometimes have an influence on policy making.[22, 23]

Independent research organizations or institutes, referred to as "think tanks," can also have a strong influence on policy making.[22, 23] Such organizations conduct research or synthesize existing information that is often summarized into reports. Some organizations have a specific ideological orientation, whereas others, which may be affiliated with universities, strive to be more independent.[22]

There are times when policy makers within one branch of government (e.g., a legislative committee) use an ad hoc or regular committee or panel of scientists to provide consultation or a recommendation on health or other issues.[36] The influence of these committees on policy makers is highly variable, depending on the purpose of the committee, specific issue, level of controversy, and recommendations provided. In some instances, the creation of expert panels serves as a tactic to delay or end consideration of a particular issue or policy decision; at other times, expert panels can be highly influential.[36]

## The Public Policy Cycle

Before deciding whether to use data for advocacy, which data to use, and how to present them, it is helpful to recognize the broad context in which advocacy occurs in terms of the public policy cycle (Figure 7.1). Although most often used in public policy making, particularly with legislators, the cycle is applicable in other settings, including advocating for public health program resources and for private policy making.

This cycle can broadly be categorized into four phases: *problem identification* (or issue recognition), *policy formulation*, *policy implementation*, and *policy evaluation*.[22, 25, 35, 36] The policy cycle involves multiple feedback loops (not shown in figure) that can result in modifications at each phase. In the problem identification phase, policy makers recognize that there is a problem

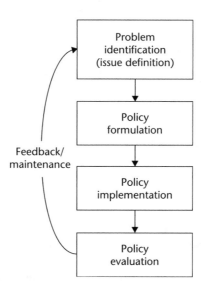

**Figure 7.1** The public policy cycle. (Sources: Birkland TA. *An Introduction to the Policy Process: Theories, Concepts, and Models of Public Policy Making.* 2nd ed. Armonk, N.Y.: M.E. Sharpe: 2005. Also Longest BB. *Health Policymaking in the United States.* 4th ed. Ann Arbor, Mich. Health Administration Press: 2005.)

or issue that should be addressed in some fashion. This may occur for a variety of reasons, such as agenda-setting efforts by prominent elected officials, growing public concern, focusing events, extensive media attention, pressure from interest groups, efforts by policy entrepreneurs, or some combination of these factors.[22, 23]

Policy formulation involves considering potential options and decisions as to what to do about the problem and, as discussed earlier in this chapter, is strongly influenced by many factors. In legislative bodies, this may result in attempts to create, amend, or kill bills. Policy implementation consists of interpretation and decision making by those responsible for carrying out what they perceive to be the intention(s) of the policy makers. After a legislative body enacts a new policy or allocates resources to a program, for example, staff members within an executive branch agency are responsible for "making it happen." This may involve developing and implementing administrative rulemaking (regulations), enforcement, and programs.[25, 35, 36]

Policy evaluation consists of informal or formal assessment of the effect(s) of the policy in a manner similar to program evaluation, for example, was it implemented, did it (or is it) achieving the desired goals? Such information then can be provided back to policy makers in the feedback loop shown in Figure 7.1, and if necessary, can be used for another problem identification or issue definition phase.

### Private Policy Making

Private policy making, as used in this chapter, refers to decisions within organizations about their own policies. Certain private policies, especially those defined by larger organizations, can have important influences on populations that may be underappreciated by many public health practitioners.[43, 44] Examples of private policy making include providing or disallowing certain health insurance benefits (e.g., cancer screening or treatment),[25] encouraging physical activity (e.g., through discounted memberships to exercise facilities),[45] or requiring drug testing of prospective or current employees.[46]

There are large differences in the policy-making environment in private organizations (Chapter 2). Such differences depend on the type of organization; organizational culture and history; and the personality, management styles, and preferences of individual leaders. There can be great variability in how private policy makers respond, or attend to, scientists themselves and public health messages in advocacy situations.

Many private organization leaders rely heavily on their "gut instincts," rather than statistical or other types of evidence when making decisions.[47] In some organizations, there is one key decision maker, thus public health–oriented organizational policies are strongly dependent on this individual's personal beliefs and preferences; in others, decisions may be much more participatory, less centralized, and more formal (Chapter 2). Compared to public policy making, decisions and implementation in private organizations can occur rapidly.

There are several examples of key private organization leaders enacting policies mainly because of the perceived social benefits, improved morale for employees, or outside pressure.[48] Regardless of whether it is a for-profit or nonprofit organization, a major concern or issue facing most private organization policy makers is the financial bottom line: how much will a new policy or program cost the organization in terms of money, especially in the short term, as a return on investment.[49] (Of course, this also occurs for public policy making but it is not always the most critical concern.) This is not surprising as private organizations must be concerned with financial decisions to survive long term.

### Communication Process and Message Delivery in Advocacy Situations

As with other situations, effective advocacy requires attention to the communication process itself, including message delivery (Table 7.4). As discussed

**Table 7.4 Communication process and message delivery recommendations for advocacy to policy makers**

**Communication process**
Conduct background research about policy makers (i.e., audience analysis)
Understand formal and informal communication processes
Consider timing
Coordinate with allies
Select best source for information and message delivery
Seek media attention
Follow up (e.g., with thank you notes)

**Message delivery**
Be brief and get to the main point(s) rapidly
Be definitive
Avoid technical jargon
Use real-world examples
Localize data and narratives
Anticipate opposition arguments and prepare responses
Provide short handouts with key points and contact information

*Source*: Brownson RC, Malone BR. Communicating public health information to policy makers. In: Nelson DE, Brownson RC, Remington PL, Parvanta C, eds. *Communicating Public Health Information Effectively: A Guide for Practitioners*. Washington, D.C.: American Public Health Association; 2002:97–114. Wallack L, Dorfman L, Jernigan D, Themba M. *Media Advocacy for Public Health*. Newbury Park, Calif.: Sage; 1993. Advocacy Institute. *By the Numbers: A Guide to the Tactical Use of Statistics for Positive Policy Change*. Washington, D.C.: Advocacy Institute; n.d.

in Chapter 2 and emphasized throughout this book, it is important to learn as much as possible about intended audiences, including policy makers, their trusted information sources, and preferred communication channels.

Internet search engines and dedicated Web sites (e.g., for legislators, members of the elected executive branch, or private organizations) can be valuable resources for obtaining information about some public or private policy makers.[13] Focus groups, in-depth interviews, and polls can be used to learn more about the opinions, knowledge, attitudes, and beliefs of the public on a specific topic or issue, and to help develop messages or arguments most likely to gain their attention and support.

There are formal and informal processes for communicating with public or private policy makers that advocates must recognize and adhere to in order to be effective. For example, legislators have formal requirements for such things as the language and time frames for introducing legislative bills and processes for presenting information at committee hearings.

Informal communication processes (unwritten rules) may play an even greater role in determining advocacy success or failure. As discussed in Chapter 2, gatekeepers for policy makers, such as top aides, executive secretaries, or administrative assistants, play a critical role in determining which people, and to what information, private or public policy makers are exposed.[13, 28, 36, 43, 47, 50] Researchers or public health practitioners will rarely interact directly with policy makers themselves, especially public policy makers.

What this means is that most communication activities geared toward policy makers will be highly dependent upon the roles and actions of gatekeepers. It is essential to understand and honor the communication preferences of gatekeepers. For example, many assistants for elected legislators are young adults (e.g., in their 20s or 30s) and likely to be quite familiar, and perhaps prefer, communicating using email or text messages and accessing information through Web sites. This underscores the importance of cultivating strong, cordial, and often long-term working relationships with gatekeepers.[13, 28, 36, 43]

Deciding when to advocate, particularly in those instances in which there is a specific opportunity such as an administrative agency or legislative hearing, can play a crucial role (e.g., choosing to advocate when a relevant focusing event has occurred or not to when policy makers are distracted by other major events; see planning phase of the OPT-In model in Chapter 5). Coordinating communication efforts with other advocates is also essential to ensure that organizations work closely together and use concordant messages.[44, 51] Given the tendency of lay audiences to base their decisions on the source who provides it (expert heuristic), it is especially important to select sources that will be perceived as trustworthy and not self-serving by policy makers (Chapter 2).

As discussed in this chapter, gaining media coverage is one of the most important ways that advocates can obtain the attention of policy makers and the public for their issue, policy, or program.[3, 15, 42] (Practical details about media advocacy in public health are provided in the suggested reading list at the end of this chapter.) Finally, an often overlooked informal communication activity is follow-up, which not only includes providing materials or other information requested by gatekeepers or policy makers themselves, but thanking them for their consideration.[13]

The fields of rhetoric and debate provide important guidance for organizing and structuring advocacy messages and for countering opposition arguments (rebuttal).[51–53] In advocacy, there is a major conclusion that supporters want their audiences to believe (e.g., a storyline). To convince audiences, the conclusion requires supportive arguments; in debate terminology, this is referred to as the premises or grounds. Arguments can be supported in several ways (e.g., appeals through authority, example, analogy, personal testimonial, or statistics).[51, 54] Numbers or statistics represent a specific means to support an argument for a conclusion.[51–54] Understanding the form(s) for presenting arguments that are more likely to be successful with intended audiences is essential.

Public health advocacy requires anticipating opposition arguments and developing strategies to counter them.[51, 53, 54] Opponents can use data or other types of information in such a way as to try to establish doubt or uncertainty about the soundness of public health advocates' arguments. Table 7.5 provides some common approaches used by opponents, and Box 7.1 contains examples of arguments and rebuttal approaches used by opponents of secondhand smoke policies.

## Scientific Data and Advocacy

Scientific evidence can influence decisions made by public and private policy makers about public health policies and programs.[3, 16, 23, 24] Before deciding what data to select for advocacy purposes, or how best to present them, it is important to consider whether scientific data even matter, that is, can they influence or persuade policy makers or the public?

The short answer is that scientific data do matter for advocacy, but not as much as scientists and other public health practitioners wish.[3, 14, 16, 22–25, 55–57] There are several reasons why this is the case. Policy making can be considered as occurring within an arena where struggles take place over ideas; after more than 2,000 years of study, it remains more an art than a science.[14, 16, 23, 55]

Policy makers are influenced by many factors, of which scientists and their findings are but one.[14, 19, 22–25, 55] The reality is that many debates about policies and programs are disagreements about values disguised as disagreements about numbers.[14, 21] It is common for groups, organizations, or individuals to use data as evidentiary matter in support of diametrically opposed positions.

**Table 7.5 Examples of common opposition strategies and arguments**

Challenge the credibility of sources or their organizations

Use scientific spokespersons (e.g., create an impression that there is controversy among scientists)

Use representatives from "front" organizations with perceived higher credibility

Provide alternative data or interpretations

Reinterpret advocates' data in a more or less favorable light in an attempt to minimize its effect

Predict adverse economic impact (e.g., too expensive, projected job losses)

Challenging data sources, methodology, analyses, or interpretation (e.g., "junk science"; a desire for "sound science")

Divide and conquer (e.g., acknowledge that *A* is a problem, but that policies or programs are needed to address problem *B* instead because it is more important)

*Source*: Remington PL, Ahrens D. Communicating public health information to private and voluntary health organizations. In: Nelson DE, Brownson RC, Remington PL, Parvanta C, eds. *Communicating Public Health Information Effectively: A Guide for Practitioners*. Washington, D.C.: American Public Health Association; 2002:115–126. Bero LA, Montini T, Bryan-Jones K, Mangurian C. Science in regulatory policy making: Case studies in the development of workplace smoking restrictions. Tob Control. 2001;10(4):329–336. Corbett E, Connors R. *Classic Rhetoric for the Modern Student*. 4th ed. New York, N.Y.: Oxford University Press; 1999. Dolnik L, Case TI, Williams KD. Stealing thunder as a courtroom tactic revisited: Processes and boundaries. *Law Hum Behav*. 2003;27:265–285. Michaels D, Monforton C. Manufacturing uncertainty: Contested science and the protection of the public's health and environment. *Am J Public Health*. 2005;95(Suppl 1):S39–S48. Ramage JD, Bean JC, Johnson J. *Writing Arguments: A Rhetoric with Readings*. 6th ed. New York, N.Y.: Pearson/Longman; 2003. Weston A. *A Rulebook for Arguments*. 3rd ed. Indianapolis, Ind.: Hackett; 2000.

**Box 7.1 Anticipating and countering common opposition arguments: Secondhand smoke laws**

Arguments used by the tobacco industry and others opposed to secondhand smoke (SHS) laws provide insights about common themes faced by public health advocates in other public health areas. The first argument against SHS laws is to question the scientific evidence. Although SHS has been confirmed by the U.S. Surgeon General, the International Agency for Research on Cancer, and others to increase the risk of certain types of cancer, heart disease, and other diseases, these research findings are commonly challenged, often by scientists with financial or other ties to the tobacco industry. Such arguments can be countered by stressing the consensus about adverse health effects reached by the scientific community, particularly among trusted individuals or organizations.

A second common argument is the alleged economic hardship associated with SHS laws, with dire predictions of doom by certain business owners or their trade associations. In El Paso, Texas, for example, restaurant owners largely accepted a strong SHS law that was enacted, but bar owners attempted to overturn the law, citing concerns about substantial

*(continued)*

273

**Box 7.1** (continued)

revenue loss. A subsequent evaluation research study found that one year after the law was passed there was no adverse economic impact. This finding of no adverse economic impact has consistently been reported by independent research studies in other geographic areas; such research can and has been used to counter dire economic predictions of proposed SHS laws elsewhere.

A third common opposition argument against SHS laws is that they pose an unnecessary infringement on individuals' rights (see Box 7.2). While it is true that SHS laws require changes in behavior by smokers (e.g., having to smoke outside), exposure to SHS can endanger the health of others. One way to counter the individual right argument is to stress that people have a right to breathe smoke-free air, and that an individual's right to smoke does not mean they are free to endanger the health of those around them.

Source: Department of Health and Human Services. *The Health Consequences of Involuntary Exposure to Tobacco Smoke: A Report of the Surgeon General.* Atlanta, Ga.: U.S. Department of Health and Human Services, Centers for Disease Control and Prevention, Office on Smoking and Health; 2006. Barnes DE, Bero LA. Why review articles on the health effects of passive smoking reach different conclusions. *JAMA.* 1998;279(19):1566–1570. Bero LA, Montini T, Bryan-Jones K, Mangurian C. Science in regulatory policy making: Case studies in the development of workplace smoking restrictions. *Tob Control* 2001;10(4):329–336. Magzamen S, Charlesworth A, Glantz SA. Print media coverage of California's Smokefree Bar Law. *Tob Control.* 2001;10:154–160. National Cancer Institute. ASSIST: Shaping the future of tobacco prevention and control. *Tob Control Monogr.* 2005;16 (NIH Pub No. 05-5645). Reynolds JH, Hobart RL, Ayala P, Eischen MH. Clean indoor air in El Paso, Texas: A case study [serial on-line]. *Prev Chronic Dis.* 2005;2(1).

For example, worldwide death data for children under 5 years of age were reported in opposite ways by UNICEF and the researchers who published the study in the journal *Lancet* in 2007.[58–61] UNICEF officials described these findings as a major public health success, with child deaths dropping to a record low of 9.7 million in 2005.[58, 59] In contrast, Christopher Murray, the study's lead author, referred to the slowing trend in the rate at which younger children were dying from 1985 to 2005 compared with 1970 to 1985 (1.3% versus 2.2% annual rates, respectively), noting that there was no cause for optimism because the expected decline of 27% from 1995 to 2015 was substantially lower than the stated goal of a 67% decline over this period.[59, 61]

Data and recommendations by scientists are often seen by program advocates and policy makers as another tool for debate and negotiation, not as "definitive truth."[14, 55, 62] Anecdotes or the concerns of individuals or groups that could be adversely affected by scientists' recommendations can also be considered by policy makers and the public as credible types of evidence.[55, 62]

Much to the chagrin of many scientists, there are many examples of policy makers and the public ignoring strong scientific evidence, and scientific consensus, concerning beneficial public health policies or programs. Even the most scientifically valid information can be trumped by other factors or individuals that are more influential or persuasive (Box 7.2).[23, 25, 55, 63, 64] Furthermore, there are policy makers and members of the public who do not trust, or even disdain, scientists and scientific reasoning; presenting data-based information or recommendations to them is unlikely to be persuasive with such individuals (Chapters 1 and 2).[23, 65, 66]

So why bother using scientific data for advocacy? Because at times, scientists and their findings can be highly influential or persuasive with policy makers and the public.[2, 14, 21, 22, 24, 38, 67] Scientists in most Westernized societies are held by many people in high esteem and have strong source credibility (Chapter 2).[23, 24, 55] They are commonly seen as independent, idealized "truth generators" who are not sullied by values and morals.

A multiyear study of federal policy making based on interviews with congressional staff, members of the executive branch (e.g., upper-level civil servants, presidential staff, and political appointees in departments), and persons outside government (e.g., journalists, lobbyists, academics) examined the perceived influence of different unofficial actors.[23] Findings from this study demonstrated that independent research organizations (including scientists) were considered to be the second-most important unofficial actor influencing public policy, surpassed only by interest groups.

Given that many policy issues are considered to be "messy," scientific data can provide the fundamental basis for advocacy by producing evidentiary matter used in the synthesis of research and the development of scientific consensus, regarding the existence of a problem, its extent, its cause(s), or the rationale for interventions or other actions (the review and synthesis step of the organize phase of the OPT-In model in Chapter 5).[2, 55, 68] All truth is not relative or subjective—some scientific findings are not easily refutable because they are based on solid research.

## Data Selection

The selection and presentation of data as part of messages for public health advocacy is the focus of the remainder of the chapter. The phases of the OPT-In framework (organize, plan, test, and integrate) discussed in Chapter 5 are applicable for advocacy. A review and synthesis of research findings leads to developing storylines (organize phase). Messages based on storylines for advocacy tend to be simple, given that the purpose for communicating with lay audiences is persuasion (part of the planning phase), often taking the

**Box 7.2** Role of other factors besides data influencing policy makers: Opposition to motorcycle helmet laws

The Federal Highway Safety Act of 1966 provided support for federal and state safety programs through the Department of Transportation, but limited funding if states did not enact motorcycle helmet laws. Although most states enacted such helmet laws, in 1976, after extensive protests by motorcycle riders, Congress amended the legislation so that federal funding was not tied to states' motorcycle helmet laws. This has resulted in some states repealing their helmet laws; helmet laws remain under contention in many states.

Scientific research has consistently shown that motorcycle helmet use reduces the risk of injury and its associated financial costs, and motorcycle helmet laws increase the use of helmets. Public opinion polls generally show that the majority of people favor motorcycle helmet laws.

Opposition to mandatory helmet laws, however, is based primarily on the loss of the right to make individual decisions about helmet use. Opponents also argue that helmets make injury to motorcyclists more likely in an accident although there is scientific consensus that this is not true. A vocal minority, led by Richard Quigley of California (photo), is highly active seeking to overturn helmet laws in many states. The differences among state motorcycle helmet laws provide a clear example that other factors besides strong scientific evidence can influence policy makers.

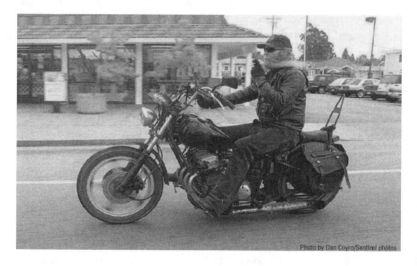

Photo by Dan Coyro/Sentinel photos

Source: Auman KM, Kufera JA, Ballesteros MF, Smialek JE, Dischinger PC. Autopsy study of motorcyclist fatalities: The effect of the 1992 Maryland motorcycle helmet use law. *Am J Public Health*. 2002 92(8):1352–1355. Bikers Rights. Biker's

*(continued)*

Rights Online. 2006 [cited 2006 April 21]; Available from HYPERLINK "http://www. bikersrights.com" www.bikersrights.com. Federal Highway Administration. *State Programs Overview.* Washington, D.C.: Federal Highway Association; 2006. Federal Highway Administration. *Community Resources: Motorcycle Safety.* Washington, D.C.: Federal Highway Association; 2006. Kraus JF, Peek C, McArthur DL, Williams A. The effect of the 1992 California motorcycle helmet use law on motorcycle crash fatalities and injuries. *JAMA.* 1994;272(19):1506–1511. Max W, Stark B, Root S. Putting a lid on injury costs: The economic impact of the California motorcycle helmet law. *J Trauma.* 1998;45(3):550–556. National Highway Traffic Safety Administration. *2003 Motor Vehicle Occupant Safety Survey.* Washington, D.C.: National Highway Traffic Safety Administration; 2003. National Highway Traffic Safety Administration. *Traffic Safety Facts. Laws. Motorcycle Helmet Use Laws.* Washington, D.C.: National Highway Traffic Safety Administration; 2004. Malikoff M. The road lawyer. *Santa Cruz Sentinel*, January 8, 2001.

form of "do this" or "don't do that" regarding a specific public health policy, program, or resource allocation.

Policy makers are the main lay audience for public health advocacy, although the public and the press may also be audiences because of their potential influence on policy makers. Understanding policy makers is crucial (Chapter 2), particularly their individual characteristics, the occupational and institutional factors under which they operate, their regular sources of information, and the communication approaches most likely to be successful in reaching them (Chapter 2; Table 7.4). Similar understanding about members of the press is essential if the press is also a target audience (Chapter 2).

The context in which communication with policy makers occurs is also important, given the formal and informal rules under which they operate (Chapter 2; earlier in this chapter). Timing of communication is a particularly important contextual consideration. Focusing events (Tables 7.1 and 7.2) can provide rare opportunities for advocacy; however, in the absence of such events an active communication strategy is necessary to gain or retain lay audience attention. Formal testing of messages and communication channels (Opt-In testing phase) is often not feasible for advocacy-oriented communication with policy makers, although message testing can sometimes be done for efforts directed toward the public (e.g., through focus groups, in-depth interviews, or public opinion polling). Last, communication efforts, and the broader integration of messages based on current scientific understanding, are important for advocacy (Opt-In integrate phase).

### Should Data Be Used at All?

Advocates must first determine the storyline they wish to convey to lay audiences. Second, they need to develop basic themes, and create messages, that will resonate with lay audiences[16]; effective advocacy depends heavily on developing such themes. Third, advocates need to determine if, or how, data would be useful to support themes.[52, 62, 68, 69]

Three basic techniques can be used to create themes: words, pictures, numbers, or some combination of the above (Chapter 4).[16] The reality is that there are many situations where data are unlikely to persuade policy makers. Photographs, other visual images, or narratives (e.g., personal stories or anecdotes) can be better choices to push forward certain themes (e.g., resources to support disease screening or treatment services); there are many such examples from journalism, legislative or private organization hearings, and other meetings.[3, 15, 70–74] One personal testimony from a credible source may be much more persuasive than strong data and scientific consensus recommendations.[51, 53, 62, 75]

### Roles of Data for Advocacy Themes

Public health data can play several roles to help communicate certain underlying advocacy themes and help to authenticate them (i.e., "these numbers demonstrate that my story is true") (Table 7.6).[16] These roles are to raise awareness, demonstrate cause and effect, predict, evaluate, and maintain awareness. The three major story themes data can support are gloom, control and hope, or success.[3, 15, 16, 51, 76, 77]

As discussed earlier, much of the work in public health advocacy involves efforts, usually long term, to raise awareness of the public and policy makers, that is, to gain their attention (Chapter 2). This occurs during the problem definition or issue awareness phase of the policy cycle (Figure 7.1).[22, 25] Descriptive data can be used to demonstrate that there is a problem, and that it is large and important enough that people should pay attention to it. Raising awareness is generally facilitated by using data as part of gloom theme (negative message framing), for example, "the growing problem of antibiotic-resistant bacteria" or "although rates have increased, there are still an estimated 10,000 children in this state who are not up-to-date with their immunizations."[3, 16] There are many variations of the gloom theme, such as decline, inequity, or disparity.[16] Such data can often be used in attempts to shame policy makers into action.

The most useful numbers to select for raising awareness among lay audiences are those that demonstrate the large magnitude or seriousness of the problem, and that are likely to be easily understood by lay audiences.[16, 52, 53] Such data generally come from public health surveillance (e.g., mortality, morbidity, number of cases), census, or administrative data sets. Administrative data, such as the number of persons receiving or needing services (e.g., unmet need), can be invaluable for program advocacy purposes.[3, 15, 16]

**Table 7.6 Potential roles for data, and types of data, for advocacy in public health**

| Role | Theme | Most useful types of data |
| --- | --- | --- |
| Raise awareness | Gloom | Surveillance, census, cost, administrative, attributable risk, trend data can be especially helpful (Descriptive) |
| Cause and effect | Control and hope | Relative or absolute risk, relative or absolute percentage change, meta-analyses, research syntheses (Analytic) |
| Predict | Control and hope | Statistical modeling, econometric modeling (Projection) |
| Evaluate | Success | Surveillance, administrative, census, cost, trend data, percentage change over time (e.g., relative or absolute change in risk or cost estimates), trend data can be especially helpful (Descriptive or Analytic) |
| Maintain awareness | Gloom or success | Surveillance, census, cost, administrative, attributable risk, trend or evaluation data |

*Source*: Stone DA. *Policy Paradox: The Art of Political Decision Making*. Rev. ed. New York, N.Y.: Norton; 2002. Blum D, Knudson M, Henig RM, eds. *A Field Guide for Science Writers: The Official Guide of the National Association of Science Writers*. 2nd ed. New York, N.Y.: Oxford University Press; 2006. Wallack L, Dorfman L, Jernigan D, Themba M. *Media Advocacy for Public Health*. Newbury Park, Calif.: Sage; 1993. Wallack LM. *News for a Change: An Advocate's Guide to Working with the Media*. Thousand Oaks, Calif.: Sage; 1999. Abelson RP. *Statistics as Principled Argument*. Hillsdale, N.J.: Lawrence Erlbaum; 1995. Cohn V, Cope L. *News and Numbers: A Guide to Reporting Statistical Claims and Controversies in Health and Other Fields*. 2nd ed. Ames, Iowa: Iowa State Press; 2001. Corbett E, Connors R. *Classic Rhetoric for the Modern Student*. 4th ed. New York, N.Y.: Oxford University Press; 1999. Ramage JD, Bean JC, Johnson J. *Writing Arguments: A Rhetoric with Readings*. 6th ed. New York, N.Y.: Pearson/Longman; 2003. Goodsell CT. *The Case for Bureaucracy: A Public Administration Polemic*. th ed. Washington, D.C.: CQ Press; 2003.

Findings from trend analyses, attributable risk estimates, or cost studies (e.g., health care costs, productivity) can also be useful for raising awareness. For advocacy purposes, big numbers are better than small numbers, official (government) numbers are better than data from other sources such as research studies, and big official numbers are best of all, provided, of course, that numbers are scientifically defensible and used in an ethical manner[16, 51, 52] (Box 7.3; note that while the Institute of Medicine is not a governmental agency, it is generally considered by scientists to be highly credible organization). If advocacy efforts are at the state or local level, then every effort should be made to use local data.[13] Simple frequencies (i.e., counts or whole number estimates) because they are larger, are generally preferred over percentages, rates, or other data for raising awareness, although relative percentage change may be of value.[36 51, 53] If rates are used, crude rates that describe what is actually happening in given geographic locations are a better choice than adjusted rates (e.g., by age) because they describe the actual magnitude or burden.[36] If trend data are used, relative percentage change

---

**Box 7.3** Using data to raise awareness: Hospital-based errors and mortality

The Institute of Medicine (IOM) issued a report in 1999 on hospital patient safety entitled *To Err Is Human*. Thanks, in part, to strong outreach efforts to major media outlets on behalf of the IOM, the findings of this report received extensive news coverage. Public and private health care organizations, and public policy makers, paid attention to this report. For example, President Clinton signed an executive order in December 1999 that required agencies of the federal government to create an activity list to improve patient safety within 90 days.

The public also attended to news stories about this IOM report: one national survey found that it was the most closely followed health policy story of the year. The rapid and broad level of interest among lay audiences about the issue of hospital patient safety spurred by this report was almost unprecedented.

One of the major factors contributing to the success of the IOM report in raising awareness was its inclusion of readily understandable data. It stated that an estimated 44,000 to 98,000 persons died each year because of preventable medical errors. This meant that medical errors were the eighth leading cause of death in the United States, exceeding the number of deaths resulting from breast cancer, AIDS, or motor vehicles. Although the report only included the estimated range of deaths, the media often chose to mention just the upper estimate of 98,000 deaths in news reports and other stories. The "98,000 deaths" number became almost an icon in and of itself, helping to magnify the seriousness of the problem and the need for action by those concerned about hospital safety.

Source: Institute of Medicine. *To Err Is Human: Building a Safer Health System.* Washington, D.C.: National Academies of Science; 2000. Ioannidis JP, Evans SJ, Gotzsche PC, et al. Better reporting of harms in randomized trials: An extension of the CONSORT statement. *Ann Intern Med.* 2004;141(10):781–788. Blendon RJ, DesRoches CM, Brodie M, et al. Views of practicing physicians and the public on medical errors. *N Engl J Med.* 2002;347(24):1933–1940. Dentzer S. Media mistakes in coverage of the Institute of Medicine's error report. *Eff Clin Pract.* 2000;3(6):305–308.

---

(increase or decrease), rather than absolute change estimates, are likely to be more effective because of their larger magnitude.

The second major use of public health data for advocacy is to demonstrate cause and effect.[36] Such data help to support a theme of control and hope and are part of the policy formulation phase of the policy cycle (Figure 7.1). They can demonstrate that, although this situation (disease or risk) was previously thought to be inevitable or random, we now know that we can control it in some fashion (e.g., through a new program, policy, screening test, treatment, medication, or diet).[16, 71, 77] Such themes are usually framed in a positive manner, that is, as a solution to a problem. The use of a control and hope theme inevitably involves some type of choice for the public and for policy makers.[16]

In contrast to raising awareness, cause-and-effect findings are usually based on analytic research. Data are usually derived from etiologic, intervention, policy, evaluation, or similar types of studies.[36] Research syntheses such as meta-analyses or evidence reviews can be invaluable.

Cause-and-effect data for advocacy usually involve relative risk estimates or some other type of change measure.[36] From an advocacy perspective, relative risk ("3 times greater risk among those not treated") or percentage relative risk ("60% reduction in cases among persons living in state *A* after the policy was implemented") data are better choices than absolute risk because they usually have larger magnitudes (Box 7.4). Similarly, if trend data are used to highlight changes over time, numbers should be presented as relative percentage change, as such values are likely to be larger than those based on absolute percentage point change (a "150% increase in the number of low income infants receiving well-baby care after the new program was instituted").

Related to the role of cause and effect is using data for prediction, that is, describing the expected effect of a policy or program.[36] Many policy debates involve projecting the effect(s) of a proposed policy or program, or of a change in an existing policy or program (Box 7.5).[16, 25] Data provide the scientific underpinnings for statements such as "if we do *X*, we believe this will be the effect on *Y*."[32] As with cause and effect, prediction usually supports a control and hope theme[16] and is part of the policy formulation phase of the policy cycle (Figure 7.1).[23]

In general, advocates use a positive frame for prediction, emphasizing the expected large magnitude and benefit(s) of a policy or program; opponents will stress just the opposite. Typically prediction involves statistical modeling projections[78]; if cost is an important factor, econometric projection models are often used. Such models may be developed anew when a legislative bill is under serious consideration; alternatively, models may already exist in the scientific literature and contribute to discussions.

Prediction, to say the least, is an inexact science. It is typically based on extending data from prior studies or other findings; sometimes attributable risk data can be used to estimate the impact of policies or programs. Some models can involve highly complex calculations and multiple assumptions about data.[36] Data most likely to be useful for prediction from an advocacy perspective involve estimated changes in frequencies (counts) or relative percentage for measures such as mortality, morbidity, risk behaviors, or number of persons receiving services (e.g., "1,000 more people each year in county

**Box 7.4** Cause-and-effect data for advocacy: Graduated driver licensing in Utah

Extensive research has demonstrated that young drivers are at greatly increased risk for motor vehicle crashes. Rates of motor vehicle crashes, based on miles driven, are about 10 times higher for drivers aged 16–17 years compared with drivers aged 30–59 years, and more than double those of drivers aged 18–19 years.

To address this problem, graduated driver licensing (GDL) policies have been developed that place driving restrictions on young drivers. These policies include mandating a learner's permit that requires that a licensed adult aged ≥21 years be in a motor vehicle with teen drivers aged 15 or 16 years for a defined number of months; a provisional license for drivers aged 16–17 years that limits nighttime driving, transporting other teenagers, requiring zero tolerance for alcohol while driving (e.g., blood alcohol concentrations of ≤.02), or mandates that drivers be motor vehicle crash- and conviction-free for a defined period; or delaying full licensure until an older age, such as 18 years. Despite state variability in the type of GDL laws, research has consistently shown that they reduce motor vehicle crash fatalities and injuries to younger teen drivers. As of 2006, more than 40 states had some type of GDL requirement.

Utah provides an excellent example of how cause-and-effect data, presented as relative risks, were effectively used to support passage of a strengthened GDL law. A GDL bill was first introduced in the Utah legislature in 1997, but received little support because it was viewed as an intrusion on parental duties. Although the state legislature enacted GDL restrictions in 1999 and 2000 related to nighttime driving restrictions and the minimum number of hours a teen must drive with an accompanying adult before full licensure, they did not address restrictions on passengers.

At the 2001 legislative session, a GDL bill was introduced that would require teen drivers be accompanied by an adult aged ≥21 years in order to have other passengers in their vehicles. Researchers and other staff at the Intermountain Injury Control Research Center played a crucial role by presenting their data, based on Utah's Crash Outcome Data Evaluation System (CODES), to policy makers during hearings and other legislative activities. They also developed and distributed a fact sheet to raise awareness among legislators and communicated findings directly to news media representatives.

Data presented to legislators and reporters showed that teenage drivers in Utah with at least one passenger were twice as likely, and teen drivers with ≥5 passengers were more than five times as likely to be cited for reckless driving than were adult drivers. Furthermore, teen drivers with

*(continued)*

282

at least one passenger were 1.5 times as likely, and teen drivers with ≥5 passengers were 2.5 times as likely to be hospitalized or die as a result of a motor vehicle crash compared with adult drivers. Data presented showed a clear linear trend: as the number of passengers that a teen driver was transporting increased, so did the risk of reckless driving, motor vehicle injury, or death. Ultimately, relative risk estimates, strengthened by the fact that they were based on Utah-specific data, were effectively communicated to legislators and reporters and contributed to this successful effort: the 2001 Utah legislature enacted a bill requiring that teenage drivers who transport passengers must have a licensed rider aged ≥21 years in their vehicles.

Source: Branche C, Williams AF, Feldman D. Graduated licensing for teens: Why everybody's doing it. *J Law Med Ethics.* 2002;30(3 Suppl):146–149. Chen IG, Durbin DR, Elliott MR, Senserrick T, Winston FK. Child passenger injury risk in motor vehicle crashes: A comparison of nighttime and daytime driving by teenage and adult drivers. *J Safety Res.* 2006;37(3):299–306. Hartling L, Wiebe N, Russell K, Petruk J, Spinola C, Klassen TP. Graduated driver licensing for reducing motor vehicle crashes among young drivers. *Cochrane Database Syst Rev.* 2004(2):CD003300. CODES U. *Passenger Limitations and Graduated Driver Licensing in Utah.* Salt Lake City, Utah: UT CODES; 2002. Williams AF. Young driver risk factors: Successful and unsuccessful approaches for dealing with them and an agenda for the future. *Inj Prev.* 2006;12(Suppl 1):i4–i8.

**Box 7.5 Use of data for prediction in advocacy: Universal preschool in California**

The David and Lucile Packard Foundation favors the adoption of state funding for universal preschool for 4-year-old children in California. To determine the estimated economic effects, they supported a RAND Corporation study on this issue. The results of the study confirmed that the expected benefits substantially exceeded the costs:

- The additional $4,300-per-child cost would result in an estimated $11,400 in benefits per child for California society.
- For every $1 invested in the program, there would be a net benefit of $2.62.
- Additional benefits would accrue to the state, such as improving the competitiveness of the state's economy and economic and social equality.

Further numeric estimates of the impacts of universal preschool based on each year for which 4 year olds completed a year of preschool were that it would result in

*(continued)*

**Box 7.5** *(continued)*

- 10,000 additional high school graduates
- 4,700 fewer abused or neglected children
- 7,300 fewer children involved in the juvenile court system
- 9,100 fewer children in special education programs.

These data were widely used in advocacy efforts, contributing to the passage of bill in 2006 with overwhelming support in the California legislature to provide increased funding for preschool education.

Source: Karoly LA, Bigelow JH. *The Economics of Investing in Universal Preschool Education in California.* Santa Monica, Calif.: RAND Corporation; 2005. Preschool California. *Governor Signs Preschool Bill.* Oakland, Calif.: Preschool California; 2006. The David and Lucile Packard Foundation. *Preschool for California's Children.* Los Altos, Calif.: The David and Lucile Packard Foundation; 2006.

*C* would receive dental care because of this program" or "there would be a 50% reduction in the number of bicycle-related head injuries if a bicycle helmet law was enacted").

The decision by advocates to select and present cost projection data (e.g., of providing services, cost effectiveness, cost benefits) to policy makers can present a dilemma. Public health policies and programs can potentially have large societal benefits but not necessarily reduce cost expenditures, especially in the short term.[2] Increases or decreases in costs and benefits depend upon the perspective of different organizations, institutions, or individuals.[2] There is no definitive answer about the decision to use cost data for advocacy purposes—it depends on the specific situation. Those who perceive they will suffer financially are likely to use cost data in opposition arguments.[21] In private policy-making settings, advocates are very likely to need to address cost issues upfront, especially in the corporate world.[49]

The fourth role for data in advocacy is evaluation (Box 7.6).[3, 16, 36] The usual underlying theme of evaluation is positively framed as success: "The *X* policy (or program) was implemented, and here are data that prove that it works (worked)."[22] Such a theme can readily be expanded (e.g., "The *X* policy (program) would be even more successful if we added new provisions, or increased resources").

It is true that policy makers may not evaluate the effect of programs in a systematic manner, if at all.[22] However, evaluation data are crucial when public health policies or programs, or the resources to support them, are challenged. Without such data, policies or programs are vulnerable to powerful opposition arguments or competing policy-maker priorities.[67]

**Box 7.6** Use of data for evaluation in advocacy: Folic acid and neural tube defect prevention

As discussed in Chapter 1 (Box 1.3) there was scientific consensus by the early 1990s that women who consumed 400 µg of folic acid before conception and during early pregnancy were much less likely to have a child born with a neural tube defect (NTD), such as spina bifida. Unfortunately, most women of childbearing age do not consume enough folic acid through dietary means. At the urging of the scientific community, the Food and Drug Administration (FDA) required manufacturers to add folic acid to enriched grain products like bread by January 1998 as a way to increase folic acid consumption. Additionally, because about half of all pregnancies in the United States are unplanned, the FDA, the Centers for Disease Control and Prevention, the March of Dimes, and other organizations recommended that all women of childbearing age take a daily multivitamin tablet with folic acid.

Subsequent evaluation research has shown the benefits of increased folic acid use among women of childbearing years. Since the new FDA requirements went into effect, there has been an estimated 25% reduction in NTDs, with the number of NTD-affected pregnancies in the United States declining from 4,000 in 1995–1996 to 3,000 in 1999–2000. Use of folic acid supplements among women of childbearing age increased from 15% in 1988 to 33% in 2005, with much of the increase occurring since 1995. Although there remains a long way to go to increase folic acid use, these evaluation data demonstrate the success of efforts to prevent NTDs and are widely used in educational efforts with health care practitioners, the public, and policy makers.

Source: Centers for Disease Control and Prevention. Spina bifida and anencephaly before and after folic acid mandate: United States, 1995–1996 and 1999–2000. *MMWR.* 2004;53:362–365. Centers for Disease Control and Prevention. Use of vitamins containing folic acid among women of childbearing age—United States, 2004. *MMWR.* 2004;53:847–950. de Jong-Van den Berg LT, Hernandez-Diaz S, Werler MM, Louik C, Mitchell AA. Trends and predictors of folic acid awareness and periconceptional use in pregnant women. *Am J Obstet Gynecol.* 2005;192(1):121–128. Mills JL, England L. Food fortification to prevent neural tube defects: Is it working? *JAMA.* 2001;285(23):3022–3023. Williams LJ, Rasmussen SA, Flores A, Kirby RS, Edmonds LD. Decline in the prevalence of spina bifida and anencephaly by race/ethnicity: 1995–2002. *Pediatrics.* 2005;116(3):580–586.

Descriptive or analytic data can be used to evaluate the success or failure of a policy or program.[36, 67] Evaluation of many public health policies and programs, particularly at the state or local level, will usually rely on descriptive data from public health surveillance or other types of routine government data collection activities.[22, 25, 36]

Showing trends can be helpful to document changes over time. As with other uses of data for advocacy, changes in frequencies (e.g., persons receiving public health–related services, number of deaths, number of injuries), relative risk, or relative percentage change are likely to be the most effective.[36] With the exception of policies or programs designed to increase the provision of services, outcome evaluation measures (e.g., changes in mortality or prevalence) are preferred over process measures (e.g., number of products distributed).[36, 67]

The last role for data in advocacy is to maintain awareness.[3, 15, 51] This means using data in attempts to keep an issue, policy, or program in the minds of the public, policy makers, or the press (Box 7.7). This role may be for the public health problem itself, a causal factor, an intervention, the projected benefits of a policy or program solution, or the benefits of an existing policy or program. This is an important phase in advocacy that can be overlooked: in the absence of sustained effort and commitment, effective public health policies and programs can be neglected, or in some instances reversed, by sustained opposition efforts.

---

**Box 7.7 Using data to maintain awareness: Breast cancer**

Without a doubt, breast cancer advocates in the United States have been remarkably successful on multiple fronts, helping to increase public and private funding for research, prevention, screening, diagnosis, and treatment. Only a few decades ago, the words "cancer" and "breast" were not acceptable to use in public discussions or debate; now the majority of women believe that breast cancer is their greatest health risk despite the fact that far more women are diagnosed, and die from, cardiovascular disease.

The effective use of data has played a key role in maintaining awareness of this disease among lay audiences. In the early 1990s, advocates compared the number of breast cancer deaths to the number of Americans killed in wars, pointing out that since the early 1970s, more women in the United States have died from breast cancer than all the men who died in World War I, World War II, and the Korean and Vietnam wars.

But the most prominent number used to maintain awareness has been the lifetime risk of women for developing breast cancer. Because recent data suggest that one in eight women will develop this disease, advocates have consistently mentioned a lifetime risk estimate in messages designed to maintain awareness and encourage women to regularly be screened for breast cancer (e.g., through mammography). Although the concept of lifetime risk is often misunderstood by lay audiences, research has shown that knowledge of the lifetime breast cancer risk estimates is high among women. This lifetime risk data estimate remains invaluable for helping maintain awareness among the public, policy makers, and the press about this issue.

*(continued)*

Source: Clarke HN, Everest MM. Cancer in the mass print media: Fear, uncertainty and the medical model. *Soc Sci Med.* 2006;62:2591–2600. Erblich J, Bovbjerg DH, Norman C, Valdimarsdottir HB, Montgomery GH. It won't happen to me: Lower perception of heart disease risk among women with family histories of breast cancer. *Prev Med.* 2000;31(6):714–721. Morris CR, Wright WE, Schlag RD. The risk of developing breast cancer within the next 5, 10, or 20 years of a woman's life. *Am J Prev Med.* 2001;20(3):214–218. Phillips KA, Glendon G, Knight JA. Putting the risk of breast cancer in perspective. *N Engl J Med.* 1999;340(2):141–144. Wells J, Marshall P, Crawley B, Dickersin K. Newspaper reporting of screening mammography. *Ann Intern Med.* 2001;135(12):1029–1037. Woloshin S, Schwartz LM, Byram SJ, Sox HC, Fischhoff B, Welch HG. Women's understanding of the mammography screening debate. *Arch Intern Med.* 2000;160(10):1434–1440. Ries L, Harkins D, Krapcho M. *SEER Cancer Statistics Review, 1975–2003.* Bethesda, MD: National Cancer Institute; 2006.

The themes that data can support for maintaining awareness are similar to those used for raising awareness or for evaluation. If advocates have not been successful in having a desired policy or program enacted or maintained, data should be selected that support a gloom theme, for example, large magnitude and importance of the problem or adverse trends. On the other hand, if a desired policy or program has been enacted and been effective, advocates should select evaluation data that highlight success, such as positive trends, other surveillance findings, or research studies. Messages supported by data may also highlight areas in which improvement is needed.

Using a few "tried and true" data items can be useful (Box 7.7), but it will be helpful to provide new data or to reformulate existing data over time to maintain awareness. The release or publication of a new report or research study by a respected source, or a relevant anniversary, provides an opportunity to put to a fresh face on an established public health issue or intervention.[16]

Specifics about what data to select depends on which of these points advocates want to emphasize. If it is to remind people of the size or importance of a public health issue or unmet need (a gloom theme), then the same approach should be used as applied to raising awareness (e.g., communicating surveillance data, trends, attributable risk estimates, or cost studies). Simple numbers, for example, frequencies (counts) or percentages, which are large and from government sources are best[16, 36]; if trend data are used, relative percentage change (increase or decrease) will be better than absolute percentage change. If evaluation data are to be used to highlight success, then changes in counts, relative risk, or relative percentage change, particularly of outcome measures, would usually be better choices.[36]

## Additional Considerations

There are a few final points to remember when selecting data for advocacy in public health. The roles for data, and themes they support (Table 7.6), can be combined to some extent to support an advocacy storyline.[16] For example, the raise awareness and cause-and-effect roles are often used together: surveillance data can be used to demonstrate the magnitude of a health problem (raising awareness through a gloom theme), followed by research findings to support a recommended action (cause and effect demonstrating a theme of control and hope).

Although stressed elsewhere in this book, it is important to mention again that the selection or omission of data involves values and ethical decisions,[18] given the temptation to oversimplify or exaggerate data to support a preferred storyline and to ignore or minimize data that are not supportive— whatever role and theme data may be used for.[16, 19]

Audience expectations play an important part in how information is understood and interpreted.[75] In some advocacy situations, such as those involving the publication or presentation of findings of a major report or study, it may be helpful to develop, frame, and communicate a message for the intended audience prior to a formal release. This can be done as a way of attempting to increase attention or interest. However, expectancy management may also be a useful strategy in situations where findings may be counterintuitive, unexpected, or likely to be framed inappropriately by opponents.[79, 80]

Depending on the findings, revealing data first that are not supportive of the underlying storyline or basic theme, that is, stealing thunder (Chapter 3 and Table 7.5), may be an approach to consider in certain situations. For example, suppose an evaluation of a health care institution's hospital infection control program by an independent organization found that there were errors in data reporting, which meant that previously reported low numbers of such infections that had been widely publicized were incorrect. Representatives of the health care institution would be much better served to release these evaluation data and other relevant information to lay audiences themselves (or perhaps in partnership with members of the evaluating organization) and acknowledge their mistakes.

Finally, opposite framing of the themes described in this section can be used, especially if public health advocates are attempting to thwart opposition attempts or arguments by others to weaken public health policies or programs.[16] Here are a few examples: "Reductions in program funding have led to a large increase in the number of persons diagnosed with tuberculosis (evaluation)"; "Relaxing workplace safety regulations would result in an estimated 3,000 additional workplace injuries in this state (prediction)."

## Data Presentation

Because advocacy is about persuasion, data need to be presented in such a manner as to fulfill their intended role and highlight the underlying storyline. Furthermore, data need to be presented in such a way as to accurately communicate scientific findings without misleading audiences (e.g., through exaggeration or minimization).

General recommendations and specific modalities for data presentation were discussed in detail in Chapter 4 and are applicable in public health advocacy situations. Because advocacy usually occurs around contested issues and attempts to influence audiences' understanding and interpretation, advocates should use words that clearly describe what data are and what they mean (interpretation).[52] Integrating words, numbers, and symbols (i.e., using titles, labels, legends, and peripheral cues for visual modalities) is important (Chapters 3 and 4). Data comparisons (e.g., trends over time, geographical differences, to established reference standards) can be beneficial because they provide contextual information to help audiences interpret findings.

Although there occasionally may be times when other data presentation formats (i.e., tables, diagrams, icons, visual scales) are used (Chapter 4), Table 7.7 lists those more likely to be effective for public health advocacy.

Research has demonstrated that simple verbal presentations of numbers can be persuasive with lay audiences,[62, 68, 75, 81, 82] as they can help support underlying advocacy themes.[51, 52, 68, 82] This may simply require explicitly stating a number ("Chronic diseases cost the United States more than $1 trillion a year,"[83] "There are more than half a million uninsured persons in our city," or "A 300% increase in hospital-acquired infections occurred over the past 20 years"). It can also be done implicitly, such as through comparative rankings ("Colorectal cancer is the second leading cause of cancer deaths among men"; "Diabetes is now the leading cause of renal failure").

No more than one or two numbers should be presented verbally, however, as using more data points tends to be confusing rather than persuasive with lay audiences because of limited quantitative literacy and cognitive burden (Chapters 3 and 4). Rounded numbers, rather than precise numbers, are easier for audiences to remember: a relative risk of 1.9 could be described as "nearly twice the risk," or a count of 4,256 described as "about 4,000." Care must be taken to choose numbers likely to be easily comprehended and meaningful to lay audiences.[62]

**Table 7.7 Recommended data presentation formats for advocacy**

One or two numbers
Verbal qualifiers
Metaphor
Narrative
Pie chart
Bar chart
Line graph
Map

Verbal qualifiers of data without presenting numbers are another viable option, for example, "small declines" or "great risk," as they help with interpretation by providing contextual information. Such qualifiers are a common way to describe trends, but can sometimes be used with comparisons (e.g., "Cigarette smoking causes more deaths than motor vehicle crashes, illegal drug use, and HIV infection combined"[84]; see also Box 7.7). Here are some examples of phrases that can be used in verbal descriptions of data: "[Program or Policy Y] resulted in a steep reduction in the number of emergency department visits," "The numbers of cases increased at a rate not seen since...," "These drastic funding cuts were associated with...," "Rapid improvement was seen after..."

Metaphors using numbers are especially valuable for communicating data for advocacy, as they can help to gain audience attention and improve comprehension (Chapter 4).[73, 85] Metaphors can transform numbers into something that people can more readily comprehend by connecting them with preexisting mental schema (Chapters 3 and 4).[85] If used, one metaphor is enough, and they work best when they are heard audibly.[86]

The key to developing a successful metaphor for advocacy is that it contains elements familiar to an audience, yet provides novel or new information.[51, 54, 86, 87] One approach used is to localize large numbers from surveillance systems or research studies, for example, "We estimate that about 1 in *xx* people in our community are affected, which is the equivalent of all the students at Jones High School." Examples of metaphors for advocacy purposes are listed in Table 7.8.

Narratives, including quotations, vignettes, personal testimony, anecdotes, and certain visual images (e.g., political cartoons) are widely used in persuasion efforts, as they can influence emotions and gain audience attention (Chapter 4).[73, 74, 88] In general, though, narratives are not a good choice for

**Table 7.8 Examples of public health metaphors for advocacy**

*Childhood violence prevention*
Child health care workers make less than $10 per hour, whereas prison
   guards are paid more than $18 per hour

*Nutrition*
A medium-sized buttered popcorn at the theater contains more artery-
   clogging fat than a bacon and eggs breakfast, a Big Mac and fries for
   lunch, and a steak dinner with all the trimmings...combined

*Sexually transmitted diseases*
Every weekend, more than 16,000 teenagers will be infected with a
   sexually transmitted disease

*Tobacco use*
Each year, more than 1 million children begin smoking; this is the
   equivalent of 33,000 classrooms per year or 90 classrooms every day

*Source*: Wallack L, Dorfman L, Jernigan D, Themba M. *Media Advocacy for Public Health*. Newbury Park, Calif.: Sage; 1993. Wallack LM. *News for a Change: An Advocate's Guide to Working with the Media*. Thousand Oaks, Calif.: Sage; 1999.

presenting data because they may detract from emotional imagery. Data should be used in narratives only to the extent that they can be integrated easily and support advocacy themes. Box 7.8 is an example of an advocacy narrative that integrates data into the main theme of cost being an important barrier in treating infant dehydration.

Visual presentations of data can also play a powerful role in advocacy. They can help to readily demonstrate magnitude, highlight changes, and make comparisons (Chapter 4). The goal of visual data presentation for advocacy is to highlight aspects that support the desired role and theme (e.g., to demonstrate cause and effect or support a gloom theme). Because of the problem of cognitive burden, it is especially critical to present only the minimal amount of data necessary, avoiding unnecessary or distracting items, such as 95% confidence interval brackets (Chapters 3 and 4). Conversely, adding contextual cues, such as text stressing key points (e.g., "a 200% increased risk"), arrows on a line graph showing when an intervention occurred and the subsequent change over time, shading or color, or comparison data (e.g., a paired bar chart, a comparison trend line) is strongly recommended, as they can help facilitate audience comprehension and interpretation (Chapters 3 and 4).[89, 90]

Pie charts, bar charts, line graphs, and maps are the four visual modalities likely to be most helpful for advocacy, as they can be created in such a way as to readily present the main message and enhance audience comprehension.[76, 90, 91] As discussed below, bar charts and line graphs are particularly good choices. (Although tables may occasionally be used for

---

**Box 7.8** Use of data in a narrative for advocacy: The cost of oral rehydration therapy

So this...woman calls up and said she has a 9-month-old baby with diarrhea and the doctor on call gave her the right advice, said go the pharmacy and buy Pedialyte®. She had Medicaid, the doctor called the pharmacy, but when she got there, they said they couldn't give it to her for free without a written prescription.

So she takes the kid home, and over the next 36 hr the baby gets worse. She doesn't call back—she should have called back. The kid appears in the emergency room 36 hr later, moribund, and dies three days later. My wife and I drove up there to that neighborhood, we went to every pharmacy. The rehydration solution costs up to $6.30 a liter. It's obscene charging this much for a product that ought to be cheaper than Coca-Cola—it has less in it.

Source: Wallack L, Dorfman L, Jernigan D, Themba M. *Media Advocacy for Public Health*. Newbury Park, Calif.: Sage; 1993:33.

advocacy, such as short-ranked lists, they are better suited for providing audiences with larger amounts of data.)

There are times when pie charts can help with advocacy, particularly for raising or maintaining awareness. Pie charts, because they represent proportions that total 100%, can be helpful for visually demonstrating magnitude when the communication objective involves the largest or smallest pie slice (Figure 7.2). For example, advocates could use a pie chart and have the largest pie slice emphasize that a particular health risk factor results in the largest mortality or morbidity number or percentage. Conversely, a small pie slice could be used to show the limited funding that a particular program receives relative to other programs.

Bar charts can be most helpful for visualizing magnitude (Figure 7.3),[89, 91] such as the actual or attributable number of individuals affected, relative risk, or relative change in percentage, including limited comparative differences. They can be used to raise awareness, demonstrate cause and effect, show evaluation findings, or maintain awareness; they are particularly valuable for showing cause-and-effect relationships. To facilitate communicating a simple and straightforward message, use as few bars as possible to minimize cognitive burden, and clearly delineate magnitude from largest to smallest (Chapter 4).

Line graphs are probably the most versatile visual modality for advocacy, as they can potentially be used to present data for all the roles and themes listed in Table 7.6. They can visually demonstrate that things are getting better, worse, or not changing (i.e., contribute to raising or maintaining awareness)

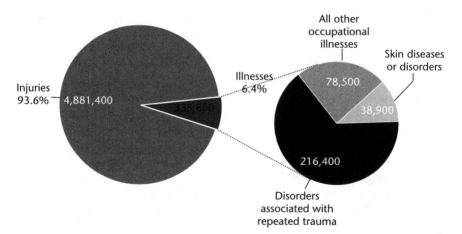

**Figure 7.2** Pie chart that could be used in advocacy to reduce repetitive trauma disorders. Illustrates the overwhelming proportion of nonfatal illnesses or injuries in U.S. private industry attributable to injury, with the portion attributable to illnesses expanded for emphasis to show the large contribution of repeated trauma disorders. (From NIOSH Publication Number 2004-146, "World Health Chart Book 2004".)

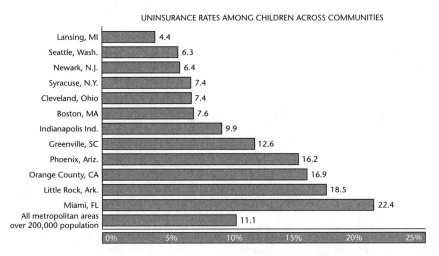

**Figure 7.3** Use of a horizontal bar chart to demonstrate differences in uninsurance among children across communities. (Source: Center for Studying Health System Change. *Issue Brief.* Washington, D.C.: Center for Studying Health System Change, Number 14; August 1998:p. 3. Reprinted with permission of the Center for Studying Health System Change, Washington DC. www.hschange.org.)

by showing trends over time. Line graphs can also be used to show cause-and-effect or evaluation findings, such as correlating the impact of an intervention with an outcome measure. As with bar charts, they can demonstrate the magnitude of an effect over time, such as in Figure 7.4 which shows the effect of vaccination on cases of measles. They are also widely used for prediction.

Maps in advocacy situations can identify geographic area(s) that are experiencing, or are at highest risk for experiencing (e.g., Figure 6.3), a particular adverse health outcome (e.g., number of cases, rates, relative risks); they can also be used to demonstrate differences in receipt of services, unmet need, or cost measures. In advocacy, this may simply involve including the names of geographic areas with higher or lower numbers or estimates, or using colors or shading to demonstrate differences as a way to help localize data (e.g., Figure 1.1). Elected representatives, such as legislators, are likely to be especially familiar with the geography of their own districts; thus maps can be particularly useful with this type of policy maker.[13]

## Conclusion

Policies and programs are important interventions to improve the health of the public. Advocacy plays a critical role in the enactment, implementation, or continuation of public health policies and programs; public health data of many kinds can assist with advocacy by providing a basis to support arguments for persuasion. As with all types of communication about data with

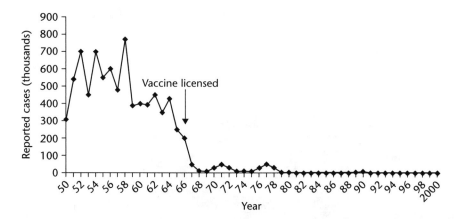

**Figure 7.4** Line graph (trend) demonstrating the effect of the measles vaccine on measles cases over several decades. (Source: Approximated from Orenstein W, Hinman AR. *A Shot at Protection: Immunizations Against Infectious Disease* In: Ward JW, Warren C. *Silent Victories: The History and Practice of Public Health in Twentieth Century America.* New York, N.Y.: Oxford University Press: 2007:p. 71)

lay audiences, decisions must be made about what numbers to select and how to most effectively present them. The problem is compounded by the reality that communicators in advocacy situations often have a limited amount of time (in the case of presentations or interviews) or space (in the case of written documents) to present their arguments. Given the level of interest and passion of advocates for their issues, special attention must be given to values and ethics underlying all public health data–related decisions.

---

**The bottom line**

There are many theories and models that provide different ways of understanding policy making and advocacy

In public health advocacy, data are most useful for (a) raising awareness, (b) demonstrating cause and effect, (c) predicting, (d) evaluating, and (e) maintaining awareness

Data can be invaluable for supporting the major advocacy themes of (a) gloom, (b) control and hope, or (c) success

Only minimal amounts of data (often one or two numbers) may be necessary to communicate to lay audiences in most advocacy situations

Metaphors containing numbers are especially valuable for communicating data for advocacy: they can transform data into mental schema familiar to audiences

Line graphs and bar charts are usually the most effective visual modalities to use in advocacy

## Further Reading

### Policy Making

Longest BB. *Health Policymaking in the United States.* 4th ed. Ann Arbor, Mich.: Health Administration Press; 2005.

McDonough JE. *Experiencing Politics: A Legislator's Stories of Government and Health Care.* Berkeley, Calif.: University of California Press; 2000.

Sabatier PA. ed. *Theories of the Political Process.* 2nd ed. Boulder, Colo.: Westview; 2007.

Stone D. *Policy Paradox: The Art of Political Decision Making.* Rev. ed. New York, N.Y.: Norton; 2002.

### Advocacy and Persuasion

Minkler M. ed. *Community Organizing and Community Building for Health.* 2nd ed. New Brunswick, N.J.: Rutgers University Press; 2004.

Smucker B. *Nonprofit Lobbying Guide: Advocating Your Cause and Getting Results.* 2nd ed. Washington, D.C.: Independent Sector; 1999.

Wallack L, Woodruff K, Dorfman L, Diaz I. *News for a Change: An Advocate's Guide to Working with the Media.* Thousand Oaks, Calif.: Sage; 1999.

Weston A. *A Rulebook for Arguments.* 3rd ed. Indianapolis, Ind.: Hackett; 2000.

## References

1. Brown LD. Knowledge and power: Health services research as a political resource. In: Ginzberg E, ed. *Health Services Research: Key to Health Policy.* Cambridge, Mass.: Harvard University Press; 1991.
2. Brownson RC, Petitti DB, eds. *Applied Epidemiology: Theory to Practice.* 2nd ed. New York, N.Y.: Oxford University Press; 2006.
3. Wallack L, Dorfman L, Jernigan D, Themba M. *Media Advocacy for Public Health.* Newbury Park, Calif.: Sage; 1993.
4. Zill N, Resnick G, McKey RH, et al. *Head Start Program Performance Measures: Second Progress Report.* Washington, D.C.: U.S. Department of Health and Human Services; 1998.
5. Bellinger DC, Bellinger AM. Childhood lead poisoning: The torturous path from science to policy. *J Clin Invest.* 2006;116(4):853–857.
6. Centers for Disease Control and Prevention. Achievements in public health, 1900–1999: Impact of vaccines universally recommended for children—United States, 1900–1998. *Morbidity and Mortality Weekly Report.* 1999;48:243–248.
7. Crombie IK, Irvine L, Elliott L, Wallace H. *Public Health Policy on Alcohol: An International Perspective.* Dundee, Scotland: University of Dundee; 2005.
8. DeRoeck D. The importance of engaging policy-makers at the outset to guide research on and introduction of vaccines: The use of policy-maker surveys. *J Health Popul Nutr.* 2004;22(3):322–330.
9. Mensah GA, Goodman RA, Zaza S, et al. Law as a tool for preventing chronic diseases: Expanding the spectrum of effective public health strategies. *Prev Chronic Dis.* 2004;1(2):A11.

10. Navarro V, Muntaner C, eds. *Political and Economic Determinants of Population Health and Well-Being: Controversies and Developments.* Amityville, N.Y.: Baywood; 2004.

11. Selig WK, Jenkins KL, Reynolds SL, Benson D, Daven M. Examining advocacy and comprehensive cancer control. *Cancer Causes Control.* 2005;16(Suppl 1):61–68.

12. Oliver TR. The politics of public health policy. *Annu Rev Public Health.* 2006;27:195–233.

13. Brownson RC, Malone BR. Communicating public health information to policy makers. In: Nelson DE, Brownson RC, Remington PL, Parvanta C, eds. *Communicating Public Health Information Effectively: A Guide for Practitioners.* Washington, D.C.: American Public Health Association; 2002:97–114.

14. McDonough JE. *Experiencing Politics: A Legislator's Stories of Government and Health Care.* Berkeley, Calif.: University of California Press; 2000.

15. Wallack LM. *News for a Change: An Advocate's Guide to Working with the Media.* Thousand Oaks, Calif.: Sage; 1999.

16. Stone DA. *Policy Paradox: The Art of Political Decision Making.* Rev. ed. New York, N.Y.: Norton; 2002.

17. Coughlin SS, Beauchamp TL. *Ethics and Epidemiology.* New York, N.Y.: Oxford University Press; 1996.

18. Guttman N. *Public Health Communication Interventions: Values and Ethical Dilemmas.* Thousand Oaks, Calif.: Sage; 2000.

19. Sabatier PA, ed. *Theories of the Political Process.* 2nd ed. Boulder, Colo.: Westview; 2007.

20. Leviton LC, Needleman CE, Shapiro MA. *Confronting Public Health Risks: A Decision Maker's Guide.* Thousand Oaks, Calif.: Sage; 1998.

21. Tesh SN. *Hidden Arguments: Political Ideology and Disease Prevention Policy.* New Brunswick, N.J.: Rutgers University Press; 1988.

22. Birkland TA. *An Introduction to the Policy Process: Theories, Concepts, and Models of Public Policy Making.* 2nd ed. Armonk, N.Y.: M.E. Sharpe; 2005.

23. Kingdon JW. *Agendas, Alternatives, and Public Policies.* 2nd ed. New York, N.Y.: Longman; 2003.

24. Lindblom CE, Woodhouse EJ. *The Policy-Making Process.* 3rd ed. Upper Saddle River, N.J.: Prentice-Hall; 2003.

25. Longest B. *Health Policymaking in the United States.* Ann Arbor, Mich.: Health Administration Press; 2005.

26. Johnson JD. *Cancer-Related Information Seeking.* Cresskill, N.J.: Hampton Press; 1997.

27. Kahneman D, Slovic P, Tversky A, eds. *Judgment under Uncertainty: Heuristics and Biases.* Cambridge, UK: Cambridge University Press; 1982.

28. Bacharach S, Lawler E. *Power and Politics in Organizations.* San Francisco, Calif.: Jossey-Bass; 1980.

29. Oliver TR. The politics of public health policy. *Annu Rev Public Health.* 2006;27:195–233.

30. Greenfield TK, Johnson SP, Giesbrecht N. The alcohol policy development process: Policymakers speak. *Contemporary Drug Problems.* 2004;31:627–654.

31. Montini T, Bero LA. Policy makers' perspectives on tobacco control advocates' roles in regulation development. *Tob Control.* 2001;10(3):218–224.

32. Petticrew M, Whitehead M, Macintyre SJ, Graham H, Egan M. Evidence for public health policy on inequalities: 1: The reality according to policymakers. *J Epidemiol Community Health.* 2004;58(10):811–816.

33. Anderson PA, Buller DB, Voeks JH, et al. Predictors of support for environmental tobacco smoke bans in state government. *Am J Prev Med.* 2006;30:292–299.

34. Bier VM. On the state of the art: Risk communication to decision-makers. *Reliab Eng Syst Saf.* 2001;71:151–157.

35. Goodsell CT. *The Case for Bureaucracy: A Public Administration Polemic.* 4th ed. Washington, D.C.: CQ Press; 2003.

36. Spasoff RA. *Epidemiologic Methods for Health Policy.* New York: Oxford University Press; 1999.

37. Frederickson HG, Smith KB. *The Public Administration Primer.* Boulder, Colo.: Westview; 2003.

38. Goldman LR. Epidemiology in the regulatory arena. *Am J Epidemiol.* 2001;154(12 Suppl):S18–S26.

39. Wilson JQ. *Bureaucracy.* Jackson, Tenn.: Perseus; 2000.

40. Dearing JW, Rogers EM. *Agenda-Setting.* Thousand Oaks, Calif.: Sage; 1996.

41. Scheufele DA, Tewksbury D. Framing, agenda setting, and priming: The evolution of three media effects models. *J Commun.* 2007;57:9–20.

42. Chapman S, Lupton D. *The Fight for Public Health: Principles and Practice of Media Advocacy.* London, UK: BMJ; 1994.

43. Morgan G. *Images of Organizations.* 2nd ed. Thousand Oaks, Calif.: Sage; 1997.

44. Remington PL, Ahrens D. Communicating public health information to private and voluntary health organizations. In: Nelson DE, Brownson RC, Remington PL, Parvanta C, eds. *Communicating Public Health Information Effectively: A Guide for Practitioners.* Washington, D.C.: American Public Health Association; 2002:115–126.

45. Matson-Koffman DM, Brownstein JN, Neiner JA, Greaney ML. A site-specific literature review of policy and environmental interventions that promote physical activity and nutrition for cardiovascular health: What works? *Am J Health Promot.* 2005;19(3):167–193.

46. Wickizer TM, Kopjar B, Franklin G, Joesch J. Do drug-free workplace programs prevent occupational injuries? Evidence from Washington State. *Health Serv Res.* 2004;39(1):91–110.

47. Harris TE. *Applied Organizational Communication: Principles and Pragmatics for Future Practice.* Mahwah, N.J.: Lawrence Erlbaum; 2002.

48. Daugherty EL. Public relations and social responsibility. In: Heath RL, ed. *Handbook of Public Relations.* Thousand Oaks, Calif.: Sage; 2004;389–401.

49. Sackett KM, Campbell-Heider N, Blyth JB. The evolution and evaluation of videoconferencing technology for graduate nursing education. *Comput Inform Nurs.* 2004;22(2):101–106.

50. Weissert CS, Weissert WG. State legislative staff influence in health policy making. *J Health Polit Policy Law.* 2000;25:1121–1148.

51. Corbett E, Connors R. *Classic Rhetoric for the Modern Student.* 4th ed. New York, N.Y.: Oxford University Press; 1999.

52. Abelson RP. *Statistics as Principled Argument.* Hillsdale, N.J.: Lawrence Erlbaum; 1995.

53. Ramage JD, Bean JC, Johnson J. *Writing Arguments: A Rhetoric with Readings.* 6th ed. New York, N.Y.: Pearson/Longman; 2004.

54. Weston A. *A Rulebook for Arguments.* 3rd ed. Indianapolis, Ind.: Hackett; 2000.

55. Garvin T. Analytical paradigms: The epistemological distances between scientists, policy makers, and the public. *Risk Anal.* 2001;21(3):443–455.

56. Sommer A. How public health policy is created: Scientific process and political reality. *Am J Epidemiol.* 2001;154(12 Suppl):S4-S6.

57. Lezine DA, Reed GA. Political will: A bridge between public health knowledge and action. *Am J Public Health.* 2007;97(11):2010–2013.

58. Bennett A. *Young Child Survival and Development: In a Child Survival Milestone, Under-Five Deaths Fall Below 10 Millions per Year.* New York, N.Y.: UNICEF; 2007.

59. Cheng M. Experts say U.N. agencies spin data. *Washington Post.* September 20, 2007.

60. Lancet. Science at WHO and UNICEF: The corrosion of trust. *Lancet.* 2007;370:1007.

61. Murray CJ, Laakso T, Shibuya K, Hill K, Lopez AD. Can we achieve Millennium Development Goal 4? New analysis of country trends and forecasts of under-5 mortality to 2015. *Lancet.* 2007;370(9592):1040–1054.

62. Reynolds RA, Reynolds JL. Evidence. In: Dillard JP, Pfau M, eds. *The Persuasion Handbook: Developments in Theory and Practice.* Thousand Oaks, Calif.: Sage; 2002:427–444.

63. Fletcher SW. Whither scientific deliberation in health policy recommendations? *Alice in Wonderland* in breast cancer screening. *N Engl J Med.* 1997;336(16):1180–1183.

64. Wagner W, Steinzor R. *Rescuing Science from Politics: Regulation and the Distortion of Scientific Research.* New York, N.Y.: Cambridge University Press; 2006.

65. Leask J, Chapman S. "The cold hard facts" immunisation and vaccine preventable diseases in Australia's newsprint media 1993–1998. *Soc Sci Med.* 2002;54(3):445–457.

66. Steel BS, Lach D, Satyal VA. Ideology and scientific credibility: Environmental policy in the American Pacific Northwest. *Public Understand Sci.* 2006;15: 481–495.

67. Rossi PH, Lipsey MW, Freeman HE. *Evaluation: A Systematic Approach.* 7th ed. Thousand Oaks, Calif.: Sage; 2004.

68. Parrott R, Silk K, Dorgan K, Condit C, Harris T. Risk communication and judgments of statistical evidentiary appeals. When a picture is not worth a thousand words. *Hum Commun Res.* 2005;32:423–452.

69. Paulos JA. *Innumeracy: Mathematical Illiteracy and Its Consequences.* New York, N.Y.: Hill & Wang; 2001.

70. Dewan S. How photos became icon of Civil Rights Movement. *New York Times.* August 28, 2005.

71. Blum D, Knudson M, Henig RM, eds. *A Field Guide for Science Writers: The Official Guide of the National Association of Science Writers.* 2nd ed. New York, N.Y.: Oxford University Press; 2006.

72. Friedman SM, Dunwoody S, Rogers CL, eds. *Communicating Uncertainty: Media Coverage of New and Controversial Science.* Mahwah, N.J.: Lawrence Erlbaum; 1999.

73. Green MC, Strange JJ, Brock TC, eds. *Narrative Impact: Social and Cognitive Foundations.* Mahwah, N.J.: Erlbaum; 2002.

74. Petraglia J. Narrative intervention in behavior and public health. *J Health Commun.* 2007;12(5):493–505.

75. O'Keefe DJ. *Persuasion: Theory and Research.* Thousand Oaks, Calif.: Sage; 2002.

76. Wainer H. *Visual Revelations: Graphical Tales of Fate and Deception from Napoleon Bonaparte to Ross Perot.* New York, N.Y.: Copernicus; 1997.

77. Cohn V, Cope L. *News and Numbers: A Guide to Reporting Statistical Claims and Controversies in Health and Other Fields.* 2nd ed. Ames, Iowa: Iowa State Press; 2001.

78. Petitti DB. *Meta-Analysis, Decision Analysis, and Cost Effectiveness Analysis: Methods for Quantitative Synthesis in Medicine.* 2nd ed. New York, N.Y.: Oxford University Press; 2000.

79. Dolnik L, Case TI, Williams KD. Stealing thunder as a courtroom tactic revisited: Processes and boundaries. *Law Hum Behav.* 2003;27:265–285.

80. Williams KD, Bourgeois MJ, Croyle RT. The effects of stealing thunder in criminal and civil trials. *Law Hum Behav.* 1993;17:597–609.

81. Allen M, Bruflat R, Fucilla R, et al. Testing the persuasiveness of evidence: Combining narrative and statistical forms. *Commun Res Rep.* 2000;17:331–336.

82. Reinard JC. Persuasion in the legal setting. In: Dillard JP, Pfau M, eds. *The Persuasion Handbook: Developments in Theory and Practice.* Thousand Oaks, Calif.: Sage; 2002:432–602.

83. Devol R, Bedroussian A, Charuwom A, et al. *An Unhealthy America: The Economic Burden of Chronic Disease—Charting a New Course to Save Lives and Increase Productivity and Economic Growth.* Santa Monica, Calif.: Milken Institute; 2007.

84. Institute of Medicine. *Growing Up Tobacco Free: Preventing Nicotine Addiction in Children and Youths.* Washington, D.C.: National Academy Press; 1994.

85. Petty RE, Cacioppo JT. *Communication and Persuasion: Central and Peripheral Routes to Attitude Change.* New York, N.Y.: Springer-Verlag; 1986.

86. Sopory P, Dillard JP. Figurative language and persuasion. In: Dillard JP, Pfau M, eds. *The Persuasion Handbook: Developments in Theory and Practice.* Thousand Oaks, Calif.: Sage; 2002:407–426.

87. Hinton GE, Anderson JA. *Parallel Models of Associative Memory.* Hillsdale, N.J.: Lawrence Erlbaum; 1981.

88. Slater MD, Rouner D. Entertainment-education and elaboration likelihood: Understanding the processing of narrative persuasion. *Commun Theory.* 2002;12:173–191.

89. Lipkus IM, Hollands JG. The visual communication of risk. *J Natl Cancer Inst Monogr.* 1999(25):149–163.

90. Tufte ER. *Visual Explanations.* Cheshire, Conn.: Graphics Press; 1997:92.

91. Ancker JS, Senathirajah Y, Kukafka R, Starren JB. Design features of graphs in health risk communication: A systematic review. *J Am Med Inform Assoc.* 2006;13(6):608–618.

# 8

# Conclusions and New Challenges

> Every activity in the area of [public understanding of science] finds
> its own particular balance between information and education on one
> hand, and advocacy and persuasion, on the other. Researchers pop-
> ularizing their work tread a fine line between sharing their enthu-
> siasm and lobbying for their particular pet project. Industry-linked
> resources for schools can easily become a straightforward exercise in
> public relations. And government information on, for example, safe
> sex can easily spill over into the party politics of "family values."
> These tensions are not always apparent: the agendas at work are
> often tacit, and the public's perceptions of, and reactions to, them are
> difficult to assess.
>
> Gregory and Miller, *Science in Public: Communication,*
> *Culture, and Credibility*[1]

## Introduction

Throughout this book, we argue that communicating data is an important, and sometimes inevitable, aspect of the ongoing diffusion of public
health research and surveillance findings among the public, the press, and
policy makers. As the global scientific enterprise continues to expand
exponentially, the quantity and complexity of scientific findings will
expand as well.

This avalanche of new information poses tremendous challenges
to communicators and their audiences. In the preceding chapters, we
described a diverse collection of ways to communicate data more effectively to lay audiences, noting, among many factors, the roles of culture
and context and the importance of source, audience, and message characteristics. In this final chapter, we recap and reflect on the implications
of previous chapters and identify some key communication challenges
facing researchers and practitioners as they strive to make data more
coherent for lay audiences.

## Epistemology: Recognizing Our Own Assumptions and Worldviews

In Chapters 1 and 2, we pointed out the cultural divide between scientists and lay audiences concerning epistemology, that is, what is considered to be knowledge and acceptable types of evidence. A careful consideration of these fundamental worldviews within a particular context is the starting point for answering questions about whether, when, and how to communicate data.

Public health communicators often presume that data should be a central component of messages without considering first whether a lay audience even considers data to be evidence. Especially within the political realm, a presumption that scientific data are the most important form of knowledge to consider (methodological empiricism) may alienate an audience whose epistemology is based on authority and principle. To complicate matters further, one's epistemology can also vary as a function of context. An individual may accept the relevance of statistics for weather forecasts or betting on baseball, but may reject his or her use in judgments about condom use or vaccine efficacy.

One of the most pervasive mistakes we have observed when scientists communicate data to other audiences is their assumption that more data are better. The communication professional is often left to determine how best to select, summarize, and explain the significance of a set of complex findings. In considering what an audience wants and needs to know, a compromise is often reached between what the scientist believes is important and what the communicator believes will engage an audience.

Successful journalists know that anecdotes can be more compelling than data, especially when the audience is not scientifically literate.[2] Therefore, the first, and most critical, decision for communication practitioners is not how to present data but whether to include data in any form. If the inclusion of data within a message is deemed appropriate for a particular audience, it is nearly always the case that less is better (Chapters 2 and 3). This demonstrates, once again, the cardinal maxim of communication: "know thy audience."

## Communication of Data Is both Art and Science

Throughout this book, we have provided an overview of relevant scientific research and made recommendations about how to better select and present data to lay audiences by identifying science-based storylines, understanding audiences, clearly delineating purpose, and choosing presentation options. But communicating about data to lay audiences, as with all other types of communication, fundamentally remains more of an art than a science because of the many different factors and other considerations involved.

For example, those who use data in attempts to persuade audiences that an important public health problem exists, describe the risk factors for the problem, or evaluate or predict the impact of interventions will tend to present limited amounts of simple data that stress larger magnitudes. The benefits of this approach when communicating data to lay audiences are that people are not overwhelmed with too much data, and frequencies (counts) and relative risk estimates, which are commonly chosen measures, are easier for lay audiences to understand. The downside is the real ethical and moral risk of selecting only those data (cherry picking) that support a strongly held belief or position.[3, 4]

Communicating data to lay audiences that are more comprehensive but more complex (e.g., absolute risk data in the form of natural frequencies) has the benefit of helping them to more accurately understand the science, especially if the data are presented and explained well; people are able to reach their own conclusions. But there is a downside to this approach because it is more cognitively burdensome, especially for persons with low levels of involvement. It also requires more work on the part of communicators who must be careful to avoid the temptation of applying the "kitchen sink" approach of giving lay audiences too much data.

Beyond the art of data communication itself, there are macro-level dialectic forces that come into play that influence the public understanding of science. There is a tendency among scientists to criticize the research of others, which can lead to inaction and the ever-present call for "more research" (Figure 8.1)

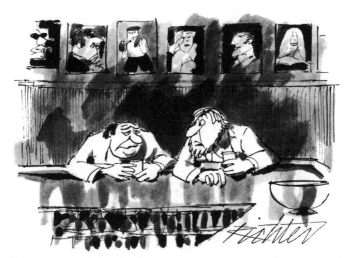

*"Then we've agreed that all the evidence isn't in, and that even if all the evidence were in, it still wouldn't be definitive."*

**Figure 8.1** The NewYorker Collection 1987 Mischa Richter from cartoonbank.com. All Rights Reserved.

As evidenced by delays in addressing important public health concerns, such as lead exposure,[5-7] cigarette smoking,[8, 9] and Reye's syndrome associated with aspirin use in children,[10-12] scientists can be too purist in their demands for unequivocal research, failing to become earlier and stronger advocates of effective public health interventions.

On the other hand, disease mongering and the hyping of health concerns, facilitated by the availability of 24-hr news media, are major forces in modern society.[13-20] They have contributed to unfounded or excessive lay audience health concerns, as well as beliefs about the effectiveness of treatment or prevention measures that have been found later to be disproved or trivial in nature—such as health risks associated with eating apples treated with the pesticide Alar,[14, 21] a link between coffee consumption and the risk of developing pancreatic cancer,[22] and alleged health benefits associated with taking vitamin E supplements to prevent cardiovascular disease or cancer.[23]

The implication is that no one "best way" exists, or could exist, that is applicable to all or even most situations when communicating with lay audiences about data. There will always be many factors to consider, and countervailing tensions operating, both of which will require communicators to make choices about whether data should be presented, what data should be selected, how data should be presented, and how much data to present.

## The Importance of Common Processes in Audience Responses to Data

From the perspective of public health communication practitioners, we believe that the public, policy makers, and the press are the three most important audiences when considering communication about scientific data. We could have included a fourth broad audience category—health information intermediaries—who are often important information sources for lay audiences.[24] Health care providers themselves are the most obvious, but there are a large number of other intermediaries. Examples include health care institutions or organizations such as the Mayo Clinic or health maintenance organizations, health insurance companies, professional health societies, nonprofit organizations such as the American Lung Association, advocacy groups, and Internet sites or search engines such as WebMD or Google Health.

We have emphasized throughout this volume the importance of considering the characteristics of specific audiences, that is, audience segmentation. Audience segmentation can be of great value for communication planning purposes,[25, 26] especially for broad-scale efforts such as health campaigns. At the same time, it is important to note that most of the fundamental psychological and communication principles and findings we have discussed apply readily to all lay and scientific audiences.

Communicator credibility, for example, is an important determinant of the persuasiveness of data-based messages across all four audiences. Audiences with low interest or issue involvement will not be motivated to understand complex data even when they are supplemented with extensive but clear explanations. In contrast, highly involved or knowledgeable audiences may expect additional data to be available, as well as information about their source and validity.

Research on biases and tendencies discussed in Chapter 3 and elsewhere has shown how pervasively we discount evidence inconsistent with our prior opinions and beliefs, recall more readily the evidence that confirms our attitudes, and are especially receptive to evidence that reinforces a positive view of ourselves.[27] Research concerning audience characteristics and biases clearly demonstrates that the task of communicating data is much more challenging if the data contradict conventional wisdom, personal beliefs, or intuition.

Therefore, one of the most important considerations in communication planning is to understand the degree of discrepancy between the data and existing lay audience beliefs (Chapters 3 and 5). Whether the purpose is to inform, persuade, or increase knowledge, a formal or informal assessment of an audience's prior beliefs can be an invaluable tool for effective communication. Because one belief or attitude is related to many others, the communicator also must consider the implications of accepting a new piece of evidence. Creating a belief that a health condition is relatively common, for example, may also lead to it being perceived as less serious.[28]

Discussions of evidence related to health disparities illustrate clearly how the meaning and context of data in relation to one's personal status and beliefs play such an important role. Traditionally, many health educators have been taught the importance of conveying health data concerning disease prevalence and susceptibility to increase the accuracy of health knowledge and risk perception among community members. Although a communicator may assume that recognition of relatively high levels of objective risk in a population will motivate action and health improvements, such data may only serve to reinforce helplessness, hopelessness, and stigma (Chapter 5).

Because health disparities data are so often descriptive rather than explanatory, members of the public, policy makers, and the media, can easily use the evidence to bolster their preexisting views about the nature of human behavior, society, or the health care system. Therefore, communication practitioners should do their best to anticipate the various interpretations of data and place them in context with other evidence that might inform those interpretations.

Data concerning racial or ethnic disparities for various types of medical treatments, use of clinical preventive services, and incidence of sexually transmitted diseases, for example, can be used to support a variety of spurious explanations unless placed within the context of data concerning disparities in income, living conditions, historical precedent, and access to quality health care. These contextual data are important for all audiences, whether they be members of the public, policy makers, or the press. In fact, scientific and political debates about the interpretation of data are often played out in arguments over what other data are relevant and whether their relationship is causal or coincidental (Chapters 3 and 7).

## Continued Growth of Lay Audience Access to Data and Other Scientific Information

Clearly, the growth of the Internet and other new communication technologies has challenged traditional concepts of health communication.[29-33] These new channels of communication provide unprecedented opportunities for individuals to directly access many types of health information, including "raw" or "preliminary" data, without the potential advantages or disadvantages of interpretation by public health practitioners, personal care health care providers, or another information intermediary.

In some ways, these changes diminish the public's reliance on health experts and the news media for health data dissemination. In addition, the ability to find, explore, and interpret data or other information from a wide and ever-growing variety of sources empowers some members of the public to question the views of health experts, policy makers, and the press about their meaning, quality, and importance. This can be seen in the rise of online blogs and "citizen journalism."[34] Another consequence of this trend is the steadily increasing expectation that data of all sorts should be made available to the widest possible audience.

Although one might argue that the rapid growth of raw data available to the public might diminish the need and importance of data presentation, we would argue quite the opposite. The public continues to express concern about the quality of health information on the Web,[35-37] while commercial and political interests grow ever more sophisticated in shaping and presenting data to serve their interests.[38] The vigorous competition among providers of business data for investors, for example, illustrates the value that users place on high quality data synthesis and presentation.

A continuing concern regarding increasing public data access is the quality of the synthesis and interpretation. Health information consumers

**Box 8.1** Benefits and burdens of the increased availability of health information

For many members of the public, the increased availability of data and other types of health information on the Internet, in the news media, and elsewhere have been a boon for increasing their knowledge about prevention and treatment (it is estimated that about 8 million adults in America go online to seek health information each day). Many people have become empowered by their growing access to information, including online access to their own medical records. This has led some to take increasingly active steps to learn more about what they can do to reduce their health risks, locate medical specialists, and investigate experimental or promising treatment options. Shared decision making is increasingly the norm in health care settings.

Cardiothoracic surgeon Tony Cosgrove of the Cleveland Clinic, Ohio, for example, reported that most of his patients in recent years had become sophisticated medical information consumers, arriving in his office with detailed knowledge about their health conditions and treatment options, much of it gleaned from their own research. Dr. Cosgrove reported that one of his patients complimented him on his home furniture—the patient had come across an article on the Internet about Cosgrove winning an architectural award for his home.

But there is another side to the widespread availability of health information. Some people not only feel overwhelmed with the amount of information available to them, but they are also burdened by the responsibility of interpreting it and making decisions for themselves. This is perhaps most evident when people need to make decisions about treatment of cancer or heart disease (Chapter 5); the Internet contains myriad Web sites where information of variable quality and credibility can be found.

But it also occurs when people consider prevention options, such as whether to use the drugs tamoxifen or raloxifene to reduce the risk of breast cancer. Furthermore, information can be easily obtained and circulated about diagnostic or screening tests, or treatments, based on preliminary research for chronic conditions such as multiple sclerosis or Alzheimer's disease. Access to the plethora of health information for some people can provide an illusion of control, raising false hopes for potential cures or promising treatments. It can cause anxiety, uncertainty, and confusion with people feeling inundated by information.

The implication of these examples is straightforward. Public health practitioners and health care providers will continue to have an important role in helping lay audiences interpret health information, and determine what the information means.

Source: Goodman E. Burdens of medical-care choices. *The Boston Globe*. April 21, 2006. Hoffman J. Awash in information, patients face a lonely, uncertain road. *The New York Times*. August 14, 2005. Noonan D. More information, please. *Newsweek*. October 29, 2007:19. Wood B. Many turn to the Web for medical advice. November 3, 2007.

are likely to be drawn to and use those data that are most informative and from sources deemed credible.[35-37] It is important to recognize that, while on one hand, some consumers seem to have an almost insatiable appetite for more health information,[39, 40] on the other hand, others can become overwhelmed with too much information and not know how best to proceed, especially when facing decisions about serious health issues (Box 8.1).[41, 42] Given the large amount of data and other health information in the public domain, there will continue to be crucial opportunities for health experts and designers to select and present data and other information that will increase the speed and efficiency with which they are used by lay audiences.

This trend in the growing availability of data and other forms of health information to lay audiences highlights the need to increase the health, science, and math literacy among all sectors of the public.[43-47] Improving all these types of literacy will require broader societal attention and investment of resources in order for lay audiences to be able to thoughtfully evaluate and use the wealth of information available to them.

## Research Challenges

Our review of research concerning the communication of data clearly illustrated that relevant findings are scattered across a wide array of journals and disciplines. Even if one focuses on quantitative literacy, a key construct for studying how and when individuals comprehend numerical concepts, relevant work can be found in education, psychology, communication, and anthropology. Scientists and practitioners would be well served by efforts to synthesize more formally the domains of evidence relevant to communicating data, such as those conducted by the Cochrane Collaboration concerning scientific evidence related to health care.

Another challenge is the ability of communication research to keep up with the rapidly changing technology and tools available for communicating data (Chapter 4). Software tools for data exploration and display have proliferated, but often lack a clear evidence base concerning their relative utility, usability, and reach. More experiments are needed to test a wide array of practical questions about user-centered design and the best ways to incorporate modern data display techniques within traditional media such as print and television. Nevertheless, the fundamentals of communication (e.g., source credibility, understanding audiences, and integrating data presentation elements) and the cognitive processes by which people process and understand data and other information will always be critical considerations regardless of the increasingly sophisticated ways that data can be presented.

Research on persuasion has focused on a wide variety of source, message, and audience factors, but the evidence concerning messages incorporating data is limited. Work is especially needed within the specific domain addressed by this volume. Investigators might consider factors that influence the credibility of the main providers of health data (such as the federal government), the circumstances under which these data are most persuasive, and the audience characteristics that determine interest in, use of, and response to public health data in particular.

In contrast to the large academic research literature on persuasion and attitude change, it is important to consider how the larger context of a health crisis can affect information processing and comprehension. In addition, research is needed on information seeking strategies and how they are shaped by the nature and format of data. Although theories and methods of cognitive psychology have advanced rapidly over the past three decades, the difficulty of translating this large body of research into practical suggestions for communicators continues to be a challenge. Applied research on communicating data can fill in the gap by providing concrete solutions to the everyday decisions faced by communication practitioners.

## Conclusion

Our attempts to review the complex issues and to research how best to communicate data remind us that many of the choices and strategies that can be considered by communication practitioners are limited only by the ethical principles adhered to by the individual. Many forms of data are highly susceptible to misuse and misinterpretation. The growing expanse of data concerning a wide range of subject matter increases the opportunities for selective choosing of only those data that conform to the biases of the communicator.

Some of the most important statistical principles and operations, such as sampling, variance, and statistical significance, continue to be poorly understood by most of the public, policy makers, and the press. As long as quantitative illiteracy is as common as it is today, the public will rely heavily on intermediaries, whose motives must be subject to as much scrutiny as the data they communicate.

Given this context, it is vital that the data essential for public discourse and decision making be as available, usable, and reliable as possible. In the case of health data, the government sector will continue to play a vital role in providing data that attempts to meet these standards. For this role to be fulfilled, appropriate resources need to be dedicated to ensure that the public, policy makers, and the media have free and rapid access to data in a variety of forms that is carefully interpreted, clearly presented, and proactively disseminated to those who need it most.

## References

1. Gregory J, Miller S. *Science in Public: Communication, Culture, and Credibility.* New York, N.Y.: Plenum Trade; 1998.
2. Blum D, Knudson M, Henig RM, eds. *A Field Guide for Science Writers: The Official Guide of the National Association of Science Writers.* 2nd ed. New York, N.Y.: Oxford University Press; 2006.
3. Nisbet MC, Mooney C. Framing science. *Science.* 2007;316(5821):56.
4. Thornton H. Patients' understanding of risk: Enabling understanding must not lead to manipulation. *BMJ.* 2003;327(7417):693–694.
5. English PC. *Old Paint: A Medical History of Childhood Lead-Paint Poisoning in the United States to 1920.* Piscataway, N.J.: Rutgers University Press; 2001.
6. Warren C. *Brush with Death: A Social History of Lead Poisoning.* Baltimore, Md.: Johns Hopkins University Press; 2001.
7. Richardson JW. *The Cost of Being Poor: Poverty, Lead Poisoning, and Policy Implementation.* New York, N.Y.: Praeger; 2005.
8. Kluger R. *Ashes to Ashes: America's Hundred-Year Cigarette War, the Public Health, and the Unabashed Triumph of Philip Morris.* New York, N.Y.: Knopf; 1997.
9. Brandt AM. *The Cigarette Century: The Rise, Fall, and Deadly Persistence of the Product that Defined America.* New York, N.Y.: Basic Books; 2007.
10. Hurwitz ES. Reye's syndrome. *Epidemiol Rev.* 1989;11:249–253.
11. Kramer MS, Lane DA. Causal propositions in clinical research and practice. *J Clin Epidemiol.* 1992;45(6):639–649.
12. Porter JD, Robinson PH, Glasgow JF, Banks JH, Hall SM. Trends in the incidence of Reye's syndrome and the use of aspirin. *Arch Dis Child.* 1990;65(8):826–829.
13. Moynihan R, Henry D. The fight against disease mongering: Generating knowledge for action. *PLoS Med.* 2006;3(4):e191.
14. Friedman SM, Dunwoody S, Rogers CL, eds. *Communicating Uncertainty: Media Coverage of New and Controversial Science.* Mahwah, N.J.: Lawrence Erlbaum; 1999.
15. Seale C. *Media and Health.* Thousand Oaks, Calif.: Sage; 2002.
16. Mazur A. *True Warnings and False Alarms: Evaluating Fears about the Health Risks of Technology 1948–1971.* Washington, D.C.: Resources for the Future; 2004.
17. Siegel M. *False Alarm: The Truth about the Epidemic of Fear.* Hoboken, N.J.: John Wiley; 2005.
18. Rifkin E, Bouwer E. *The Illusion of Certainty: Health Benefits and Risks.* New York, N.Y.: Springer; 2007.
19. Deyo RA, Patrick DL. *Hope or Hype: The Obsession with Medical Advances and the High Cost of False Promises.* New York, N.Y.: AMACOM, American Management Association; 2005.
20. Taubes G. Do we really know what makes us healthy? *New York Times.* September 16, 2007;1–16.

21. Lomborg B. *The Skeptical Environmentalist: Measuring the Real State of the World*. Cambridge, UK: Cambridge University Press; 2001.

22. Tavani A, La Vecchia C. Coffee and cancer: A review of epidemiological studies, 1990–1999. *Eur J Cancer Prev*. 2000;9(4):241–256.

23. Pham DQ, Plakogiannis R. Vitamin E supplementation in cardiovascular disease and cancer prevention: Part 1. *Ann Pharmacother*. 2005;39(11):1870–1878.

24. Remington PL, Ahrens D. Communicating public health information to private and voluntary health organizations. In: Nelson DE, Brownson RC, Remington PL, Parvanta C, eds. *Communicating Public Health Information Effectively: A Guide for Practitioners*. Washington, D.C.: American Public Health Association; 2002:115–126.

25. Rice RE, Atkin CK eds. *Public Communication Campaigns*. 3rd ed. Thousand Oaks, Calif.: Sage; 2001.

26. Maibach EW, Weber D, Massett H, Hancock GR, Price S. Understanding consumers' health information preferences: Development and validation of a brief screening instrument. *J Health Commun*. 2006;11:717–736.

27. Dillard JP, Pfau M, eds. *The Persuasion Handbook: Development in Theory and Practice*. Thousand Oaks, Calif.: Sage; 2002.

28. Croyle RT, Ditto PH. Illness cognition and behavior: An experimental approach. *J Behav Med*. 1990;13(1):31–52.

29. Mazur D. *The New Medical Conversation: Media, Patients, Doctors, and the Ethics of Scientific Communication*. Oxford, UK: Rowman & Littlefield; 2003.

30. Rains SA. Perceptions of traditional information sources and use of the World Wide Web to seek health information: Findings from the Health Information National Trends Survey. *J Health Commun*. 2007;12:667–680.

31. Stone JH. Communication between physicians and patients in the era of E-medicine. *N Engl J Med*. 2007;356(24):2451–2454.

32. Hesse BW, Shneiderman B. eHealth research from the user's perspective. *Am J Prev Med*. 2007;32(5 Suppl):S97-S103.

33. LaVenture M. Using the power of googling and health informatics to improve public health practice. *Am J Prev Med*. 2007;33(1):75–76.

34. Gillmor D. *We the Media: Grassroots Journalism by the People, for the People*. Sebastopol, Calif.: O'Reilly Media; 2004.

35. Bates BR, Romina S, Ahmed R, Hopson D. The effect of source credibility on consumers' perceptions of the quality of health information on the Internet. *Med Inform Internet Med*. 2006;31(1):45–52.

36. Cline RJW, Haynes KM. Consumer health information seeking on the Internet: The state of the art. *Health Educ Res*. 2001;16(6):671–692.

37. Wathen CN. Believe it or not: factors influencing credibility on the Web. *J Am Soc Inform Sci Technol*. 2002;53:134–144.

38. Davis JJ, Cross E, Crowley J. Pharmaceutical websites and the communication of risk information. *J Health Commun*. 2007;12(1):29–39.

39. Noonan D. More information, please. *Newsweek*. 2007;150:19.

40. Wood B. Many turn to the Web for medical advice. *Copley News Service*, La Jolla, CA; November 2, 2007.

41. Goodman E. Burdens of medical-care choices. *The Boston Globe*. April 21, 2006.

42. Hoffman J. Awash in information, patients face a lonely, uncertain road. *The New York Times*. August 14, 2005.

43. Nielsen-Bohlman L, Panzer AM, Kindig DA, eds. *Health Literacy: A Prescription to End Confusion*. Washington, D.C.: National Academy Press; 2004.

44. Paulos JA. *Innumeracy: Mathematical Illiteracy and Its Consequences*. New York, N.Y.: Hill & Wang; 2001.

45. Weigold ME. Communicating science: A review of the Literature. *Sci Commun*. 2001;23:164–193.

46. von Roten FC. Do we need a public understanding of statistics? *Public Understand Sci*. 2006;15:243–249.

47. National Mathematics Advisory Panel. *Foundations for Success: The Final Report of the National Mathematics Advisory Panel*. Washington, D.C.: U.S. Department of Education; 2008.

# Index